THE PHARMACEUTICAL RECIPE BOOK

THIRD EDITION

(R.B. III)

BY AUTHORITY OF THE
AMERICAN PHARMACEUTICAL ASSOCIATION

PREPARED BY THE COMMITTEE ON RECIPE BOOK
OF THE AMERICAN PHARMACEUTICAL ASSOCIATION

PUBLISHED BY
THE AMERICAN PHARMACEUTICAL ASSOCIATION
1943

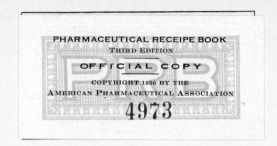

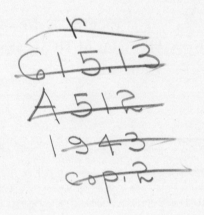

PRINTED IN THE UNITED STATES OF AMERICA

CONTENTS

iii

PREFACE

"The Recipe Book represents the outcome of an effort of the American Pharmaceutical Association to place in the hands of the practicing pharmacist a reliable and comprehensive book of recipes applicable to his business. It is hoped this book will eventually assume the same serviceable and dignified position that the National Formulary has attained in its particular field." The foregoing introductory of the preface to the First Edition of the Recipe Book expressed a hope which has been given assurance by the favorable reception given to the first and second editions.

The preparation of a third edition of the Recipe Book was necessitated by the demand for it after the second edition had been exhausted. Moreover, a revision was prompted by the appearance of the U. S. Pharmacopœia XII and the National Formulary VII, deletions from which were to be included, and a continued desire on the part of the Association to extend the usefulness of the Recipe Book. Suggestions made by physicians, pharmacists, dentists, chiropodists, veterinarians and others for additional formulas contributed to this extensive revision.

The General Principles Followed in the Compilation of the Work

1. Scope.—The purpose of the Recipe Book is to supply definite formulas for preparations, other than those contained in official books, that are frequently called for in retail and hospital pharmacies, or which are required in the manufacture of products relative to which the pharmacist may be called upon for advice, or which he may be required to supply.

2. Arrangement of Subject Matter.—The contents of each part of the Recipe Book are arranged in alphabetical sequence, the English title being accepted as the primary title, and the Latin title when included to appear as a synonym. The Recipe Book is departmentized as follows:

I. Pharmaceutical Formulas.
    a. Pharmaceutical and Hospital Formulas.
    b. Preparations for Use by Diabetics.
    c. Dental.
    d. Podiatry.
    e. Veterinary.
II. Flavoring Extracts and Imitation Flavors.
III. Certified Coal Tar Dyes.
IV. Cosmetics.
V. Technical and Miscellaneous.
VI. Table of Average Doses.
VII. Antidotes for Poisons.

VIII.   Table of Solubilities and Table of Equivalents for Preparing Percentage
            Solutions.
  IX.   Table of Synonyms.
   X.   Latin Terms and Abbreviations.
  XI.   Vitamin Synopsis.

   3. Admissions.—Any formula, if it is reliable and worthy, may be admitted to
the Recipe Book.   All of the formulas deleted from the U. S. Pharmacopœia XI and
N.F. VI have been included in the third edition of the Recipe Book; formulas of
prior official books have been included only where a definite use for them has been
shown.

   4. Therapeutic Authority Disclaimed.—The Recipe Book makes no claim regarding the remedial action of any drug or preparation, and does not assume any
responsibility for the therapeutic value of the formulas, nor for the doses specified.
The doses stated are the average doses and are based upon generally accepted practice.

   5. Tolerances.—Tolerance figures for standards, physical constants, etc., have
not been given with a range, but the Committee of Revision of the Recipe Book
has decided that a tolerance of 10 per cent above or below the figure given will be
permitted.   This range shall be inclusive and is not to be exceeded.

   6. Nomenclature.—The titles of preparations represent, as far as possible, the
leading ingredients in the formula and the therapeutically suggestive titles have
been eliminated.   Common names or synonyms of such preparations may, however,
be found in the index.   The source of Hospital formulas is given in such cases where
the source could be definitely ascertained.

   7. Quality of Ingredients.—In all formulas, the ingredients that are official in
the U.S.P. XII or N.F. VII must be of the official strength, quality and purity.
Galenicals listed as ingredients, the formulas for which are not included in the official
books, are specified as "R.B." and formulas for them are to be found in this edition
of the Recipe Book.

   Cooperation and Assistance: The Committee acknowledges and expresses its
thanks for the assistance rendered by present and former members of the Committee
on Recipe Book and by other pharmacists in connection with this revision.
   Thanks are also due the following, outside of the Committee, for their contribu-
tion of specialized formulas to this edition: M. J. Stoklosa, D. A. Clarke, and H. L.
Goldwag.   Appreciation is also extended to Mrs. R. Tannenbaum and S. W.
Goldstein for their valuable services.
   The Federal Food, Drug and Cosmetic Administration has given valuable as-
sistance in the matter of revising titles.
   Thanks are extended to the American Dental Association and to the American
Veterinary Medical Association for their aid in connection with Dental Formulas and
Veterinary Formulas appearing in this edition of the Recipe Book.
   The committee expresses its thanks to H. J. Amsterdam of the Columbia Uni-
versity College of Pharmacy and to M. W. Green of the American Pharmaceutical
Association Laboratory for their assistance in the preparation of Recipe Book III.

Dr. E. F. Kelly has the special gratitude of the chairman and Committee for the hearty coöperation he has given at all times.

THE COMMITTEE ON RECIPE BOOK

J. Leon Lascoff, Chairman

J. K. ATTWOOD	W. H. GLOVER	C. L. O'CONNELL
I. A. BECKER	WM. GRAY	J. L. POWERS
F. E. BIBBINS	L. D. HAVENHILL	R. W. RODMAN
H. M. BURLAGE	S. L. HILTON	G. C. SCHICKS
C. J. CLAYTON	H. E. KENDIG	O. U. SISSON
E. F. COOK	J. F. McCLOSKEY	R. L. SWAIN
M. G. deNAVARRE	C. E. McCORMICK	R. E. TERRY
BERNARD FANTUS*	G. A. MOULTON	H. A. K. WHITNEY
R. P. FISCHELIS	J. C. MUNCH	C. P. WIMMER
E. N. GATHERCOAL		

* Deceased.

HISTORICAL INTRODUCTION

The American Pharmaceutical Association has ever been alive to the desirability of collecting and making accessible to retail pharmacists the formulas of preparations not included in any official compendia.

As early as 1856 a committee was appointed by the president to collect unofficial formulas and report them to the Association. The efforts of that committee and other committees continuing its work led eventually to the issuance of the present-day National Formulary. The enactment of the Food and Drugs Act made the National Formulary in addition to the United States Pharmacopœia official standard publications, and this fact made the publication of a book containing the formulas for remedies not included in the two official books a pressing necessity. Professor Henry P. Hynson, of Baltimore, had the foresight to urge upon the American Pharmaceutical Association the publication of such a book. In 1909, he wrote, as follows:

> "I trust I may be pardoned for presuming to present to the Members of the Council for consideration and discussion at Los Angeles, the propriety of the American Pharmaceutical Association publishing a general druggists' recipe book.
> "I consider this an important matter just now, because it must be apparent to everyone that the coming editions of both the United States Pharmacopœia and National Formulary must be more restricted, more scientific and much more works of standards than ever before and they cannot become such unless many eliminations are made, and to make these eliminations possible there must be some receptacle provided for them. It seems to me that the American Pharmaceutical Association would be wise to act quickly in the matter and publish a book which should not be, in any way, under government control or subject to criticism by anyone who is not actively engaged in pharmaceutical pursuits."

The proposition of Professor Hynson, together with letters from Leo Eliel and Otto Raubenheimer, on the same subject, were referred to the Committee on Standards for Non-Official Drugs and Chemical Products for consideration and report at the Los Angeles meeting of the Association. In addition, the Council recommended that the Committee named above devote its early attention to the compilation of a list of useful recipes for druggists' use.

At the Richmond meeting in 1910, the Committee on Unofficial Standards reported that it was not expedient at that time to compile a recipe book, as the committee felt that its efforts should be restricted to establishing correct standards for simples in the then forthcoming N.F. IV, and this undertaking would require all of the time of the committee.

At the same meeting, however, the question was agitated again. Among a number of recommendations to the Association made in the address of the Chairman of the Section of Pharmacy and Dispensing, Professor Otto Raubenheimer included one in which he recommended the publication of a recipe book, stating that the practical pharmacists of the country were in favor of such a book. In addition, Professor Raubenheimer addressed a communication to the Council suggesting that the matter be put into the hands of a "Committee on A. Ph. A. Recipe Book." This suggestion was brought officially before the Council in the form of a motion made by Mr. Franklin M. Apple. According to that motion, seconded by Mr. Leonard A. Seltzer, a committee consisting of Messrs. Hynson and Raubenheimer, the General Secretary, the Secretary of the Council and the Chairman of the Finance Committee were to constitute a special committee to investigate the advisability of the Association publishing a pharmacists' recipe book; to define its scope and character, and submit plans and details for the consideration of the Council and the Association.

The motion was amended by George M. Beringer, seconded by Ambrose Hunsberger, to read that a committee of five be appointed for the purpose. The motion passed the Council and the Association, and the following were appointed to constitute the first committee: Messrs. O. Raubenheimer, M. I. Wilbert, F. M. Apple, Theo. D. Wetterstroem and J. M. Good. The committee immediately set out to collect useful formulas, and at the end of the first year about 120 formulas had been contributed.

At the request of Chairman Raubenheimer the original committee of five was enlarged in 1915 to fifteen members, namely: Messrs. Scoville, Nixon (succeeded by Glover), Wimmer, Thum, Becker, Roehr, Roemer (succeeded by Spalding), Cook, Gray, Wetterstroem, Utech, Cliffe, Hynson (succeeded by LaWall), Wilbert and Raubenheimer as chairman. This committee, divided into seven sub-committees, in 1916 compiled Formulas No. 115 to No. 390 and during 1917 Formulas No. 391 to No. 642. These Formulas were published in the Journal of the A. Ph. A. as a special Department of "Pharmaceutical Formulas" and were copied to a considerable extent by other domestic and foreign pharmaceutical journals. Chairman Raubenheimer also compiled an Index of all the Formulas from February, 1912, up to December, 1916, which was published separately in Vol. V, Jour. A. Ph. A., and another index of the Formulas published during 1917 in Vol. VI.

Requests were then sent out for formulas which might be suitable for inclusion. These formulas were printed in the Journal of the A. Ph. A. each month. In 1916, one year after the Committee had been considerably enlarged and made into a standing committee of the Association, the number of formulas contributed numbered about 625. Several colleges offered their assistance in compounding and trying out the formulas submitted.

In May, 1920, in Washington, a new committee was appointed and J. Leon Lascoff was elected Chairman. This committee was later enlarged until it finally consisted of twenty-five members.

This group was sub-divided into several working committees, each with its respective chairman. In this way each member came in direct contact with the sort of work which interested him. Bulletins, voting sheets and formulas admitted for publication were sent to each of the members, and valuable criticism, many corrections and a number of new suggestions were received.

In April, 1921, the first set of Pharmaceutical Formulas, numbers 643 to 654, was published in the Journal of the A. Ph. A.; in May, formulas 655 to 667, in June, 668 to 683, and in July, 684 to 697, inclusive. More formulas appeared in the August and September numbers.

In 1924, at the Buffalo meeting of the American Pharmaceutical Association, Chairman J. Leon Lascoff turned over a collection of formulas to the Association, and also exhibited a large number of preparations with which he and other committee members had experimented.

This collection of formulas, as yet unedited, represented a total of over fifteen hundred. At the same meeting, Professor Ivor Griffith was elected Editor and was requested to assemble and arrange the formulas for publication.

A careful study of these recipes showed the need for a reconsideration of their suitability for inclusion in the book, whereupon a Committee on Scope was appointed. This committee deleted some formulas which had outlived their usefulness and supplied others which were more modern to fill the gaps.

During this interval many other up-to-date formulas were introduced and the completed manuscript was turned over by the Editor to the Council of the Association at the Philadelphia Convention, September, 1926. It was favorably received by the Council and the Committee on Publication was authorized to secure bids on its publication.

The Historical Introduction, published in the first edition of the Recipe Book, closed with a report made at the meeting of the American Pharmaceutical Association held in Philadelphia, September, 1926. Editor Ivor Griffith reported that the Book was nearing completion.

The report was presented at the General Sessions of the American Pharmaceutical Association held in St. Louis, August, 1927, that the contract for the manufacture, the agency and sale of the Recipe Book, First Edition, had been awarded to J. B. Lippincott Company. In Council Letter No. 7, February 1, 1928, a request was made by Editor Ivor Griffith and Chairman J. Leon Lascoff that a meeting of the Sub-Committee on Scope of the Committee on Recipe Book be held in New York, N. Y., during February, 1928. It was submitted that a final review of the text was desirable. Council Letter No. 9, published in the March Journal of the A. Ph. A. for 1928, reported the approval of the meeting which had been held February 14th and 15th. In addition to the members of the Sub-Committee on Scope, the following attended: Messrs. DuMez, Eberle, Fischelis, Griffith, Hilton, Kelly, Lascoff, Raubenheimer, Scoville and Wimmer. J. Leon Lascoff acted as Chairman and Ivor Griffith as Secretary.

The progress of the Recipe Book was reviewed, and the text studied in considerable detail. It was decided to omit assay processes for extracts, fluidextracts and wines in general, therapeutic terms and statements from the text, and to include introductory chapters to certain important groups of preparations for which such chapters had not been provided. The inclusion of a statement of the average alcoholic content of preparations was considered, but was not thought feasible at that time. A more complete classification was worked out, and the Editor was authorized to make necessary corrections and bring about uniformity in arrangement of formulas, wording of directions, titles, etc. The former titles may be found in the Index with appropriate references to the new titles.

The Committee on Recipe Book, at that time, was composed of the following: Chairman, J. Leon Lascoff; Editor, Ivor Griffith; I. A. Becker, C. J. Clayton, E. F. Cook, M. A. Davis, Bernard Fantus, R. P. Fischelis, E. N. Gathercoal, R. R. Gerstner, W. H. Glover, William Gray, L. D. Havenhill, S. L. Hilton, W. W. Horne, F. B. Kilmer, H. A. Langenhan, H. L. Meredith, F. W. Nitardy,

Otto Raubenheimer, C. M. Roehr, Thomas Roach, W. L. Scoville, J. K. Thum, P. H. Utech, C. P. Wimmer. Of these the following have ceased their labors: H. L. Meredith, P. H. Utech, F. B. Kilmer, Bernard Fantus and W. L. Scoville.

The first edition of the Pharmaceutical Recipe Book was brought to conclusion with 777 Pharmaceutical Formulas, 373 Hospital Formulas, 34 Dental Formulas, 66 Diagnostic Reagents and Clinical Tests, 28 Veterinary Formulas, 45 Photographic Formulas, 184 Cosmetic Formulas, 45 Flavoring Formulas, 69 Technical Formulas— a total of 1621 formulas.

At the Portland, Maine, meeting it was reported that progress in line with the action of the Conference held in New York had been made, and that proofs of approximately half of the Book had been distributed. Announcement was made in March, 1929, that the Recipe Book had been completed; the first copy was designated as a memorial volume honoring Prof. Henry P. Hynson, the father of the movement. The ceremonial of the presentation, under the auspices of the Baltimore Branch of the A. Ph. A., was part of the program at the Rapid City meeting.

On March 18, 1929, Chairman Lascoff gave a brief summary of the activities connected with the Recipe Book and presented to President H. A. B. Dunning, of the A. Ph. A., the original manuscripts which form part of the basis of the Recipe Book. This material was placed on exhibition at the meeting of the A. Ph. A. at Rapid City and there presented to the Association for its museum in Washington.

A second copy of the Book was presented to Chairman Lascoff by the American Pharmaceutical Association.

A third copy of the Recipe Book was formally presented to Editor Ivor Griffith on behalf of the American Pharmaceutical Association. In due procedure copies of the publication were also given to Joseph W. E. Harrisson, Reba Kancher, Edward Hughes and Millicent R. LaWall, who had assisted Editor Griffith in his work.

Chairman Lascoff in behalf of the Committee expressed thanks for coöperation in giving publicity to the Recipe Book to the *Druggists' Circular*, the *Practical Druggist*, the *Chicago Retail Druggists Association News*, the *N. A. R. D. Journal*, the *Journal of the A. Ph. A.* and others.

At a meeting of the American Pharmaceutical Association in Miami, Fla., the Chairman, J. Leon Lascoff, presented a comprehensive report of the sales of the Recipe Book together with a number of new formulas for the succeeding edition of the Recipe Book. A system of revision was prepared at the Miami meeting, and the Association by-laws were amended by an addition to Chapter VIII which placed the Recipe Book on the same basis as the National Formulary. The matter of another edition of the Recipe Book was discussed, and it was deemed advisable to prepare a revised edition rather than correct the first.

The work of revision, preparatory to the issuance of Recipe Book II, was begun in 1932.

Early in 1933, Bulletins containing formulas for the new Recipe Book were sent out for criticism and review. An extensive display of preparations prepared according to the Recipe Book was exhibited at the Madison meeting.

The favorable reception of the Recipe Book was evidenced when in May of 1934 Chairman Lascoff reported that practically all of the copies of the Recipe Book I had been sold and that it was necessary to proceed with the issuing of the second printing. The Council Letter of July 19 announced that the contract for printing and binding Recipe Book II had been awarded to the Mack Printing Co., Easton, Pa.

Chairman Lascoff submitted a complete report relative to the activities of the Chairman's office and the Committee. He reported that the formulas for the Recipe Book were being edited and corrected for typographical errors, and that he was experimenting with new formulas and testing out composition and methods for others.

Several meetings held under the Chairman's directions for discussing the revision were attended by E. N. Gathercoal, E. F. Kelly, S. L. Hilton and E. G. Eberle.

These sessions were helpful in perfecting the work of revision and bringing about early publication. The volume contains nearly 2000 formulas.

At the annual meeting of the American Pharmaceutical Association in Dallas, Texas, in August 1936, it was decided to begin the revision of Recipe Book III. This was found necessary in order to bring the Recipe Book up to date to conform with the changes being made in the new issues of the U. S. Pharmacopœia XII and National Formulary VII, and in order to include the deletions from the last editions of the official books. Chairman J. Leon Lascoff advised that there were many new formulas which would be valuable to the retail practicing pharmacist if included in the Recipe Book.

A new Committee was appointed and work was started on Recipe Book III. On July 18, 1938, the first Bulletin went forward to the Committee.

At each of the subsequent annual meetings of the American Pharmaceutical Association, a meeting of the Recipe Book Committee was called. The Chairman presented a report of the progress of the R.B. III, and a review of formulas presented to date. At all these meetings, a number of preparations of R.B. III were displayed by the Chairman for review and inspection.

At the Richmond meeting in 1940, all new formulas submitted to date were reviewed by the Recipe Book Committee.

On November 7, 1941, the last Bulletin, No. 19, with the 330th new formula of Recipe Book III went forward to the Committee for their vote.

A three-day meeting of the Committee on Scope was held at the Columbia University College of Pharmacy on December 18, 19 and 20, 1941, to review the old and new formulas to be included in R.B. III. The members of the Committee on Scope present at this meeting were: F. E. Bibbins, H. M. Burlage, E. Fullerton Cook, R. P. Fischelis, Samuel L. Hilton, E. F. Kelly, James C. Munch, C. Leonard O'Connell, George C. Schicks, R. L. Swain, R. E. Terry, C. P. Wimmer and J. Leon Lascoff who served as Chairman of this Committee.

Several sections of the Recipe Book have been completely revised for this new edition. These include sections on Podiatry, Dental, Veterinarian and Cosmetic formulas.

New sections which have been added to Recipe Book III are:

1. Latin Terms and Abbreviations.
2. Table of Synonyms.
3. Table of Certified Coal Tar Dyes.
4. Vitamin Synopsis.
5. Formulas and Preparations for Use by Diabetics.
6. Tables for Preparing Percentage Solutions.
7. Preparations for Ophthalmic Use.
8. American Pharmaceutical Association "Code of Ethics."

LIST OF ABBREVIATIONS

Austral. Ph. F.	Australian Pharmaceutical Formulary, 1925
B.P.	British Pharmacopœia, 1898, 1914, 1932
B.P.C.	British Pharmaceutical Codex, 1911, 1923, 1934
Can. Ph. J.	Canadian Pharmaceutical Journal
Cod. Fr.	Codex Française, 1927
D.A.B.	Deutsches Arzneibuch, III, IV, V, VI; 1895, 1900, 1910, 1925
D.M.	Dieterich's Manual
E.B.	Erganzungsbuch (supplement to D.A.B.), III, IV; 1906, 1916
Ext. Ph.	Extra Pharmacopœia, XX, XXI; 1932, 1935, 1936, 1938
F. Ital.	Farmacopea Ufficiale del Regno d'Italia, V. 1929
F.M.G.	Formulæ Magistrales Germanicæ (Berlin Formulary)
J. A. Ph. A.	Journal American Pharmaceutical Association
Lux. F.	Luxemburg Formulary
N.D.A.	National Dental Association (Accepted Dental Remedies)
N.F.	National Formulary, III, IV, V, VI
N.N.R.	New and Non-Official Remedies, American Medical Association, 1928–1941
P.F.	Pharmaceutical Formulas, 10th Edition, 1929
Ph. Aust.	Pharmacopœia Austriaca, 1906
Ph. Belg.	Pharmacopœia Belge, IV, 1930
Ph. Dan.	Pharmacopœia Danica, 1907, 1925
Ph. Helv.	Pharmacopœia Helvitica, 1907, 1934
Ph. Ross.	Pharmacopœia Rossica, 1910, 1925
Ph. Svec.	Pharmacopœia Svecica, X, 1925
R.B.	Recipe Book, I, II, 1929, 1936
R.P.P.	Remington's Practice of Pharmacy
U.S.P.	United States Pharmacopœia, VIII, IX, X, XI

HOSPITALS

B.N.Y.	Bellevue and Allied Hospitals, New York
E.H.P.	Episcopal Hospital, Philadelphia
G.H.N.Y.	German Hospital and Dispensary, New York
L.H.F.	Lankenau Hospital Formulary, Philadelphia
N.Y.H.F.	New York Hospital Formulary
N.Y.P.G.H.	New York Post Graduate Hospital
P.H.C.	Presbyterian Hospital, Chicago
P.H.N.Y.	Presbyterian Hospital, New York
S. and C.H.N.Y.	Skin and Cancer Hospital, New York
S.H.F.	Stetson Hospital Formulary, Philadelphia
U.C.H.	University of California Hospital Formulary, San Francisco
V.C.N.Y.	Vanderbilt Hospital and Clinics, New York

CODE OF ETHICS
of the
American Pharmaceutical Association

The Pharmacist and the Public

Pharmacy has for its primary object the service which it can render to the public in safeguarding the handling, sale, compounding and dispensing of medicinal substances. The practice of pharmacy demands knowledge, skill and integrity on the part of those engaged in it. Pharmacists are required to pass certain educational tests in order to qualify under the laws of our states. The states thus restrict the practice of pharmacy to those persons who by reason of special training and qualifications are able to qualify under regulatory requirements and grant to them privileges necessarily denied to others.

In return the states expect the Pharmacist to recognize his responsibility to the community and to fulfill his professional obligations honorably and with due regard for the physical and moral well-being of society.

The Pharmacist should uphold the approved legal standards of the United States Pharmacopœia and the National Formulary for articles which are official in either of these works, and should, as far as possible, encourage the use of these official drugs and preparations and discourage the use of objectionable nostrums.* He should sell and dispense only drugs of the best quality for medicinal use and for filling prescriptions.

He should neither buy, sell nor use sub-standard drugs for uses which are in any way connected with medicinal purposes.

The Pharmacist should be properly remunerated by the public for his knowledge and skill when used in its behalf in compounding prescriptions, and his fee for such professional work should take into account the time consumed and the great responsibility involved as well as the cost of the ingredients.

The Pharmacist should not sell or dispense powerful drugs and poisons to persons not properly qualified to administer or use them, and should use every proper precaution to safeguard the public from poisons and from all habit-forming medicines.

The Pharmacist, being legally entrusted with the dispensing and sale of narcotic drugs and alcoholic liquors, should merit this responsibility by upholding and conforming to the laws and regulations governing the distribution of these substances.

The Pharmacist should seek to enlist and merit the confidence of his patrons and when this confidence is won it should be jealously guarded and never abused by extortion or misrepresentation or in any other manner.

---

* An objectionable nostrum is one which does not meet the requirements of the Commission on Proprietary Medicines of the American Pharmaceutical Association.

The Pharmacist should consider the knowledge which he gains of the ailments of his patrons and their confidences regarding these matters, as entrusted to his honor, and he should never divulge such facts unless compelled to do so by law.

The Pharmacist should hold the health and safety of his patrons to be of first consideration; he should make no attempt to prescribe or treat diseases or strive to sell drugs or remedies of any kind simply for the sake of profit.

He should keep his pharmacy clean, neat and sanitary in all its departments and should be well supplied with accurate measuring and weighing devices and other suitable apparatus for the proper performance of his professional duties.

It is considered inimical to public welfare for the Pharmacist to have any clandestine arrangement with any physician in which fees are divided or in which secret prescriptions are concerned.

The Pharmacist should primarily be a good citizen, and should uphold and defend the laws of the state and nation. He should inform himself concerning the laws, particularly those relating to food and drug adulteration and those pertaining to health and sanitation and should always be ready to coöperate with the proper authorities having charge of the enforcement of the laws.

The Pharmacist should be willing to join any constructive effort to promote the public welfare and he should regulate his public and private conduct and deeds so as to entitle him to the respect and confidence of the community in which he practices.

The Pharmacist and the Physician

The Pharmacist even when urgently requested so to do should always refuse to prescribe or attempt diagnoses. He should, under such circumstances, refer applicants for medical aid to a reputable, legally qualified Physician. In cases of extreme emergency as in accident or sudden illness on the street in which persons are brought to him pending the arrival of a Physician such prompt action should be taken to prevent suffering as is dictated by humanitarian impulses and guided by scientific knowledge and common sense.

The Pharmacist should not, under any circumstances, substitute one article for another, or one make of an article for another in a prescription, without the consent of the Physician who wrote it. No change should be made in a Physician's prescription except such as is essentially warranted by correct pharmaceutical procedure, nor any that will interfere with the obvious intent of the prescriber, as regards therapeutic action.

He should follow the Physician's directions explicitly in the matter of refilling prescriptions, copying the formula upon the label or giving a copy of the prescription to the patient. He should not add any extra directions or caution or poison labels without due regard for the wishes of the prescriber, providing the safety of the patient is not jeopardized.

Whenever there is doubt as to the interpretation of the Physician's prescription or directions, he should invariably confer with the Physician in order to avoid a possible mistake or an unpleasant situation.

He should never discuss the therapeutic effect of a Physician's prescription with a patron nor disclose details of composition which the Physician has withheld, suggesting to the patient that such details can be properly discussed with the prescriber only.

When an obvious error or omission in a prescription is detected by the Pharmacist, he should protect the interests of his patron and also the reputation of the Physician by conferring confidentially upon the subject, using the utmost caution and delicacy in handling such an important matter.

The Pharmacist and Pharmacy

The Pharmacist should strive to perfect and enlarge his professional knowledge. He should contribute his share toward the scientific progress of his profession and encourage and participate in research investigation and study. He should associate himself with pharmaceutical organizations whose aims are compatible with this code of ethics and to whose membership he may be eligible. He should contribute his share of time, energy and expense to carry on the work of these organizations and promote their welfare. He should keep himself informed upon professional matters by reading current pharmaceutical and medical literature.

He should perform no act, nor should he be a party to any transaction, which will bring discredit to himself or to his profession or in any way bring criticism upon it, nor should he unwarrantedly criticize a fellow Pharmacist or do anything to diminish the trust reposed in the practitioners of pharmacy.

The Pharmacist should expose any corrupt or dishonest conduct of any member of his profession which comes to his certain knowledge, through those accredited processes provided by the civil laws or the rules and regulations of pharmaceutical organizations, and he should aid in driving the unworthy out of the calling.

He should not accept agencies for objectionable nostrums nor allow his name to be used in connection with advertisements or correspondence for furthering their sale.

He should courteously aid a fellow Pharmacist who may request advice or professional information or who, in an emergency, needs supplies.

He should not aid any person to evade legal requirements regarding character, time or practical experience by carelessly or improperly endorsing or approving statements relating thereto.

He should not imitate the labels of his competitors or take any other unfair advantage of merited professional or commercial success. When a bottle or package of a medicine is brought to him to be refilled, he should remove all other labels and place his own thereon unless the patron requests otherwise.

He should not fill orders which come to him by mistake, being originally intended for a competitor.

He should deal fairly with manufacturers and wholesale druggists from whom he purchases his supplies; all goods received in error or excess and all undercharges should be promptly reported as are shortages and overcharges.

He should earnestly strive to follow all proper trade regulations and rules, promptly meet all obligations and closely adhere to all contracts and agreements.

THE PHARMACEUTICAL RECIPE BOOK

PHARMACEUTICAL FORMULAS
PART I-A

PHARMACEUTICAL AND HOSPITAL FORMULAS

AMPULS

For directions for the preparation of ampuls and standards for ampul glass reference should be made to the National Formulary VII, pages 29–38, and to the United States Pharmacopœia XII, pages 219–222, 567–571, 606–607, 609–610 and 614–620.   Herein will be found detailed directions for conducting such operations as the cleansing and sterilization of empty glass ampuls, the preparation of ampul solutions, the filling of ampuls, the sterilization of the filled ampuls and the testing of the ampuls for sterility.   The pharmacist takes grave responsibility when he prepares solutions for parenteral use, and it is highly important that such materials meet the general requirements for *ampuls* in the National Formulary and for *injections* in the United States Pharmacopœia.

AMPULS OF ATROPINE SULFATE
(R.P.P.)

A sterile solution in isotonic solution of sodium chloride containing atropine sulfate 0.0006 Gm. in each cc.

Atropine Sulfate.	0.6 Gm.
Isotonic Solution of Sodium Chloride, a sufficient quantity,	
To make	1000 cc.

Prepare the solution, adjust to a slightly acid reaction with fiftieth-normal sulfuric acid, filter and fill 1-cc. cleansed ampuls according to the requirements (see N.F. VII, pages 29–34).   Sterilize by Process F (see N.F. VII, page 36).

AVERAGE DOSE—1 CC.

1

AMPULS OF CALCIUM CACODYLATE
(R.P.P.)

A sterile aqueous solution containing calcium cacodylate 0.045 Gm. in each cc.

Calcium Cacodylate . . . .   **45 Gm.**

Ampul Water, a sufficient quantity,
                                                                    _____
                            To make . . . .   **1000 cc.**

Prepare the solution, filter and fill 1-cc. cleansed ampuls according to the requirements (see N.F. VII, pages 29–34). Sterilize by Process C (see N.F. VII, page 35).

AVERAGE DOSE—1 cc.

AMPULS OF IRON ARSENITE (SOLUBLE)
(R.P.P.)

A sterile aqueous solution containing iron arsenite and ammonium citrate 0.06
Gm. in each cc.

Iron Arsenite and Ammonium Citrate . . . .   **60 Gm.**

Quinine and Urea Hydrochloride . . . .   **10 Gm.**

Diluted Solution of Ammonia, a sufficient quantity,

Ampul Water, a sufficient quantity,
                                                                    _____
                            To make . . . .   **1000 cc.**

Prepare the solution by dissolving the iron arsenite and ammonium citrate and the
quinine and urea hydrochloride separately and then pouring the second solution into
the first while stirring rapidly. Add diluted solution of ammonia gradually until
the solution is but slightly acid, filter and fill 1-cc. cleansed ampuls according to the
requirements (see N.F. VII, pages 29–34). Sterilize by Process D (see N.F. VII,
page 35).

AVERAGE DOSE—1 cc.

AMPULS OF IRON ARSENITE AND STRYCHNINE
R.B. II.

A sterile aqueous solution containing iron arsenite and ammonium citrate
0.045 Gm., strychnine nitrate 0.001 Gm. and quinine and urea hydrochloride
0.005 Gm. in each cc.

Iron Arsenite and Ammonium Citrate . . . .   **45 Gm.**

Strychnine Nitrate . . . .   **1 Gm.**

Quinine and Urea Hydrochloride . . . .   **5 Gm.**

Ampul Water, a sufficient quantity,
                                                                    _____
                            To make . . . .   **1000 cc.**

Dissolve the quinine and urea hydrochloride in sufficient ampul water to produce
500 cc. and the iron arsenite and ammonium citrate and strychnine nitrate in a second
portion of ampul water to produce 500 cc. Pour the first solution into the second
while stirring rapidly. Filter and fill 1-cc. cleansed ampuls according to the requirements (see N.F. VII, pages 29–34). Sterilize by Process F (see N.F. VII, page 36).

AVERAGE DOSE—1 cc.

AMPULS OF IRON CACODYLATE
(R.P.P.)

A sterile aqueous solution containing iron cacodylate 0.03 Gm. in each cc.

Iron Cacodylate	30 Gm.
Ampul Water, a sufficient quantity,	
To make	1000 cc.

Prepare the solution by adding the iron cacodylate to boiling ampul water and immediately cool; filter and fill 1-cc. cleansed ampuls according to the requirements (see N.F. VII, pages 29–34). Sterilize by Process C (see N.F. VII, page 35).

AVERAGE DOSE—1 cc.

To prepare a solution containing iron cacodylate 0.0125 Gm. in each cc., use 12.5 Gm. for 1000 cc. of solution, filter and fill 1-cc. cleansed ampuls according to the requirements (see N.F. VII, pages 29–34). Sterilize by Process C (see N.F. VII, page 35).

AVERAGE DOSE—1 cc.

NOTE—Some samples of iron cacodylate, while differing imperceptibly from others so far as can be determined chemically, cause extreme irritation at the site of injection. The solution should be made as nearly neutral as possible by using diluted solution of ammonia or solution of citric acid as required.

AMPULS OF MERCURIC OXYCYANIDE
(R.P.P.)

A sterile aqueous solution containing mercuric oxycyanide 0.0015 Gm. in each cc.

Mercuric Oxycyanide.	1.5 Gm.
Ampul Water, a sufficient quantity,	
To make	1000 cc.

Prepare the solution, filter and fill 1-cc. cleansed ampuls according to the requirements (see N.F. VII, pages 29–34). Sterilize by Process F (see N.F. VII, page 36).

AVERAGE DOSE—1 cc.

AMPULS OF SODIUM GLYCEROPHOSPHATE, STRYCHNINE CACODYLATE AND IRON CACODYLATE

Ampuls of Glycerophosphate Compound
(R.B. II)

A sterile aqueous solution containing sodium glycerophosphate 0.1 Gm., strychnine cacodylate 0.0005 Gm., iron cacodylate 0.01 Gm. and chlorobutanol 0.005 Gm. in each cc.

Sodium Glycerophosphate.	100 Gm.
Strychnine Cacodylate	0.5 Gm.
Iron Cacodylate	10 Gm.
Chlorobutanol	5 Gm.
Ampul Water, a sufficient quantity,	
To make	1000 cc.

Prepare the solution, filter and fill 1-cc. cleansed ampuls according to the requirements (see N.F. VII, pages 29–34).   Sterilize by Process F (see N.F. VII, page 36).

AVERAGE DOSE—1 cc.

AROMATIC SULFURIC ACID
Acidum Sulfuricum Aromaticum
(U.S.P. XI)

Sulfuric Acid	114 cc.
Fluidextract of Ginger	10 cc.
Oil of Cinnamon	1 cc.
Alcohol, a sufficient quantity,	
To make	1000 cc.

Add the sulfuric acid gradually, and with great caution, to 700 cc. of alcohol and allow the mixture to cool.   Then mix with it the fluidextract of ginger and the oil of cinnamon and add enough alcohol to make the product measure 1000 cc.

AVERAGE DOSE—Metric, 0.5 cc.—Apothecaries, 8 minims.

BALSAMS

BALSAM OF BENZOIC AND TANNIC ACIDS
(Lux. F.)

Benzoic Acid	10 Gm.
Tannic Acid	50 Gm.
Glycerin	40 cc.
Alcohol	250 cc.
Rose Water, a sufficient quantity,	
To make	1000 cc.

Dissolve the benzoic and tannic acids in the alcohol, add the glycerin and sufficient rose water to make the product measure 1000 cc.

BALSAM OF POTASSIUM IODIDE AND CAMPHOR
(R.B. I)

Hard Soap, in powder	60 Gm.
Potassium Iodide	30 Gm.
Camphor	15 Gm.
Tincture of Benzoin	60 cc.
Glycerin	60 cc.
Rose Water or Distilled Water	60 cc.
Alcohol, a sufficient quantity,	
To make	1000 cc.

Dissolve the potassium iodide in the glycerin and rose water.   Dissolve the hard soap and camphor in 700 cc. of alcohol and add the tincture of benzoin and the potassium iodide solution.   Lastly, add sufficient alcohol to make the product measure 1000 cc.

BATHS

The temperature for a medicinal bath is 35° to 40° C. (slightly lower for an effervescent bath). The weights of medicaments given below are for 114 liters (30 gallons) of water, since this is approximately the usual quantity for a bath.

ALKALINE BATH
Balneum Alkalinum
(B.P.C. 1934)

Monohydrated Sodium Carbonate . . . .   65 Gm.

BORIC ACID BATH
Balneum Acidi Borici
(B.P.C. 1923)

Boric Acid . . . .   175 Gm.

EFFERVESCENT BATH
Balneum Effervescens
(B.P.C. 1934)

Sodium Bicarbonate . . . .   460 Gm.
Sodium Bisulfate. . . . .   230 Gm.

Dissolve the sodium bicarbonate in the bath water and add the sodium bisulfate just before use.

SULFURATED BATH SALTS
Sal Sulfuratum pro Balneo
(Lux. F.)

Monohydrated Sodium Carbonate . . . .   920 Gm.
Sublimed Sulfur. . . . .   40 Gm.
Potassium Chromate . . . .   10 Gm.
Distilled Water . . . .   30 cc.
                        To make about . . . .   1000 Gm.

Dissolve the potassium chromate in the distilled water and mix well with the other ingredients, then melt the mass in a covered crucible, only about half filled. Pour the fused mass on a cold marble slab and, after cooling, break the finished product into pieces.

Keep in well-closed bottles.

CAPSULES

ACETYLSALICYLIC ACID AND ACETOPHENETIDIN CAPSULES WITH CAFFEINE AND CODEINE
(P.H.N.Y.)

Acetylsalicylic Acid   30   Gm.
Acetophenetidin (Phenacetin)   18   Gm.
Caffeine   3   Gm.
Codeine . . . .   0.7 Gm.

To make . . . .   100 Capsules

Triturate the ingredients together until mixed intimately and then pack into capsules of appropriate size.

Each capsule contains 0.007 Gm. ($\frac{1}{10}$ grain) of codeine.

AVERAGE DOSE—1 capsule.

CAPSULES OF THEOPHYLLINE ETHYLENEDIAMINE, EPHEDRINE AND PHENOBARBITAL
(U.C.H.)

Theophylline Ethylenediamine   20   Gm.
Ephedrine Sulfate . . . .   2.5 Gm.
Phenobarbital . . . .   1.5 Gm.

To make . . . .   100 Capsules

Mix the ingredients intimately and then pack into capsules of appropriate size.

AVERAGE DOSE—1 capsule.

A.P.A.C. CAPSULES
(R.B. II)

Acetylsalicylic Acid . . . .   30 Gm.
Acetophenetidin (Phenacetin) . . . .   12 Gm.
Acetanilid . . . .   6 Gm.
Caffeine . . . .   3 Gm.

To make . . . .   100 Capsules

Triturate the ingredients together until mixed intimately and then pack into capsules of appropriate size.

AVERAGE DOSE—1 capsule.

ARSENIC, IRON, QUININE AND STRYCHNINE CAPSULES
(B.N.Y.)

Arsenic Trioxide . . . .   0.25 Gm.
Strychnine Sulfate . . . .   0.12 Gm.
Exsiccated Ferrous Sulfate   20   Gm.
Quinine Sulfate   3   Gm.
Ipecac, in fine powder . . . .   0.30 Gm.

To make . . . .   100 Capsules

Triturate the ingredients together until mixed intimately and then pack into capsules of appropriate size.

AVERAGE DOSE—1 capsule.

Each capsule contains 0.0025 Gm. ($\frac{1}{24}$ grain) of arsenic trioxide, and 0.0012 Gm. ($\frac{1}{50}$ grain) of strychnine sulfate.

COMPOUND CAPSULES OF BELLADONNA AND PHENOBARBITAL
(U.C.H.)

Extract of Belladonna	1.5 Gm.
Phenobarbital Sodium	2 Gm.
Sodium Bicarbonate	30 Gm.
To make	100 Capsules

Mix the ingredients intimately and then pack into capsules of appropriate size.

AVERAGE DOSE—1 capsule.

C.A.P. CAPSULES
I
(P.H.N.Y.)

Citrated Caffeine	6 Gm.
Acetanilid	12 Gm.
Acetophenetidin (Phenacetin)	18 Gm.
To make	100 Capsules

Triturate the ingredients together until mixed intimately and then pack into capsules of appropriate size.

AVERAGE DOSE—1 capsule.

II
(B.N.Y.)

Citrated Caffeine	12 Gm.
Acetanilid	20 Gm.
Acetophenetidin (Phenacetin)	30 Gm.
To make	100 Capsules

Triturate the ingredients together until mixed intimately and then pack into capsules of appropriate size.

AVERAGE DOSE—1 capsule.

NUX VOMICA, CASCARA, AND IRON CAPSULES
Hematinic Capsules

Extract of Nux Vomica	0.8 Gm.
Extract of Cascara Sagrada	2.8 Gm.
Exsiccated Ferrous Sulfate	28.8 Gm.
To make	100 Capsules

Triturate the ingredients together until mixed intimately and then pack into capsules of appropriate size.

AVERAGE DOSE—1 capsule three times a day.

IRON, QUININE, AND NUX VOMICA CAPSULES
(B.N.Y.)

Saccharated Ferrous Carbonate	12	Gm.
Quinine Sulfate	12	Gm.
Extract of Nux Vomica	1.6	Gm.
Extract of Gentian	6	Gm.
To make	100	Capsules

Triturate the ingredients together until mixed intimately and then pack into capsules of appropriate size.

AVERAGE DOSE—1 capsule.

METHENAMINE AND SALOL CAPSULES WITH METHYLTHIONINE CHLORIDE
(G.H.N.Y.)

Methylthionine Chloride	5 Gm.
Phenyl Salicylate	30 Gm.
Methenamine	30 Gm.
To make	100 Capsules

Triturate the ingredients together until mixed intimately and then pack into capsules of appropriate size.

AVERAGE DOSE—1 capsule.

SALICYLATE—CARBONATE CAPSULES
(U.C.H.)

Sodium Salicylate	30 Gm.
Sodium Bicarbonate	30 Gm.
To make	100 Capsules

Mix the powders intimately and then pack into capsules of appropriate size.

AVERAGE DOSE—1 to 3 capsules.

SALOL, ACETOPHENETIDIN AND QUININE CAPSULES
(B.N.Y.)

Phenyl Salicylate	12 Gm.
Acetophenetidin	12 Gm.
Quinine Sulfate	12 Gm.
To make	100 Capsules

Triturate the ingredients together until mixed intimately and then pack into capsules of appropriate size.

AVERAGE DOSE—1 capsule.

SOFT CAPSULES OF SALOL AND CASTOR OIL
(N.Y.H.F.)

Phenyl Salicylate	30 Gm.
Castor Oil	30 cc.
To make	100 Soft Capsules

Dissolve the phenyl salicylate in the castor oil with the aid of gentle heat and divide into 100 soft capsules.

AVERAGE DOSE—1 capsule.

CERATES

ASEPTIC WAX
Ceratum Aseptica
(B.P.C. 1934)

White Wax	875 Gm.
Expressed Almond Oil or Persic Oil	125 cc.
Salicylic Acid	10 Gm.
To make about	1000 Gm.

Melt the wax with the oil and strain through muslin, add the salicylic acid and heat for half an hour on a water bath. Pour while hot into dry, sterile bottles.

Keep covered with an aqueous solution (1 in 500) of mercury bichloride.

Aseptic wax is used to arrest hemorrhage from cranial bones by smearing the wax over the bleeding surface.

CAMPHOR CERATE
Ceratum Camphoræ
(N.F. V)

Camphor Liniment	100 Gm.
White Wax	350 Gm.
White Petrolatum	150 Gm.
Benzoinated Lard	400 Gm.
To make	1000 Gm.

Melt the white wax, add the white petrolatum, then the benzoinated lard, and continue the heat until the mixture is liquefied. Add the camphor liniment and stir the mixture until it congeals.

PETROLATUM CERATE

Ceratum Paraffini

Paraffin Cerate

(B.P.C. 1923)

Yellow Wax.	62 Gm.
Petrolatum	938 Gm.
To make	1000 Gm.

Melt together and stir constantly as the mixture cools.

Petrolatum cerate can be incorporated with half its weight of water.

This cerate may be prepared with the yellow or white varieties of beeswax and petrolatum; if required as a basis of a white ointment the white beeswax and white petrolatum should be employed.

COLLODIONS

CANTHARIDAL COLLODION

Collodium Cantharidatum

Blistering Collodion, Vesicating Collodion

(U.S.P. IX)

Cantharides, in fine powder	600 Gm.
Glacial Acetic Acid.	50 cc.
Flexible Collodion,	
Acetone, of each, a sufficient quantity,	
To make	1000 cc.

Mix the cantharides with 550 cc. of acetone, to which the glacial acetic acid has been added, and set the mixture aside in a closely covered container for 24 hours. Then transfer it to a percolator and percolate with acetone until the drug is practically exhausted. Reduce the percolate by distillation on a water bath, in a tared flask, to 150 Gm. and, when cold, dissolve this concentrated extract in sufficient flexible collodion to make the product measure 1000 cc. Finally allow the solution to stand for several hours, decant the clear liquid from any sediment which may have deposited, and transfer the product to containers, which must be well closed.

Keep in a cool place, remote from fire.

IODINE COLLODION

Collodium Iodi

Collodium Iodatum

(N.F. IV)

Iodine, in powder	50 Gm.
Flexible Collodion, a sufficient quantity,	
To make	1000 cc.

Add the iodine to the flexible collodion in a bottle and agitate the mixture frequently until the iodine is dissolved.

Keep in a cool place, remote from fire.

CONFECTIONS

COMPOUND CONFECTION OF GUAIAC
Confectio Guaiaci Composita
Compound Confection of Guaiac with Rhubarb and Sulfur

Chelsea Pensioner
(B.P.C. 1934)

Guaiac, in fine powder	10 Gm.
Rhubarb, in fine powder	20 Gm.
Potassium Bitartrate	75 Gm.
Sublimed Sulfur	145 Gm.
Myristica, in fine powder	10 Gm.
Honey	740 Gm.
To make	1000 Gm.

Mix the guaiac, rhubarb, potassium bitartrate, myristica and sublimed sulfur and add gradually to the honey with constant trituration; mix thoroughly.

AVERAGE DOSE—Metric, 4 to 8 Gm.—Apothecaries, 1 to 2 drachms.

LAXATIVE CONFECTION
Confectio Laxativa
Household Physic

Prunes, deprived of seed	240 Gm.
Dates, deprived of seed	240 Gm.
Seedless Raisins	220 Gm.
Fig	240 Gm.
Senna, in fine powder	60 Gm.
To make	1000 Gm.

Pass the ingredients through a meat chopper to produce a uniform paste. Keep in a well-covered jar in a cool place.

AVERAGE DOSE—Metric, 15 to 30 Gm.—Apothecaries, ½ to 1 ounce.

CONFECTION OF ROSE
Confectio Rosæ
(N.F. V)

Rose, in fine powder	80 Gm.
Sucrose, in fine powder	640 Gm.
Honey	120 Gm.
Stronger Rose Water	160 cc.
To make about	1000 Gm.

Rub the rose with the stronger rose water, previously heated to 65° C., add gradually the sucrose and honey and knead the mixture until a uniform mass is obtained.

CONFECTION OF SENNA
Confectio Sennæ
Confection of Senna and Cassia Fistula
(N.F. V)

Senna, in fine powder.	100 Gm.
Cassia Fistula, bruised	160 Gm.
Tamarind.	100 Gm.
Prunes, deprived of seeds	70 Gm.
Fig, bruised	120 Gm.
Sucrose, in fine powder.	555 Gm.
Oil of Coriander	5 Gm.
Distilled Water, a sufficient quantity,	
To make	1000 Gm.

Digest the cassia fistula, tamarind, prune and fig with 500 cc. of distilled water in a covered vessel, on a water bath, for 3 hours. Pass the pulpy mass through a meat chopper and then through a muslin cloth. Mix the residue with 150 cc. of distilled water, digest the mixture for a short time, then treat it as before and add the strained product to the pulpy mass first obtained. Then, by means of a water bath, dissolve the sucrose in the mixture and evaporate it, in a tared vessel, until it weighs 895 Gm. Lastly, add the senna and the oil of coriander, and incorporate them thoroughly with the other ingredients while they are yet warm.

AVERAGE DOSE—Metric, 4 Gm.—Apothecaries, 1 drachm.

CORDIALS

BLACKBERRY CORDIAL
Cordiale Rubi Fructus
(N.F. IV)

Cinnamon, in No. 40 powder	20 Gm.
Clove, in No. 40 powder	5 Gm.
Myristica, freshly grated	5 Gm.
Purified Talc	15 Gm.
Syrup of Blackberry Fruit, R.B.	750 cc.
Diluted Alcohol, a sufficient quantity,	
To make	1000 cc.

Pack the mixed drugs firmly in a cylindrical glass percolator and percolate with diluted alcohol until the percolate measures 250 cc.; to this add the syrup of blackberry fruit, mix, add the purified talc and filter.

AVERAGE DOSE—Metric, 8 cc.—Apothecaries, 2 fluidrachms.

CURAÇAO CORDIAL

Cordiale Curassao

Elixir of Curaçao

(N.F. III)

Spirit of Curaçao, R.B. . . . . 16 cc.
Orris, in fine powder . . . . 4 Gm.
Alcohol . . . . 250 cc.
Citric Acid . . . . 7 Gm.
Syrup . . . . 500 cc.
Purified Talc . . . . 15 Gm.
Distilled Water, a sufficient quantity,

To make . . . . 1000 cc.

Mix the spirit of curaçao with the alcohol, add the orris, the purified talc and 185 cc. of distilled water. Allow the mixture to stand 12 hours, occasionally agitating; then pour it on a wetted filter, returning the first portions of the filtrate until it runs through clear, and pass enough distilled water through the filter to make the filtrate measure 500 cc. In this dissolve the citric acid, and finally add the syrup.

AVERAGE DOSE—Metric, 15 cc.—Apothecaries, 4 fluidrachms.

MEDICATED CREAMS

BISMUTH CREAM I

Bismuth, Zinc Oxide and Boric Acid Cream

(R.B. II)

Zinc Oxide . . . . 80 Gm.
Starch . . . . 80 Gm.
Bismuth Subnitrate. 80 Gm.
Boric Acid . . . . 120 Gm.
Liquid Petrolatum, heavy . . . . 80 Gm.
Rose Water or Distilled Water . . . . 120 cc.
Solution of Calcium Hydroxide. . . . . 240 cc.
Wool Fat . . . . 30 Gm.
Paraffin Ointment, R.B. . . . . 170 Gm.

To make about . . . . 1000 Gm.

Rub the powders with the paraffin ointment and wool fat until thoroughly incorporated. Add slowly the liquid petrolatum and solution of calcium hydroxide, then incorporate the rose water.

BISMUTH CREAM II

Bismuth and Zinc Oxide Cream

(R.B. II)

Bismuth Subnitrate	16 Gm.
Zinc Oxide	32 Gm.
Bentonite	30 Gm.
Olive Oil or Peanut Oil	500 cc.
Solution of Calcium Hydroxide, a sufficient quantity,	
To make	1000 cc.

Emulsify the olive oil or peanut with 450 cc. of solution of calcium hydroxide by thorough shaking. Triturate the powders with this and add sufficient solution of calcium hydroxide to make the product measure 1000 cc.

COAL TAR CREAM

Carbonis Cream

(U.C.H.)

Solution of Coal Tar	80 cc.
Stearic Acid	150 Gm.
Alcohol	120 cc.
Potassium Hydroxide	7 Gm.
Glycerin	50 cc.
Water, a sufficient quantity,	
To make	1000 Gm.

Heat the stearic acid to 80° C. with 300 cc. of water on a water bath and add the potassium hydroxide previously dissolved in water. Remove from the heat and stir until the stearic acid is completely saponified; add the glycerin and the mixture of coal tar solution and alcohol shaking or stirring continuously. Lastly add sufficient water to make the product weigh 1000 Gm. Stir until a uniform cream results.

SULFUR CREAM

(R.B. II)

Precipitated Sulfur	125 Gm.
Glycerin	125 Gm.
Rose Water Ointment	750 Gm.
To make	1000 Gm.

Rub the precipitated sulfur to a smooth paste with the glycerin, then incorporate it with the rose water ointment.

CREAM FOR WATERPROOFING THE SKIN

(Arch. Dermatology & Syphilology)

White Wax	10 Gm.
Hydrous Wool Fat	5 Gm.
Sulfonated Olive Oil, 75 per cent	10 Gm.
Petrolatum, a sufficient quantity,	
To make	100 Gm.

Triturate the ingredients together until mixed intimately and then pack into capsules of appropriate size.

AVERAGE DOSE—1 capsule.

SOFT CAPSULES OF SALOL AND CASTOR OIL
(N.Y.H.F.)

Phenyl Salicylate	30 Gm.
Castor Oil	30 cc.
To make	100 Soft Capsules

Dissolve the phenyl salicylate in the castor oil with the aid of gentle heat and divide into 100 soft capsules.

AVERAGE DOSE—1 capsule.

CERATES

ASEPTIC WAX
Ceratum Aseptica
(B.P.C. 1934)

White Wax	875 Gm.
Expressed Almond Oil or Persic Oil	125 cc.
Salicylic Acid	10 Gm.
To make about	1000 Gm.

Melt the wax with the oil and strain through muslin, add the salicylic acid and heat for half an hour on a water bath. Pour while hot into dry, sterile bottles.

Keep covered with an aqueous solution (1 in 500) of mercury bichloride.

Aseptic wax is used to arrest hemorrhage from cranial bones by smearing the wax over the bleeding surface.

CAMPHOR CERATE
Ceratum Camphoræ
(N.F. V)

Camphor Liniment	100 Gm.
White Wax	350 Gm.
White Petrolatum	150 Gm.
Benzoinated Lard	400 Gm.
To make	1000 Gm.

Melt the white wax, add the white petrolatum, then the benzoinated lard, and continue the heat until the mixture is liquefied. Add the camphor liniment and stir the mixture until it congeals.

PETROLATUM CERATE
Ceratum Paraffini

Paraffin Cerate
(B.P.C. 1923)

Yellow Wax.	62 Gm.
Petrolatum	938 Gm.
To make	1000 Gm.

Melt together and stir constantly as the mixture cools.

Petrolatum cerate can be incorporated with half its weight of water.

This cerate may be prepared with the yellow or white varieties of beeswax and petrolatum; if required as a basis of a white ointment the white beeswax and white petrolatum should be employed.

COLLODIONS

CANTHARIDAL COLLODION
Collodium Cantharidatum

Blistering Collodion, Vesicating Collodion
(U.S.P. IX)

Cantharides, in fine powder	600 Gm.
Glacial Acetic Acid.	50 cc.
Flexible Collodion,	
Acetone, of each, a sufficient quantity,	
To make	1000 cc.

Mix the cantharides with 550 cc. of acetone, to which the glacial acetic acid has been added, and set the mixture aside in a closely covered container for 24 hours. Then transfer it to a percolator and percolate with acetone until the drug is practically exhausted. Reduce the percolate by distillation on a water bath, in a tared flask, to 150 Gm. and, when cold, dissolve this concentrated extract in sufficient flexible collodion to make the product measure 1000 cc. Finally allow the solution to stand for several hours, decant the clear liquid from any sediment which may have deposited, and transfer the product to containers, which must be well closed.

Keep in a cool place, remote from fire.

IODINE COLLODION
Collodium Iodi

Collodium Iodatum
(N.F. IV)

Iodine, in powder	50 Gm.
Flexible Collodion, a sufficient quantity,	
To make	1000 cc.

Add the iodine to the flexible collodion in a bottle and agitate the mixture frequently until the iodine is dissolved.

Keep in a cool place, remote from fire.

Melt together the wax, wool fat and petrolatum and add the sulfonated olive oil; stir until cool and uniformly mixed.

NOTE—This cream is useful to waterproof the skin when there is prolonged contact of the hands with water.

ZINC CREAM
Cremor Zinci
(B.P.C. 1934)

Zinc Oxide	320 Gm.
Wool Fat	80 Gm.
Expressed Oil of Almond or Persic Oil	320 cc.
Solution of Calcium Hydroxide, a sufficient quantity,	
To make.	1000 Gm.

Triturate the zinc oxide with the almond oil, and incorporate the wool fat and sufficient solution of calcium hydroxide to make the product weigh 1000 Gm.

ZINC AND ALUMINUM CREAM
(R.B. II)

Wool Fat.	100 Gm.
Olive Oil or Peanut Oil	400 cc.
Zinc Oxide	100 Gm.
Purified Talc	100 Gm.
Solution of Aluminum Acetate	28 cc.
Solution of Calcium Hydroxide, a sufficient quantity,	
To make	1000 cc.

Melt the wool fat and mix it with the olive oil. Next, incorporate the zinc oxide and talc. Then add the solution of aluminum acetate. Finally, add sufficient solution of calcium hydroxide to make 1000 cc.

DECOCTIONS

COMPOUND DECOCTION OF SARSAPARILLA
Decoctum Sarsaparillæ Compositum
(N.F. IV)

Sarsaparilla, cut and bruised	100 Gm.
Sassafras, in No. 20 powder.	20 Gm.
Guaiac Wood, rasped.	20 Gm.
Glycyrrhiza, cut and bruised	20 Gm.
Mezereum, cut and bruised	10 Gm.
Distilled Water, a sufficient quantity,	
To make	1000 cc.

Add the sarsaparilla and guaiac wood to 1000 cc. of distilled water in a suitable vessel and boil the mixture for 30 minutes, replacing the water lost by evaporation. Then add the sassafras, glycyrrhiza and mezereum, cover the vessel and macerate the mixture for 2 hours.   Finally strain, and add enough cold distilled water through the strainer to make the product measure 1000 cc.

AVERAGE DOSE—Metric, 120 cc.—Apothecaries, 4 fluidounces.

ZITTMANN'S DECOCTION
(B.P.C. 1923)

Sarsaparilla, cut	40	Gm.
Sucrose	2.5	Gm.
Alum	2.5	Gm.
Mild Mercurous Chloride	1.5	Gm.
Red Mercuric Sulfide	0.5	Gm.
Fennel, bruised	1.5	Gm.
Anise, bruised	1.5	Gm.
Senna, cut	10	Gm.
Glycyrrhiza, in coarse powder	5	Gm.
Distilled Water, a sufficient quantity,		
To make	1000	cc.

Macerate the sarsaparilla with 1000 cc. of distilled water for 24 hours at 35° to 40° C., add the sucrose and alum, stir well and then add the mild mercurous chloride and the red mercuric sulfide previously enclosed in a piece of linen.   Heat on a water bath with frequent stirring for 3 hours.   Add the fennel, anise, senna and glycyrrhiza, heat again for 15 minutes, strain and express.   After 1 hour, decant the clear liquid and add sufficient distilled water to make the product measure 1000 cc.

Dispense with a "shake well" label.

AVERAGE DOSE—Metric, 60 cc.—Apothecaries, 2 fluidounces.

DOUCHES

ALUM AND ZINC SULFATE DOUCHE WITH PHENOL
(B.N.Y.)

Alum	4	Gm.
Zinc Sulfate	4	Gm.
Liquefied Phenol	5	cc.
Glycerin	125	cc.
Distilled Water, a sufficient quantity,		
To make	1000	cc.

Dissolve the alum and zinc sulfate in 500 cc. of distilled water.   Then add the liquefied phenol, which has been previously mixed with the glycerin, and sufficient distilled water to make the product measure 1000 cc.

BORIC ACID AND ZINC SULFATE DOUCHE
(B.N.Y.)

Boric Acid . . . . 34 Gm.
Zinc Sulfate. . . . . 4 Gm.
Alcohol . . . . 68 cc.
Distilled Water, a sufficient quantity,

       To make . . . . 1000 cc.

Dissolve the boric acid and zinc sulfate in 900 cc. of distilled water, add the alcohol and filter. Then add sufficient distilled water to make the product measure 1000 cc.

DOUCHE POWDERS

POWDER OF ALUM AND BORIC ACID WITH ZINC AND COPPER SULFATES
(R.B. II)

Alum,
Zinc Sulfate,
Cupric Sulfate,
Boric Acid, of each, an equal weight.

Reduce the ingredients to a fine powder, mix intimately and pass through a No. 60 sieve.

For preparing douches, 1 teaspoonful is dissolved in a quart of water.

ASTRINGENT DOUCHE POWDER
(R.B. I)

Sodium Borate . . . . 575 Gm.
Exsiccated Alum. . . . . 400 Gm.
Phenol . . . . 5 Gm.
Thymol. . . . . 5 Gm.
Menthol . . . . 5 Gm.
Eucalyptol . . . . 5 cc.
Methyl Salicylate . . . . 5 cc.

      To make . . . . 1000 Gm.

Mix intimately and pass through a No. 60 sieve.
For preparing douches, 1 to 2 teaspoonfuls are dissolved in a quart of water.

ALUM AND ZINC DOUCHE POWDER
(P.H.N.Y.)

Alum, in fine powder,
Zinc Sulfate, in fine powder, of each, an equal weight.

Mix intimately and pass through a No. 60 sieve.
For preparing douches, 1 teaspoonful is dissolved in a quart of water.

BORAX, ALUM AND MENTHOL DOUCHE POWDER
(R.B. II)

Menthol, in fine powder	3 Gm.
Alum, in fine powder	45 Gm.
Sodium Borate	465 Gm.
Sodium Bicarbonate	487 Gm.
To make	1000 Gm.

Mix intimately and pass through a No. 60 sieve.

For preparing douches, 1 teaspoonful is dissolved in a quart of water.

BORO-TANNIC DOUCHE POWDER
(B.N.Y.)

Boric Acid, in fine powder,
Tannic Acid, in fine powder, of each, an equal weight.

Mix thoroughly and pass through a No. 60 sieve.

For preparing douches, 1 teaspoonful is dissolved in a quart of water.

PHENOLATED DOUCHE POWDER WITH ALUM AND BORIC ACID
(P.H.N.Y.)

Oil of Peppermint	40 cc.
Liquefied Phenol	80 cc.
Alum, in fine powder	200 Gm.
Boric Acid, in fine powder	680 Gm.
To make about	1000 Gm.

Mix the alum and boric acid, then incorporate the oil of peppermint and liquefied phenol.   Finally pass the powder through a No. 40 sieve.

For preparing douches, 1 teaspoonful is dissolved in a quart of water.

MEDICATED NASAL DROPS

NASAL DROPS

CAUTION—*Frequent or excessive use of these preparations may cause damage to the lungs.   Do not use for infants or small children without the advice of a physician.*

I
(R.B. II)

Oil of Eucalyptus	10 cc.
Oil of Dwarf Pine Needles	10 cc.
Menthol	1 Gm.
Light Liquid Petrolatum, a sufficient quantity,	
To make	1000 cc.

Dissolve the menthol in the liquid petrolatum and add the oils.

II
(R.B. II)

Thymol. . . . .   5 Gm.
Camphor . . . .   5 Gm.
Menthol . . . .   5 Gm.
Light Liquid Petrolatum, a sufficient quantity,

               To make . . . .   1000 cc.

Triturate the thymol, camphor and menthol together until liquefied and then add gradually sufficient liquid petrolatum to make the product measure 1000 cc.

MILD PROTEIN SILVER AND EPHEDRINE NOSE DROPS
(R.B. II)

Mild Protein Silver . . . .   30 Gm.
Ephedrine Sulfate . . . .   10 Gm.
Glycerin . . . .   60 cc.
Distilled Water, a sufficient quantity,

               To make . . . .   1000 cc.

Dissolve the mild protein silver and ephedrine sulfate separately, each in 200 cc. of distilled water, and mix the solutions. Add the glycerin and sufficient distilled water to make the product measure 1000 cc.

NOTE—These drops should be freshly prepared.

EFFERVESCENT SALTS

EFFERVESCENT ARTIFICIAL VICHY SALT WITH LITHIUM
Sal Vichyanum Factitium Effervescens cum Lithio

Pulvis Salis Vichyani Factitii Effervescens cum Lithio
(N.F. IV)

Artificial Vichy Salt, dried and powdered . . . .   250 Gm.
Lithium Citrate, dried and powdered . . . .   85 Gm.
Sodium Bicarbonate . . . .   445 Gm.
Tartaric Acid, dried and powdered . . . .   125 Gm.
Citric Acid, in effloresced crystals . . . .   250 Gm.

            To make about . . . .   1000 Gm.

Prepare an effervescent salt by either of the general processes (see N.F. VII, page 361).

AVERAGE DOSE—Metric, 6 Gm.—Apothecaries, 1½ drachms.

EFFERVESCENT CITRATED CAFFEINE
Caffeina Citrata Effervescens
(U.S.P. IX)

Citrated Caffeine.	40 Gm.
Sodium Bicarbonate	570 Gm.
Tartaric Acid, dried and powdered	300 Gm.
Citric Acid, in effloresced crystals	195 Gm.
To make about	1000 Gm.

Prepare an effervescent salt by either of the general processes (see N.F. VII, page 361).

AVERAGE DOSE—Metric, 4 Gm.—Apothecaries, 1 drachm.

EFFERVESCENT SALT OF POTASSIUM BROMIDE
Sal Potassii Bromidi Effervescens
Pulvis Potassii Bromidi Effervescens (N.F. III)
(N.F. IV)

Potassium Bromide, dried	166 Gm.
Sodium Bicarbonate	530 Gm.
Tartaric Acid, dried and powdered	204 Gm.
Citric Acid, in effloresced crystals	250 Gm.
To make about	1000 Gm.

Prepare an effervescent salt by either of the general processes (see N.F. VII, page 361).

AVERAGE DOSE—Metric, 6 Gm.—Apothecaries, 1½ drachms.

EFFERVESCENT SALINE LAXATIVE
Buckeye Saline Laxative
(R.B. I)

Potassium Sulfate, dried	10 Gm.
Sodium Chloride, dried	90 Gm.
Sodium Bicarbonate	180 Gm.
Sodium Sulfate, dried.	220 Gm.
Magnesium Sulfate, dried	125 Gm.
Sodium Phosphate, dried	250 Gm.
Tartaric Acid, dried.	125 Gm.
To make about	1000 Gm.

Mix the ingredients, except the sodium bicarbonate, and dry to constant weight at about 100 to 110° C. Cool, add the sodium bicarbonate and mix thoroughly.

AVERAGE DOSE—Metric, 6 Gm.—Apothecaries, 1½ drachms.

ELECTUARIES

APERIENT ELECTUARY
(R.B. II)

Senna, in fine powder	115 Gm.
Potassium Bitartrate	55 Gm.
Tamarind	230 Gm.
Syrup of Manna, R.B.	600 Gm.
To make	1000 Gm.

Triturate the solid ingredients with the syrup of manna until homogeneous.

AVERAGE DOSE—Metric, 15 Gm.—Apothecaries, 4 drachms.

LENITIVE ELECTUARY
Electuarium Lenitivum

Senneslatwerge, Electuaire lenitif
(Ph. Helv. IV)

Tamarind	400	Gm.
Syrup	300	Gm.
Senna, in fine powder	200	Gm.
Potassium Bitartrate	100	Gm.
Alcohol	1	cc.
Methyl Parahydroxybenzoate	0.1	Gm.
To make about	1000	Gm.

Add to the tamarind and syrup, the solution of methyl parahydroxybenzoate in the alcohol, then mix in the other ingredients thoroughly.

AVERAGE DOSE—Metric, 15 Gm.—Apothecaries, 4 drachms.

ELIXIRS

The elixirs for which formulas are given should, without exception, be perfectly clear when dispensed.

No class of preparations calls for greater care in the selection of the ingredients than does that of the elixirs; this is particularly true with reference to the flavoring substances, mainly volatile oils, which must be absolutely fresh and of the finest quality if satisfactory products are to be obtained.

On mixing the ingredients for any particular elixir a cloudy liquid is usually obtained, which will not immediately filter clear through paper. After standing several hours filtration becomes easier and the liquid usually comes through perfectly clear. This procedure is recommended. When a clear product is not obtained in this way, or when immediate results are needed, there may be added to each 1000 cc. of the turbid liquid 10 Gm. to 20 Gm. of purified talc; the mixture must be well shaken and preferably allowed to stand for a time, then filtered, the first portions of filtrate being returned to the filter until it comes through perfectly clear.

Elixirs must not be exposed to extremes of temperature, nor to direct sunlight. Preserve them in tightly stoppered bottles at the ordinary room temperature.

COMPOUND ACETANILID ELIXIR
Elixir Acetanilidi Compositum
(R.B. II)

Acetanilid.	20 Gm.
Caffeine.	2 Gm.
Sodium Bromide.	60 Gm.
Aromatic Elixir, a sufficient quantity,	
To make	1000 cc.

Dissolve, and filter if necessary.

AVERAGE DOSE—Metric, 4 cc.—Apothecaries, 1 fluidrachm.

COMPOUND ELIXIR OF ALMOND
Elixir Amygdalæ Compositum
(N.F. VI)

Vanillin	1	Gm.
Oil of Bitter Almond	0.5	cc.
Orange Flower Water	150	cc.
Alcohol	50	cc.
Syrup	400	cc.
Distilled Water, a sufficient quantity,		
To make.	1000	cc.

Dissolve the oil of bitter almond and the vanillin in the alcohol; add the syrup, the orange flower water, and sufficient distilled water in several portions, shaking the mixture thoroughly after each addition, to make the product measure 1000 cc.; then filter until the product is clear.

NOTE—This elixir is used as a vehicle.

ELIXIR OF AMINOACETIC ACID

Aminoacetic Acid	120 Gm.
Distilled Water.	500 cc.
Elixir of Orange, a sufficient quantity,	
To make.	1000 cc.

Dissolve the acid in the distilled water and add the elixir of orange.

ELIXIR OF AMINOPYRINE AND PHENOBARBITAL
(U.C.H.)

Elixir of Aminopyrine	500 cc.
Elixir of Phenobarbital, a sufficient quantity,	
To make.	1000 cc.

Mix.

AVERAGE DOSE—Metric, 4 cc.—Apothecaries, 1 fluidrachm.

ELIXIR OF ANISE
Elixir Anisi
(N.F. V)

Anethol.	3.5	cc.
Oil of Fennel	0.5	cc.
Spirit of Benzaldehyde	12	cc.
Alcohol.	50	cc.
Syrup.	625	cc.
Distilled Water, a sufficient quantity,		
To make	1000	cc.

Mix the anethol, oil of fennel, spirit of benzaldehyde and alcohol, add the syrup and sufficient distilled water to make the product measure 1000 cc. and filter.

AVERAGE DOSE—For Infants: Metric, 1 cc.—Apothecaries, 15 minims.

AQUEOUS ELIXIR
Elixir Aquosum
(N.F. VI)

Vanillin	1	Gm.
Oil of Bitter Almond	0.3	cc.
Oil of Fennel.	0.2	cc.
Chloroform	0.6	cc.
Glycerin	50	cc.
Orange Flower Water	200	cc.
Syrup	400	cc.
Purified Talc.	10	Gm.
Distilled Water, a sufficient quantity,		
To make.	1000	cc.

Dissolve the vanillin in the orange flower water and add the glycerin, in which the oils and the chloroform have been mixed. Then add the syrup and finally enough distilled water to make the product measure 1000 cc. Shake well until solution is effected. Add the talc, set aside for about six hours, and then filter.

NOTE—This elixir is used as a vehicle.

ELIXIR OF BELLADONNA AND SODIUM BROMIDE
(U.C.H.)

Tincture of Belladonna	125	cc.
Sodium Bromide	250	Gm.
Aromatic Elixir, a sufficient quantity,		
To make.	1000	cc.

Dissolve the sodium bromide in the aromatic elixir and gradually add the tincture of belladonna, then filter if necessary.

AVERAGE DOSE—Metric, 4 cc.—Apothecaries, 1 fluidrachm.

COMPOUND ELIXIR OF BLACKBERRY
Elixir Rubi Compositum
(N.F. IV)

Rubus, in moderately coarse powder	16 Gm.
Nutgall, in moderately coarse powder.	16 Gm.
Cinnamon, in moderately coarse powder.	16 Gm.
Clove, in moderately coarse powder	4 Gm.
Mace, in moderately coarse powder.	2 Gm.
Ginger, in moderately coarse powder	2 Gm.
Syrup of Blackberry Fruit, R.B.	750 cc.
Diluted Alcohol, a sufficient quantity,	
To make	1000 cc.

Prepare 250 cc. of a tincture from the mixed drugs by Process P (see N.F. VII, page 439) using diluted alcohol as the menstruum.   To this add the syrup of blackberry fruit and mix thoroughly; set aside for several days and filter.

AVERAGE DOSE—Metric, 15 cc.—Apothecaries, 4 fluidrachms.

ELIXIR OF CALCIUM BROMIDE
Elixir Calcii Bromidi
(N.F. IV)

Calcium Bromide.	85 Gm.
Diluted Hydrobromic Acid	4 cc.
Syrup	200 cc.
Distilled Water	460 cc.
Aromatic Elixir, a sufficient quantity,	
To make	1000 cc.

Dissolve the calcium bromide in the distilled water to which the diluted hydrobromic acid has been added, add the syrup and sufficient aromatic elixir to make the product measure 1000 cc.   Filter.

AVERAGE DOSE—Metric, 4 cc.—Apothecaries, 1 fluidrachm.

ELIXIR OF CALCIUM HYPOPHOSPHITE
Elixir Calcii Hypophosphitis
(N.F. IV)

Calcium Hypophosphite.	35 Gm.
Hypophosphorous Acid	4 cc.
Aromatic Elixir, a sufficient quantity,	
To make	1000 cc.

Dissolve the calcium hypophosphite in 750 cc. of aromatic elixir to which the hypophosphorous acid has been added; add sufficient aromatic elixir to make the product measure 1000 cc. and filter.

AVERAGE DOSE—Metric, 8 cc.—Apothecaries, 2 fluidrachms.

COMPOUND ELIXIR OF CASCARA SAGRADA
Elixir Cascaræ Sagradæ Compositum

Elixir Rhamni Purshianæ Compositum, Laxative Elixir
(N.F. V)

Aromatic Fluidextract of Cascara Sagrada.	125 cc.
Fluidextract of Senna	75 cc.
Fluidextract of Juglans, R.B.	65 cc.
Aromatic Elixir, a sufficient quantity,	
To make	1000 cc.

Mix and filter.

AVERAGE DOSE—Metric, 4 cc.—Apothecaries, 1 fluidrachm.

ELIXIR OF FOUR CHLORIDES
Elixir Chloridorum

Elixir of Chlorides
(N.F. V)

Mercury Bichloride	0.275	Gm.
Solution of Arsenous Acid	16.5	cc.
Tincture of Ferric Chloride	83	cc.
Diluted Hydrochloric Acid	83	cc.
Compound Spirit of Orange	10	cc.
Syrup	250	cc.
Alcohol	200	cc.
Distilled Water, a sufficient quantity,		
To make	1000	cc.

Dissolve the mercuric bichloride in the diluted hydrochloric acid, add the solution of arsenous acid and the tincture of ferric chloride. Mix the compound spirit of orange with the alcohol, add the syrup, the first solution and then sufficient distilled water to make the product measure 1000 cc. and filter.

Preserve the elixir in dark amber-colored bottles.

AVERAGE DOSE—Metric, 4 cc.—Apothecaries, 1 fluidrachm.

One average dose contains about:

0.0011 Gm. or 164 grains of Mercury Bichloride.
0.00065 Gm. or 1/100 grain of Arsenic Trioxide.
0.043 Gm. or 3/5 grain of Ferric Chloride.
0.332 cc. or 4 3/4 minims of Diluted Hydrochloric Acid.

COMPOUND ELIXIR OF CHLORAL AND POTASSIUM BROMIDE
Elixir Chloralis et Potassii Bromidi Compositum
Elixir of Bromide and Chloral

Chloral Hydrate	250 Gm.
Potassium Bromide	250 Gm.
Extract of Hyoscyamus	2 Gm.
Sucrose	210 Gm.
Caramel	12 Gm.
Pumice, in fine powder	20 Gm.
Distilled Water, a sufficient quantity,	
To make	1000 cc.

Triturate the extract in a mortar with the pumice, gradually added, until they are thoroughly mixed. Dissolve the chloral hydrate in 175 cc. of distilled water, and the potassium bromide in 450 cc. of distilled water and gradually add each of these solutions, with constant trituration, to the mixture of the extract and pumice. Add the sucrose and the caramel to this mixture, agitate until the sucrose is dissolved, and set the product aside during 24 hours. Then filter, and add sufficient distilled water through the filter to make the product measure 1000 cc. Mix well.

AVERAGE DOSE—Metric, 4 cc.—Apothecaries, 1 fluidrachm.

One average dose, metric, contains 1 Gm. each of Chloral Hydrate and Potassium Bromide, and represents 0.008 Gm. of Extract of Hyoscyamus.

ELIXIR OF CINCHONA ALKALOIDS AND HYPOPHOSPHITES
Elixir Cinchonæ Alkaloidorum et Hypophosphitum
Elixir Cinchonæ et Hypophosphitum, Elixir of Calisaya and Hypophosphites
(N.F. IV)

Calcium Hypophosphite	17.5 Gm.
Sodium Hypophosphite	17.5 Gm.
Hypophosphorous Acid	8 cc.
Distilled Water	125 cc.
Elixir of Cinchona Alkaloids, a sufficient quantity,	
To make	1000 cc.

Dissolve the hypophosphites in the distilled water, to which the hypophosphorous acid has been added, then add sufficient of the elixir to make the product measure 1000 cc. and filter.

AVERAGE DOSE—Metric, 8 cc.—Apothecaries, 2 fluidrachms.

ELIXIR OF CINCHONA ALKALOIDS AND IRON
Elixir Cinchonæ Alkaloidorum et Ferri

Ferrated Elixir of Calisaya, Alkaloidal
(N.F. V)

Soluble Ferric Phosphate	35 Gm.
Distilled Water	60 cc.
Elixir of Cinchona Alkaloids, a sufficient quantity,	
To make	1000 cc.

Dissolve the soluble ferric phosphate in the distilled water with the aid of heat, and add sufficient elixir to make the product measure 1000 cc. and filter.
Preserve in amber-colored bottles.

AVERAGE DOSE—Metric, 8 cc.—Apothecaries, 2 fluidrachms.

ELIXIR OF CINCHONA ALKALOIDS, IRON AND CALCIUM LACTOPHOSPHATE
Elixir Cinchonæ Alkaloidorum, Ferri et Calcii Lactophosphatis

Elixir Cinchonæ, Ferri et Calcii Lactophosphatis,
Elixir of Calisaya, Iron and Lactophosphate of Lime
(N.F. IV)

Syrup of Calcium Lactophosphate	500 cc.
Potassium Citrate	30 Gm.
Elixir of Cinchona Alkaloids and Iron, R.B., a sufficient quantity,	
To make	1000 cc.

Dissolve the potassium citrate in 450 cc. of elixir of cinchona alkaloids and iron, add the syrup and finally sufficient elixir to make the product measure 1000 cc.

AVERAGE DOSE—Metric, 8 cc.—Apothecaries, 2 fluidrachms.

DAFFY'S ELIXIR

Senna	175 Gm.
Caraway, powdered	25 Gm.
Coriander, powdered	25 Gm.
Raisins, seedless	100 Gm.
Diluted Alcohol, a sufficient quantity,	
To make	1000 cc.

Macerate the mixed drugs with the diluted alcohol for a period of 7 days and filter.

AVERAGE DOSE—Metric, 8, cc.—Apothecaries, 2 fluidrachms.

AROMATIC ELIXIR OF ERIODICTYON
Elixir Eriodictyi Aromaticum
Aromatic Elixir of Yerba Santa, Elixir Corrigens
(N.F. V)

Fluidextract of Eriodictyon	60 cc.
Syrup.	500 cc.
Pumice, in fine powder	30 Gm.
Magnesium Carbonate	10 Gm.
Compound Elixir of Taraxacum	440 cc.
To make about	1000 cc.

Triturate the fluidextract with the pumice and the magnesium carbonate and add the elixir gradually, followed by the syrup. Shake the mixture frequently during 2 hours, allow it to stand 12 or more hours and filter.

AVERAGE DOSE—Metric, 4 cc.—Apothecaries, 1 fluidrachm.

ELIXIR OF FERRIC HYPOPHOSPHITE
Elixir Ferri Hypophosphitis
(N.F. IV)

Ferric Hypophosphite.	16.5 Gm.
Potassium Citrate	21.5 Gm.
Distilled Water	35 cc.
Aromatic Elixir, a sufficient quantity,	
To make	1000 cc.

Dissolve the potassium citrate in the distilled water, add the ferric hypophosphite and heat the mixture gently until a clear solution is obtained. Add sufficient aromatic elixir to make the product measure 1000 cc. and filter.

AVERAGE DOSE—Metric, 4 cc.—Apothecaries, 1 fluidrachm.

ELIXIR OF FERRIC PHOSPHATE
Elixir Ferri Phosphatis
(N.F. IV)

Soluble Ferric Phosphate	35 Gm.
Distilled Water	60 cc.
Aromatic Elixir, a sufficient quantity,	
To make	1000 cc.

Dissolve the soluble ferric phosphate in the distilled water with the aid of heat, add sufficient aromatic elixir to make the product measure 1000 cc. and filter.

AVERAGE DOSE—Metric, 4 cc.—Apothecaries, 1 fluidrachm.

ELIXIR OF FERRIC PYROPHOSPHATE
Elixir Ferri Pyrophosphatis
Elixir of Pyrophosphate of Iron
(N.F. IV)

Soluble Ferric Pyrophosphate	35 Gm.
Distilled Water	60 cc.
Aromatic Elixir, a sufficient quantity,	
To make	1000 cc.

Dissolve the soluble ferric pyrophosphate in the distilled water, with the aid of heat, add sufficient aromatic elixir to make the product measure 1000 cc. and filter.

AVERAGE DOSE—Metric, 4 cc.—Apothecaries, 1 fluidrachm.

NOTE—A color change occurs in this elixir which does not affect its medicinal value.

ELIXIR OF FERROUS LACTATE
Elixir Ferri Lactatis
(N.F. IV)

Ferrous Lactate	17.5 Gm.
Potassium Citrate	52.5 Gm.
Distilled Water	120 cc.
Aromatic Elixir, a sufficient quantity,	
To make	1000 cc.

Dissolve the ferrous lactate and potassium citrate in the distilled water with the aid of gentle heat. Add sufficient aromatic elixir to make the product measure 1000 cc. and filter.

AVERAGE DOSE—Metric, 4 cc.—Apothecaries, 1 fluidrachm.

ELIXIR OF GLYCEROPHOSPHATE AND NUX VOMICA
Compound Glycerophosphate Elixir with Nux Vomica
(N.Y.H.F.)

Sodium Glycerophosphate	80 Gm.
Tincture of Nux Vomica.	80 cc.
Aromatic Elixir, a sufficient quantity,	
To make	1000 cc.

Dissolve the sodium glycerophosphate in 500 cc. of the aromatic elixir, add the tincture of nux vomica and sufficient aromatic elixir to make the product measure 1000 cc.

AVERAGE DOSE—Metric, 4 cc.—Apothecaries, 1 fluidrachm.

NOTE—This preparation is not to be confused with Compound Elixir of Glycerophosphates, N.F. VII.

AROMATIC ELIXIR OF GLYCYRRHIZA
Elixir Glycyrrhizæ Aromaticum
Aromatic Elixir of Licorice
(N.F. IV)

Fluidextract of Glycyrrhiza 125   cc.
Oil of Clove . . . . 0.75 cc.
Oil of Cinnamon . . . . 0.75 cc.
Oil of Myristica . . . . 0.50 cc.
Oil of Fennel . . . . 1.50 cc.
Purified Talc 20   Gm.
Aromatic Elixir, a sufficient quantity,

To make 1000   cc.

Triturate the oils with the purified talc, add gradually the fluidextract and sufficient aromatic elixir to make 1000 cc. Allow the mixture to stand overnight and filter, returning the first portions of the filtrate until it passes through clear. Add sufficient aromatic elixir through the filter to make the product measure 1000 cc.

AVERAGE DOSE—Metric, 8 cc.—Apothecaries, 2 fluidrachms.

ELIXIR OF HOP
Elixir Humuli
(N.F. IV)

Fluidextract of Humulus . . . . 125 cc.
Tincture of Vanilla . . . . 30 cc.
Compound Elixir of Taraxacum . . . . 125 cc.
Purified Talc . . . . 20 Gm.
Aromatic Elixir, a sufficient quantity,

To make . . . . 1000 cc.

Triturate the fluidextract of humulus with the purified talc, add gradually the compound elixir of taraxacum, tincture of vanilla and sufficient aromatic elixir to make 1000 cc. Set aside overnight and filter, returning the first portions of the filtrate until it passes through clear. Finally add sufficient aromatic elixir through the filter to make the product measure 1000 cc.

AVERAGE DOSE—Metric, 8 cc.—Apothecaries, 2 fluidrachms.

ELIXIR OF HYDRASTIS
(L.H.F.)

Fluidextract of Hydrastis . . . . 100 cc.
Aromatic Elixir, a sufficient quantity,

To make . . . . 1000 cc.

Mix.

AVERAGE DOSE—Metric, 4 cc.—Apothecaries, 1 fluidrachm.

COMPOUND HYDRASTIS AND VIBURNUM ELIXIR
(L.H.F.)

Viburnum Opulus, in fine powder	150 Gm.
Hydrastis, in fine powder	100 Gm.
Jamaica Dogwood, in coarse powder	75 Gm.
Pulsatilla, in coarse powder	25 Gm.
Compound Spirit of Orange	15 cc.
Glycerin	150 cc.
Sucrose.	150 Gm.
Diluted Alcohol, a sufficient quantity,	
To make	1000 cc.

Moisten the powdered drugs with 200 cc. of diluted alcohol, macerate for 24 hours, then pack firmly in a percolator, pour on diluted alcohol and allow percolation to proceed until the percolate measures 685 cc. Add the glycerin and sucrose, agitate until solution has been effected, then add the compound spirit of orange and sufficient diluted alcohol to make the product measure 1000 cc.

AVERAGE DOSE—Metric, 8 cc.—Apothecaries, 2 fluidrachms.

ELIXIR OF HYPOPHOSPHITES COMPOUND
Elixir Hypophosphitum Compositum
(R.B. II)

Calcium Hypophosphite.	50 Gm.
Sodium Hypophosphite	20 Gm.
Potassium Hypophosphite.	20 Gm.
Hypophosphorous Acid	5 cc.
Distilled Water	420 cc.
Glycerin	30 cc.
Compound Spirit of Cardamom	1 cc.
Aromatic Elixir, a sufficient quantity,	
To make	1000 cc.

Dissolve the hypophosphites in the distilled water to which the acid has been added, then add the glycerin, compound spirit of cardamom and sufficient aromatic elixir to make the product measure 1000 cc., and filter.

AVERAGE DOSE—Metric, 8 cc.—Apothecaries, 2 fluidrachms.

ELIXIR OF HYPOPHOSPHITES AND IRON
Elixir Hypophosphitum et Ferri
(R.B. II)

Calcium Hypophosphite.	20 Gm.
Sodium Hypophosphite	20 Gm.
Potassium Hypophosphite.	10 Gm.
Ferric Hypophosphite.	10 Gm.
Potassium Citrate	15 Gm.
Hypophosphorous Acid	5 cc.
Distilled Water	250 cc.
Syrup. . . . .,	250 cc.
Aromatic Elixir, a sufficient quantity,	
To make	1000 cc.

Dissolve the ferric hypophosphite and the potassium citrate in 50 cc. of warm distilled water and add the syrup.   Dissolve the other hypophosphites in the remainder of the distilled water and mix the two solutions.   Finally add the acid and sufficient aromatic elixir to make the product measure 1000 cc. and filter.

Store in dark amber-colored bottles.

AVERAGE DOSE—Metric, 8 cc.—Apothecaries, 2 fluidrachms.

ELIXIR OF LITHIUM BROMIDE
Elixir Lithii Bromidi
(N.F. IV)

Lithium Bromide.	85 Gm.
Syrup.	200 cc.
Distilled Water	460 cc.
Aromatic Elixir, a sufficient quantity,	
To make	1000 cc.

Dissolve the lithium bromide in the distilled water, add the syrup and sufficient aromatic elixir to make the product measure 1000 cc. and filter.

AVERAGE DOSE—Metric, 8 cc.—Apothecaries, 2 fluidrachms.

ELIXIR OF LITHIUM CITRATE
Elixir Lithii Citratis
(N.F. IV)

Lithium Citrate	85 Gm.
Aromatic Elixir, a sufficient quantity,	
To make	1000 cc.

Dissolve and filter.

AVERAGE DOSE—Metric, 8 cc.—Apothecaries, 2 fluidrachms.

ELIXIR OF LITHIUM SALICYLATE
Elixir Lithii Salicylatis
(N.F. IV)

Lithium Salicylate . . . . 85 Gm.
Aromatic Elixir, a sufficient quantity,

            To make . . . .   1000 cc.

     Dissolve and filter.

AVERAGE DOSE—Metric, 8 cc.—Apothecaries, 2 fluidrachms.

ELIXIR OF ORANGE

Tincture of Sweet Orange Peel . . . . 30 cc.
Aromatic Elixir, a sufficient quantity,

            To make . . . .   1000 cc.

     Mix, and filter if necessary.

ELIXIR OF OVOLECITHIN
Elixir of Lecithin
(B.P.C. 1934)

Ovolecithin (Lecithin) . . . . 18.3   Gm.
Yolk of Egg 125   cc.
Glycerin 350   cc.
Tincture of Lemon . . . . 18.75 cc.
Distilled Water, a sufficient quantity,

            To make 1000   cc.

     Triturate the ovolecithin with the yolk of egg added gradually to form a smooth cream; add the glycerin and tincture of lemon; then add gradually, with constant stirring, sufficient distilled water to make the product measure 1000 cc.

AVERAGE DOSE—Metric, 4 to 16 cc.—Apothecaries, 1 to 4 fluidrachms.

ELIXIR OF PARALDEHYDE
Elixir Paraldehydi
(Ext. Ph. 1920)

Saccharin. . . . . 1 Gm.
Oil of Bitter Orange . . . . 8 cc.
Oil of Cinnamon. . . . . 4 cc.
Paraldehyde . . . . 240 cc.
Alcohol . . . . 500 cc.
Glycerin, a sufficient quantity,

            To make . . . .   1000 cc.

     Dissolve the saccharin in the alcohol, add the paraldehyde and the oils and then sufficient glycerin to make the product measure 1000 cc. Filter.

AVERAGE DOSE—Metric, 4 to 12 cc.—Apothecaries, 1 to 3 fluidrachms.

PEPTO-LACTIC ELIXIR
(R.B. I)

Glycerite of Pepsin.	215 cc.
Diluted Hydrochloric Acid	20 cc.
Lactic Acid	2 cc.
Solution of Amaranth	5 cc.
Aromatic Elixir, a sufficient quantity,	
To make	1000 cc.

Mix.

AVERAGE DOSE—Metric, 8 cc.—Apothecaries, 2 fluidrachms.

ELIXIR OF POTASSIUM ACETATE
Elixir Potassii Acetatis
(N.F. IV)

Potassium Acetate	85 Gm.
Aromatic Elixir, a sufficient quantity,	
To make	1000 cc.

Dissolve and filter.

AVERAGE DOSE—Metric, 15 cc.—Apothecaries, 4 fluidrachms.

ELIXIR OF POTASSIUM ACETATE AND JUNIPER
Elixir Potassii Acetatis et Juniperi
(N.F. IV)

Potassium Acetate	85 Gm.
Fluidextract of Juniper	125 cc.
Purified Talc	20 Gm.
Aromatic Elixir, a sufficient quantity,	
To make	1000 cc.

Mix the fluidextract of juniper with 750 cc. of aromatic elixir, in which the potassium acetate has been dissolved, and add sufficient aromatic elixir to make 1000 cc. Add the purified talc, allow the mixture to stand for 12 hours with occasional agitation and filter, returning the first portions of the filtrate until it passes through clear. Finally add sufficient aromatic elixir to make the product measure 1000 cc.

AVERAGE DOSE—Metric, 15 cc.—Apothecaries, 4 fluidrachms.

ELIXIR OF RHUBARB
Elixir Rhei
(R.B. II)

Fluidextract of Rhubarb.	40 cc.
Tincture of Bitter Orange Peel	50 cc.
Tincture of Cardamom, R.B.	40 cc.
Sherry Wine.	370 cc.
Glycerin	125 cc.
Syrup.	200 cc.
Alcohol	70 cc.
Cinnamon Water, a sufficient quantity,	
To make	1000 cc.

Mix, and filter if necessary.

AVERAGE DOSE—Metric, 8 cc.—Apothecaries, 2 fluidrachms.

RINGELMANN'S ELIXIR
Elixir Ringelmanni

Elixir e Succo Liquiritæ, Elixir Regis Daniæ
(R.B. II)

Pure Extract of Glycyrrhiza	200 Gm.
Oil of Fennel	5 cc.
Oil of Anise.	5 cc.
Diluted Solution of Ammonia	6 cc.
Alcohol.	182 cc.
Distilled Water, a sufficient quantity,	
To make	1000 cc.

Dissolve the extract in 600 cc. of distilled water, add to the diluted solution of ammonia and set aside for 36 hours. Add the solution of the oils in the alcohol, shake well and let stand for 8 days. Decant the clear portion and filter the remainder in a well-covered funnel so as to avoid loss of ammonia, adding sufficient distilled water through the filter to make the product measure 1000 cc.

AVERAGE DOSE—Metric, 8 cc.—Apothecaries, 2 fluidrachms.

ELIXIR OF SACCHARIN
Elixir Saccharini

Elixir of Gluside
(B.P.C. 1934)

Saccharin.	50 Gm.
Sodium Bicarbonate	30 Gm.
Alcohol, 90 per cent	125 cc.
Distilled Water, a sufficient quantity,	
To make	1000 cc.

Add the saccharin to the sodium bicarbonate previously dissolved in 800 cc. of distilled water; when effervescence ceases add the alcohol, filter and wash the filter with sufficient distilled water to make the product measure 1000 cc.

AVERAGE DOSE—Metric, 0.3 to 1.25 cc.—Apothecaries, 5 to 20 minims.

ELIXIR OF SALICYLIC ACID
Elixir Acidi Salicylici
(N.F. III)

Salicylic Acid	85 Gm.
Potassium Citrate	125 Gm.
Glycerin	500 cc.
Aromatic Elixir, a sufficient quantity,	
To make	1000 cc.

Dissolve the potassium citrate in the glycerin with the aid of gentle heat. Add the salicylic acid and continue the heat until it is dissolved. Then add sufficient aromatic elixir to make the product measure 1000 cc. and filter.

AVERAGE DOSE—Metric, 4 cc.—Apothecaries, 1 fluidrachm.

NOTE—This elixir should be freshly prepared.

ELIXIR OF SODIUM HYPOPHOSPHITE
Elixir Sodii Hypophosphitis
(N.F. IV)

Sodium Hypophosphite	35 Gm.
Hypophosphorous Acid	4 cc.
Aromatic Elixir, a sufficient quantity,	
To make	1000 cc.

Dissolve the sodium hypophosphite in 825 cc. of aromatic elixir. Add the acid and sufficient aromatic elixir to make the product measure 1000 cc. and filter.

AVERAGE DOSE—Metric, 4 cc.—Apothecaries, 1 fluidrachm.

COMPOUND ELIXIR OF TERPIN HYDRATE, CREOSOTE AND CODEINE
Elixir Terpini Hydratis, Creosoti et Codeinæ
(R.B. I)

Terpin Hydrate	10	Gm.
Creosote	4	cc.
Codeine Sulfate	1.2	Gm.
Syrup of Wild Cherry	400	cc.
Aromatic Elixir, as ufficient quantity,		
To make	1000	cc.

Dissolve the terpin hydrate and codeine sulfate in 500 cc. of aromatic elixir, add the other ingredients and sufficient aromatic elixir to make the product measure 1000 cc.

AVERAGE DOSE—Metric, 4 cc.—Apothecaries, 1 fluidrachm.

ELIXIR OF ZINC VALERATE
Elixir Zinci Valeratis
Elixir Zinci Valerianatis
(N.F. IV)

Zinc Valerate	18 Gm.
Citric Acid	60 Gm.
Alcohol.	125 cc.
Spirit of Benzaldehyde	10 cc.
Compound Tincture of Cudbear	15 cc.
Stronger Solution of Ammonia,	
Distilled Water,	
Aromatic Elixir, of each, a sufficient quantity,	
To make	1000 cc.

Dissolve the citric acid in 50 cc. of distilled water, neutralize with the stronger solution of ammonia and add sufficient distilled water to make 100 cc. of solution. Add 250 cc. of aromatic elixir and the alcohol, and dissolve the zinc valerate in this mixture. Then add the spirit of benzaldehyde, the compound tincture of cudbear, and finally sufficient aromatic elixir to make the product measure 1000 cc. and filter.

AVERAGE DOSE—Metric, 4 cc.—Apothecaries, 1 fluidrachm.

EMULSIONS

Emulsification—The preparation of pharmaceutical emulsions, whether of fixed or volatile oils, is generally most satisfactorily and expeditiously accomplished with acacia as the emulsifying agent. It is essential that the oil, the acacia and the water shall primarily be in definite proportion to each other. This proportion is 4 parts of fixed oil, 1 part of acacia and 2 parts of water (liquids by measure, solids by weight). The oil and the acacia, in fine powder, are well mixed by trituration in a perfectly dry mortar; the water is then added in one portion and the whole is triturated briskly until a thick, creamy emulsion is produced; the sides of the mortar should be carefully scraped, and the mixture again thoroughly triturated so as to insure complete emulsification of the oil. The other ingredients may then be added gradually; first the flavoring, then the syrup and the water necessary to make the required volume. Alcoholic liquids are added last, and must be mixed previously with a portion of the water. When available, it is advisable to use an homogenizer.

Under ordinary conditions, emulsions are prone to deteriorate on standing and they should be freshly prepared when required. If they are intended to be kept for any length of time they must be suitably preserved and kept in a cool, dark place. Frequently they may be preserved by replacing 70 cc. (per 1000 cc. of emulsion) of water by an equal volume of alcohol, which is added last, in small portions, the emulsion being shaken after each addition. The addition of 0.1 per cent of methyl parahydroxybenzoic acid aids in the preservation of emulsions.

Flavoring—No single aromatic can be suggested that would be acceptable under all circumstances for all emulsions; the selection of the most suitable flavoring must be left to the prescriber or dispenser.

The following have been found to be useful, the quantities given being intended for 1000 cc. of finished emulsion:

1. Methyl Salicylate.   4   cc.
2. Methyl Salicylate.   2   cc.
   Oil of Sassafras   2   cc.
3. Compound Spirit of Orange . . . .   1.5 cc.
4. Methyl Salicylate.   2   cc.
   Benzaldehyde . . . .   0.25 cc.
   Oil of Coriander . . . .   0.25 cc.
5. Methyl Salicylate. . . . .   1.50 cc.
   Oil of Sassafras . . . .   1.50 cc.
   Benzaldehyde . . . .   0.25 cc.
6. Methyl Salicylate. . . . .   2.5 cc.
   Benzaldehyde . . . .   2.5 cc.

NOTE—Emulsions should always be dispensed with a "shake well" label.

EMULSION OF ALMOND
Emulsum Amygdalæ
Milk of Almond
(U.S.P. IX)

Sweet Almond. . . . .   60 Gm.
Acacia, in fine powder . . . .   10 Gm.
Sucrose. . . . .   30 Gm.
Distilled Water, a sufficient quantity,
                    To make . . . .   1000 cc.

Blanch the almonds, add the acacia and sucrose and beat them in a mortar until thoroughly mixed. Add 900 cc. of distilled water, very gradually at first, and triturate until a uniform mixture results. Strain, and wash the mortar and strainer with sufficient distilled water to make the product measure 1000 cc. Mix thoroughly.

NOTE—This emulsion should be freshly prepared.

EMULSION OF ASAFETIDA
Emulsum Asafoetida
Milk of Asafetida
(U.S.P. XI)

Asafetida, in tears or selected pieces . . . .   40 Gm.
Distilled Water, a sufficient quantity,
                    To make . . . .   1000 cc.

Rub the asafetida in a mortar with 900 cc. of distilled water, at first very gradually added, until a uniform emulsion results. Then strain the mixture into a graduated vessel and rinse the mortar and strainer with enough distilled water to make the product measure 1000 cc. Mix thoroughly.

AVERAGE DOSE—Metric, 15 cc.—Apothecaries, 4 fluidrachms.

EMULSION OF ASPIDIUM
Emulsum Aspidii
(N.Y.P.G.H.)

Oleoresin of Aspidium . . . .   250 Gm.
Mucilage of Acacia, a sufficient quantity,

To make . . . .   1000 cc.

Add the oleoresin of aspidium gradually with constant trituration to 250 cc. of the mucilage of acacia. Then incorporate sufficient mucilage of acacia to make the product measure 1000 cc.

AVERAGE DOSE—Metric, 15 cc.—Apothecaries, 4 fluidrachms.

NOTE—This is a single dose to be given once a day.

EMULSION OF BENZYL BENZOATE
(R.B. II)

Benzyl Benzoate, 20 per cent alcoholic solution . . . .   40 cc.
Acacia, in fine powder . . . .   20 Gm.
Compound Tincture of Cardamom . . . .   500 cc.
Aromatic Syrup of Eriodictyon, a sufficient quantity,

To make . . . .   1000 cc.

Incorporate the solution of benzyl benzoate into a heavy mucilage made by triturating the acacia with a small quantity of the syrup. Continue the trituration with the addition of sufficient syrup to make 500 cc. Finally, add the compound tincture of cardamom and mix thoroughly by shaking.

AVERAGE DOSE—Metric, 8 cc.—Apothecaries, 2 fluidrachms.

EMULSION OF AROMATIC CASCARA SAGRADA IN MINERAL OIL

Aromatic Fluidextract of Cascara Sagrada . . . .   94 cc.
Emulsifying Agent, a sufficient quantity,
Heavy Liquid Petrolatum, a sufficient quantity,

To make . . . .   1000 cc.

Prepare a primary emulsion of the liquid petrolatum, preferably with an homogenizer, and add the fluidextract to the prepared emulsion with agitation.

AVERAGE DOSE—Metric, 15 to 30 cc.—Apothecaries, ½ to 1 fluidounce.

NOTE—The least expensive emulsifying agent to use is either Acacia or Agar.

EMULSION OF CASTOR OIL
Emulsum Olei Ricini
(N.F. V)

Castor Oil. . . . .   350 cc.
Acacia, in fine powder. . . . .   90 Gm.
Tincture of Vanilla. . . . .   25 cc.
Syrup. . . . .   200 cc.
Distilled Water, a sufficient quantity,

To make . . . .   1000 cc.

Triturate the acacia with the castor oil in a dry mortar until uniformly mixed, then add 180 cc. of distilled water and triturate lightly and rapidly until the oil is completely emulsified.   Incorporate the syrup and tincture gradually and finally add sufficient distilled water to make the product measure 1000 cc.   Mix thoroughly.

AVERAGE DOSE—Metric, 45 cc.—Apothecaries, 1½ fluidounces.

EMULSION OF COAL TAR
Emulsum Picis Carbonis
(Cod. Fr.)

Solution of Coal Tar . . . .   200 cc.
Distilled Water . . . .   800 cc.

To make . . . .   1000 cc.
Mix.

This emulsion is diluted with about 10 volumes of water for ordinary use.

EMULSION OF COD LIVER OIL WITH CALCIUM LACTOPHOSPHATE
Emulsum Olei Morrhuæ cum Calcii Lactophosphate
(N.F. IV)

Cod Liver Oil . . . .   500 cc.
Calcium Lactophosphate . . . .   50 Gm.
Lactic Acid . . . .   16 cc.
Acacia, in fine powder . . . .   125 Gm.
Syrup of Tolu Balsam . . . .   100 cc.
Flavoring (see R.B. page 38),
Distilled Water, a sufficient quantity,

To make . . . .   1000 cc.

Triturate the acacia with the cod liver oil in a dry mortar until uniformly mixed, then add at once 250 cc. of distilled water and triturate the mixture rapidly until complete emulsification results.   Dissolve the calcium lactophosphate in 65 cc. of distilled water with the aid of the lactic acid and incorporate the solution with the emulsion just prepared, adding the flavoring, the syrup of tolu balsam and sufficient distilled water to make the product measure 1000 cc.   Mix thoroughly.

AVERAGE DOSE—Metric, 15 cc.—Apothecaries, 4 fluidrachms.

NOTE—This emulsion must be freshly prepared.

EMULSION OF COD LIVER OIL WITH CALCIUM PHOSPHATE
Emulsum Olei Morrhuæ cum Calcii Phosphate
Emulsion of Cod Liver Oil with Phosphate of Lime
(N.F. IV)

Cod Liver Oil	500 cc.
Acacia in fine powder	125 Gm.
Tribasic Calcium Phosphate	35 Gm.
Syrup of Tolu Balsam	100 cc.
Flavoring (see R.B. page 38),	
Distilled Water, a sufficient quantity,	
To make	1000 cc.

Triturate the acacia with the cod liver oil in a dry mortar until uniformly mixed, then add at once 250 cc. of distilled water and triturate lightly and rapidly until the oil is completely emulsified. Then incorporate the flavoring, the syrup of tolu balsam and precipitated calcium phosphate, previously mixed, and lastly sufficient distilled water to make the product measure 1000 cc. Mix thoroughly.

AVERAGE DOSE—Metric, 15 cc.—Apothecaries, 4 fluidrachms.

NOTE—This emulsion must be freshly prepared.

EMULSION OF COD LIVER OIL WITH CREOSOTE
(V.C.N.Y.)

Creosote	15 cc.
Emulsion of Cod Liver Oil, a sufficient quantity,	
To make	1000 cc.

Add the emulsion of cod liver oil gradually to the creosote with continuous trituration.

AVERAGE DOSE—Metric, 8 cc.—Apothecaries, 2 fluidrachms.

IRISH MOSS EMULSION OF COD LIVER OIL WITH HYPOPHOSPHITES
(R.B. I)

Cod Liver Oil	400 cc.
Mucilage of Chondrus	450 cc.
Calcium Hypophosphite	10 Gm.
Sodium Hypophosphite	5 Gm.
Potassium Hypophosphite	5 Gm.
Syrup of Citric Acid	100 cc.
Distilled Water, a sufficient quantity,	
To make	1000 cc.

Emulsify the cod liver oil in a capacious mortar with the mucilage. Add the syrup of citric acid, in which the salts have been dissolved, and finally sufficient distilled water to make the product measure 1000 cc.

AVERAGE DOSE—Metric, 15 cc.—Apothecaries, 4 fluidrachms.

NOTE—This preparation is not to be confused with Emulsion of Cod Liver Oil with Hypophosphites, N.F. VII.

EMULSION OF COD LIVER OIL WITH WILD CHERRY
Emulsum Olei Morrhuæ cum Pruno Virginiana
(N.F. IV)

Cod Liver Oil	500 cc.
Acacia, in fine powder	125 Gm.
Fluidextract of Wild Cherry	65 cc.
Syrup of Tolu Balsam	100 cc.
Flavoring (see R.B. page 38),	
Distilled Water, a sufficient quantity,	
To make	1000 cc.

Triturate the cod liver oil in a capacious mortar with the acacia, then add at once 250 cc. of distilled water and triturate lightly and rapidly until the oil is completely emulsified. Incorporate gradually the fluidextract and syrup, previously mixed with a portion of the remaining distilled water, and finally add sufficient distilled water to make the product measure 1000 cc. Mix thoroughly.

AVERAGE DOSE—Metric, 15 cc.—Apothecaries, 4 fluidrachms.

EMULSION OF CREOSOTE CARBONATE
Mistura Creosoti Carbonatis
(B.N.Y.)

Creosote Carbonate	75 cc.
Tragacanth, in fine powder	8 Gm.
Alcohol	60 cc.
Compound Spirit of Orange	65 cc.
Syrup	250 cc.
Distilled Water, a sufficient quantity,	
To make	1000 cc.

Mix the creosote carbonate, tragacanth and syrup in a mortar by vigorous trituration. Add the alcohol, compound spirit of orange and sufficient distilled water to make the product measure 1000 cc.

AVERAGE DOSE—Metric, 4 cc.—Apothecaries, 1 fluidrachm.

EMULSION OF CREOSOTE CARBONATE WITH MALT AND HYPOPHOSPHITES
(N.Y.P.G.H.)

Creosote Carbonate . . . .   38 Gm.
Compound Syrup of Hypophosphites . . . .   400 cc.
Extract of Malt, a sufficient quantity,

To make . . . .   1000 cc.

Add the compound syrup of hypophosphites gradually to the creosote carbonate while triturating vigorously. Then add sufficient extract of malt to make the product measure 1000 cc. Agitate the mixture thoroughly.

AVERAGE DOSE—Metric, 8 cc.—Apothecaries, 2 fluidrachms.

COMPOUND EMULSION OF KAOLIN

Kaolin   120   Gm.
Aluminum Hydroxide . . . .   5.5 Gm.
Liquid Petrolatum   200   cc.
Acacia   50   Gm.
Peppermint Water, a sufficient quantity,

To make   1000   cc.

Add the acacia to the liquid petrolatum and triturate; pour into a bottle, add 100 cc. of peppermint water and shake vigorously until an emulsion is obtained. Add the remaining peppermint water to which has been added previously the kaolin, and aluminum hydroxide.

THOMSON'S EMULSION OF LINSEED OIL

Linseed Oil . . . .   300 cc.
Glycerin . . . .   15 cc.
Syrup . . . .   200 cc.
Diluted Hydrocyanic Acid . . . .   5 cc.
Oil of Cinnamon . . . .   5 cc.
Methyl Salicylate . . . .   5 cc.
Mucilage of Chondrus . . . .   470 cc.

To make . . . .   1000 cc.

Emulsify the linseed oil with the mucilage of chondrus. Add the syrup and the other ingredients and mix thoroughly.

AVERAGE DOSE—Metric, 15 to 30 cc.—Apothecaries, ½ to 1 fluidounce.

COMPOUND EMULSION OF MAGNESIUM TRISILICATE AND KAOLIN

Magnesium Trisilicate	108	Gm.
Kaolin	44	Gm.
Aluminum Hydroxide	5.5	Gm.
Liquid Petrolatum	200	cc.
Acacia	50	Gm.
Peppermint Water, a sufficient quantity,		
To make	1000	cc.

Add the acacia to the liquid petrolatum and triturate; pour into a bottle, add 100 cc. of peppermint water and shake vigorously until an emulsion is obtained. Add the remaining peppermint water to which has been added previously the kaolin, aluminum hydroxide and magnesium trisilicate.

EMULSION OF PETROLATUM
Emulsum Petrolati
Emulsum Petrolei
(N.F. V)

Petrolatum	225 Gm.
Expressed Almond Oil or Persic Oil	225 cc.
Acacia, in fine powder	125 Gm.
Syrup	100 cc.
Tincture of Lemon	15 cc.
Distilled Water, a sufficient quantity,	
To make	1000 cc.

Triturate the melted petrolatum with the expressed almond oil in a warm, dry mortar, add the acacia and triturate until it is uniformly mixed. Then add 250 cc. of warm distilled water and triturate lightly and rapidly until the oil is completely emulsified. Now add the syrup and the tincture, previously mixed, and sufficient distilled water to make the product measure 1000 cc. Mix thoroughly.

AVERAGE DOSE—Metric, 15 cc.—Apothecaries, 4 fluidrachms.

EMULSION OF LIQUID PETROLATUM
Emulsum Petrolati Liquidi
(R.B. II)

Heavy Liquid Petrolatum	500	cc.
Agar	10	Gm.
Acacia, in fine powder	40	Gm.
Alcohol	60	cc.
Vanillin	0.05	Gm.
Saccharin	0.05	Gm.
Distilled Water, a sufficient quantity,		
To make	1000	cc.

Place the agar in a suitable container, graduated to 350 cc., and boil it with about 400 cc. of distilled water for about 20 minutes, or until it has dissolved. Continue the heat, if necessary, until the solution measures 350 cc., allow to cool to about 45° C., stirring frequently to prevent the formation of an agar film on the surface and adding additional distilled water, if necessary, to maintain the volume. Emulsify 160 cc. of the liquid petrolatum with the acacia and 80 cc. of distilled water. Then add the remainder of the liquid petrolatum in portions, emulsifying each portion thoroughly and adding the agar solution in portions as required to maintain the proper consistence. Dissolve the vanillin and saccharin in the alcohol, and add the resulting solution gradually to the emulsion.

AVERAGE DOSE—Metric, 15 cc.—Apothecaries, 4 fluidrachms.

EMULSION OF LIQUID PETROLATUM WITH HYPO-PHOSPHITES
Emulsio Liquidi Petrolei cum Hypophosphitibus
(B.P.C. 1934)

Heavy Liquid Petrolatum	500 cc.
Calcium Hypophosphite	18 Gm.
Sodium Hypophosphite	18 Gm.
Acacia, in fine powder	125 Gm.
Tragacanth, in fine powder	10 Gm.
Oil of Cinnamon	2 cc.
Elixir of Saccharin, R.B.	3 cc.
Distilled Water, a sufficient quantity,	
To make	1000 cc.

Triturate the liquid petrolatum and the oil of cinnamon with the acacia and tragacanth, add all at once 300 cc. of distilled water, and stir until emulsified. Dissolve the hypophosphites in 300 cc. of distilled water and add the solution to the emulsion with constant trituration; finally add the elixir of saccharin and sufficient distilled water to make the product measure 1000 cc.

AVERAGE DOSE—Metric, 4 to 15 cc.—Apothecaries, 1 to 4 fluidrachms.

ENEMAS
ASAFETIDA ENEMA
(S.H.F.)

Tincture of Asafetida	70 cc.
Enema of Starch, R.B.	930 cc.
To make	1000 cc

Mix.

AVERAGE DOSE—Metric, 60 to 120 cc.—Apothecaries, 2 to 4 fluidounces.

BARIUM SULFATE ENEMA
(S.H.F.)

Barium Sulfate . . . .   200 Gm.
Mucilage of Acacia. . . . .   165 cc.
Enema of Starch, R.B., a sufficient quantity,

To make . . . .   1000 cc.

Mix.

AVERAGE DOSE—Metric, 250 to 500 cc.—Apothecaries, 8 to 16 fluidounces.

EPSOM SALT ENEMA
Enema Magnesii Sulfatis
(B.P.C. 1934)

Magnesium Sulfate. . . . .   50 Gm.
Olive Oil . . . .   100 cc.
Mucilage of Starch, R.B., a sufficient quantity,

To make . . . .   1000 cc.

Dissolve the magnesium sulfate in the mucilage of starch and incorporate the olive oil by vigorous agitation.

AVERAGE DOSE—Metric, 600 cc.—Apothecaries, 20 fluidounces.

GLUCOSE ENEMA
Enema Dextrosi
(S.H.F.)

Dextrose . . . .   60 Gm.
Isotonic Solution of Sodium Chloride, a sufficient quantity,

To make . . . .   1000 cc.

Dissolve.

AVERAGE DOSE—Metric, 250 cc.—Apothecaries, 8 fluidounces.

ALKALINE GLUCOSE ENEMA
Enema Dextrosi Alkalinum
(S.H.F.)

Sodium Bicarbonate . . . .   10 Gm.
Glucose Enema, R.B., a sufficient quantity,

To make . . . .   1000 cc.

Dissolve.

AVERAGE DOSE—Metric, 250 cc.—Apothecaries, 8 fluidounces.

1-2-3 ENEMA
Enema of Magnesium Sulfate
(U.C.H.)

Magnesium Sulfate . . . .   200 Gm.
Glycerin . . . .   400 cc.
Water, a sufficient quantity,

To make . . . . 1000 cc.

Dissolve the magnesium sulfate in 500 cc. of water, add the glycerin, and finally add sufficient water to make 1000 cc.

AVERAGE DOSE—Metric, 150 cc.—Apothecaries, 5 fluidounces.

COMPOUND SOAP ENEMA
Enema Saponis Compositum
(S.H.F.)

Soft Soap. . . . .   50 Gm.
Glycerin . . . .   12 cc.
Water, a sufficient quantity,

To make . . . . 1000 cc.

Dissolve the soft soap in 500 cc. of water, add the glycerin, and finally add sufficient water to make 1000 cc.

AVERAGE DOSE—Metric, 250 to 500 cc.—Apothecaries, 8 to 16 fluidounces.

STARCH ENEMA
Enema Amyli
Clysmus Amyli
(Cod. Fr.)

Starch . . . .   30 Gm.
Water, a sufficient quantity,

To make . . . . 1000 cc.

Mix the starch thoroughly with 200 cc. of cold water. Then add 800 cc. of boiling water and stir vigorously. When sufficiently cooled it is ready for use.

AVERAGE DOSE—Metric, 300 to 600 cc.—Apothecaries, 10 to 20 fluidounces.

NOTE—This enema should be freshly prepared.

TURPENTINE ENEMA
Enema Terebinthinæ
(S.H.F.)

Rectified Oil of Turpentine . . . .   20 cc.
Castor Oil . . . .   60 cc.
Enema of Starch, R.B., a sufficient quantity,

To make . . . . 1000 cc.

Incorporate the oils with the enema of starch by vigorous agitation.

AVERAGE DOSE—Metric, 150 to 250 cc.—Apothecaries, 5 to 8 fluidounces.

EXTRACTS

FERRATED EXTRACT OF APPLES
Extractum Ferri Pomatum
Ferri Malas Crudus, Crude Malate of Iron
(N.F. V)

Reduced Iron . . . .   40 Gm.
Fresh Apple Juice . . . .   1000 cc.
Water, a sufficient quantity.

Mix the fresh apple juice with the iron in an enameled or porcelain vessel, and heat on a water bath until no more gas is given off, adding a little water from time to time to make up any loss by evaporation. Dilute the liquid with distilled water to make 1000 cc. and set it aside for a few days. Then filter and evaporate the filtrate in an enameled or porcelain vessel on a water bath to the consistence of a pilular extract.

AVERAGE DOSE—Metric, 0.6 Gm.—Apothecaries, 10 grains.

EXTRACT OF HEMATOXYLON
Extractum Hæmatoxyli
(N.F. V)

Hematoxylon, rasped. . . . .   1000 Gm.
Water . . . .   10000 cc.

Macerate the hematoxylon with the water for 48 hours. Then boil the mixture (avoiding the use of iron vessels) until one-half of the water has evaporated; strain the decoction while hot and evaporate the strained liquid to dryness.

AVERAGE DOSE—Metric, 1 Gm.—Apothecaries, 15 grains.

FLUIDEXTRACTS

FLUIDEXTRACT OF CUBEB
Fluidextractum Cubebæ
(N.F. V)

Prepare the Fluidextract from cubeb, in moderately coarse powder, by Process A (see N.F. VII, page 167). Use alcohol as the menstruum, macerate the drug 48 hours, and percolate at a moderate rate.

AVERAGE DOSE—Metric, 1 cc.—Apothecaries, 15 minims.

FLUIDEXTRACT OF EUCALYPTUS
Fluidextractum Eucalypti
(U.S.P. IX)

Prepare the Fluidextract from eucalyptus, in coarse powder, by Process A (see N.F. VII, page 167). Use a mixture of 3 volumes of alcohol and 1 volume of water as the menstruum, macerate the drug 48 hours, and percolate at a moderate rate.

AVERAGE DOSE—Metric, 2 cc.—Apothecaries, 30 minims.

FLUIDEXTRACT OF JUGLANS
Fluidextractum Juglandis
(N.F. V)

Prepare the Fluidextract from juglans, in moderately coarse powder, by Process B (see N.F. VII, page 168). Use a mixture of 1 volume of glycerin, 5 volumes of alcohol and 4 volumes of water as Menstruum I and diluted alcohol as Menstruum II; macerate the drug 48 hours, and percolate slowly.

AVERAGE DOSE—Metric, 4 cc.—Apothecaries, 1 fluidrachm.

FLUIDEXTRACT OF MEZEREUM
Fluidextractum Mezerei
(N.F. V)

Prepare the Fluidextract from mezereum, in moderately coarse powder, by Process A (see N.F. VII, page 167). Use a mixture of 2 volumes of alcohol and 1 volume of water as the menstruum, macerate the drug 48 hours, and percolate slowly.

FLUIDEXTRACT OF PILOCARPUS
Fluidextractum Pilocarpi
Fluidextract of Jaborandi
(U.S.P. IX)

Prepare the Fluidextract from pilocarpus, in moderately coarse powder, by Process A, as modified for assayed fluidextracts (see N.F. VII, page 167). Use a mixture of 2 volumes of alcohol and 1 volume of water as the menstruum, macerate the drug 48 hours, and percolate at a moderate rate.

Adjust the Fluidextract to make each 100 cc. of the finished product contain 0.55–0.65 Gm. of the alkaloids of pilocarpus, as determined by assay, using the menstruum for dilution, if necessary.

AVERAGE DOSE—Metric, 2 cc.—Apothecaries, 30 minims.

FLUIDEXTRACT OF RUBUS
Fluidextractum Rubi
(N.F. V)

Prepare the Fluidextract from rubus, in moderately coarse powder, by Process A (see N.F. VII, page 167). Use diluted alcohol as the menstruum, macerate the drug 48 hours, and percolate slowly.

AVERAGE DOSE—Metric, 1 cc.—Apothecaries, 15 minims.

AROMATIC FLUIDEXTRACT OF SENNA
Fluidextractum Sennæ Aromaticum

Senna, in No. 40 powder	1000 Gm.
Sucrose	500 Gm.
Oil of Coriander	1 cc.
Alcohol,	
Diluted Alcohol,	
Distilled Water, of each, a sufficient quantity,	
To make	1000 cc.

Extract the senna by percolation with alcohol until exhausted and reject this alcoholic percolate which contains the resin or griping principle. Remove the senna from the percolator, dry it and then prepare a fluidextract by percolation with diluted alcohol by Process A (see N.F. VII, page 167). Evaporate the alcohol from the fluidextract on a water bath, dissolve the sucrose in the remaining portion, and add sufficient distilled water to make the product measure 1000 cc. Lastly, add the oil of coriander and mix thoroughly.

AVERAGE DOSE—Metric, 2 cc.—Apothecaries, ½ fluidrachm.

NOTE—This preparation contains very little or no alcohol. It has the strength of a fluidextract with the properties of a syrup, and is therefore especially adapted for children.

COMPOUND FLUIDEXTRACT OF TRIFOLIUM
Fluidextractum Trifolii Compositum
(N.F. VI)

Trifolium	215 Gm.
Glycyrrhiza	215 Gm.
Berberis	108 Gm.
Cascara Amarga	108 Gm.
Lappa	108 Gm.
Phytolacca	108 Gm.
Stillingia	108 Gm.
Xanthoxylum	30 Gm.
To make	1000 cc.

Prepare the Fluidextract from the mixed drugs, in moderately coarse powder, by Process A (see N.F. VII, page 167). Use a mixture of 1 volume of alcohol and 3 volumes of water as the menstruum, macerate the mixed drugs for 24 hours, and percolate at a moderate rate.

AVERAGE DOSE—Metric, 4 cc.—Apothecaries, 1 fluidrachm.

GARGLES

A.B.C. GARGLE POWDER
(N.Y.P.G.H.)

Alum, in fine powder,
Sodium Borate,
Potassium Chlorate, of each, an equal weight.

Mix thoroughly and pass through a No. 60 sieve several times.
For use, 4 Gm. (60 grains) is dissolved in 120 cc. (4 fluidounces) of warm water.

ALUM GARGLE
(R.B. I)

Alum, in fine powder	50 Gm.
Honey	500 Gm.
Compound Infusion of Rose, R.B., a sufficient quantity,	
To make	1000 cc.

Triturate the alum with 300 cc. of the infusion until a homogeneous paste is obtained. Add the honey and mix thoroughly. Finally add sufficient infusion to make the product measure 1000 cc. Shake well to dissolve.

For use, this gargle is diluted with an equal volume of water.

ALUM AND POTASSIUM CHLORATE GARGLE
(V.C.N.Y.)

Alum.	20 Gm.
Potassium Chlorate.	40 Gm.
Glycerin	20 cc.
Distilled Water, a sufficient quantity,	
To make	1000 cc.

Dissolve.
For use, this gargle is diluted with 7 volumes of water.

ASTRINGENT GARGLE
(Curtis)

Tannic Acid. . . . .   12 Gm.
Glycerin . . . .   60 cc.
Liquefied Phenol . . . .   11 cc.
Distilled Water, a sufficient quantity,
              To make . . . .   1000 cc.

Dissolve the tannic acid and phenol in the glycerin and about 500 cc. of distilled water.   Add sufficient distilled water to make the product measure 1000 cc.

For use, this gargle is diluted with an equal volume of water.

COMPOUND BORIC ACID GARGLE
(P.H.N.Y.)

Boric Acid . . . .   33 Gm.
Antiseptic Solution, N.F.   265 cc.
Solution of Hydrogen Peroxide . . . .   265 cc.
Distilled Water, a sufficient quantity,
              To make . . . .   1000 cc.

Dissolve the boric acid in the antiseptic solution to which 400 cc. of distilled water has been added.   Add the solution of hydrogen peroxide and sufficient distilled water to make the product measure 1000 cc.

For use, this gargle is diluted with 4 volumes of water.

NOTE—This gargle must be freshly prepared.

CHLORINE GARGLE
(V.C.N.Y.)

Hydrochloric Acid . . . .   5 cc.
Potassium Chlorate, in powder . . . .   80 Gm.
Syrup of Citric Acid . . . .   80 cc.
Glycerin . . . .   20 cc.
Distilled Water, a sufficient quantity,
              To make . . . .   1000 cc.

Add the hydrochloric acid to the potassium chlorate contained in a liter bottle. When the reaction is evident add 500 cc. of distilled water and shake to dissolve the chlorine.   Then add the syrup of citric acid and glycerin and sufficient distilled water to make the product measure 1000 cc.

For use, this gargle is diluted with 1 or more volumes of water.

IODINE AND PHENOL GARGLE
(R.B. II)

Tincture of Iodine	60 cc.
Liquefied Phenol	22 cc.
Glycerin	180 cc.
Solution of Amaranth	30 cc.
Distilled Water, a sufficient quantity,	
To make	1000 cc.

Dissolve the liquefied phenol in the glycerin and add 500 cc. of distilled water. Add the tincture of iodine and solution of amaranth and sufficient distilled water to make the product measure 1000 cc.

For use, this gargle is diluted with 10 volumes of water.

PEROXIDE GARGLE
(N.Y.P.G.H.)

Antiseptic Solution, N.F.	200 cc.
Solution of Hydrogen Peroxide	465 cc.
Peppermint Water, a sufficient quantity,	
To make	1000 cc.

Mix the solution of hydrogen peroxide with 300 cc. of peppermint water, and add the antiseptic solution and sufficient peppermint water to make the product measure 1000 cc.

For use, this gargle is diluted with 4 volumes of water.

NOTE—This gargle must be freshly prepared.

PHENOL GARGLE
Gargarisma Phenolis
(R.B. I)

Liquefied Phenol.	35 cc.
Spirit of Peppermint	35 cc.
Glycerite of Tannic Acid	35 cc.
Glycerin, a sufficient quantity,	
To make	1000 cc

Mix.

For use, this gargle is diluted with an equal volume of water.

COMPOUND SAGE GARGLE
(V.C.N.Y.)

Alum.	30 Gm.
Sage, in coarse powder	60 Gm.
Honey	120 Gm.
Distilled Water, a sufficient quantity,	
To make	1000 cc.

Add 850 cc. of boiling distilled water to the alum, sage and honey. Set aside until cool. Filter and add sufficient distilled water to make the product measure 1000 cc.

For use, this gargle is diluted with an equal volume of water.

SALICYLIC ACID GARGLE
(V.C.N.Y.)

Salicylic Acid	13 Gm.
Sodium Borate.	26 Gm.
Tincture of Myrrh	60 cc.
Distilled Water, a sufficient quantity,	
To make	1000 cc.

Dissolve the sodium borate in 500 cc. of distilled water, add the salicylic acid and dissolve. Add the tincture of myrrh gradually, and finally sufficient distilled water to make the product measure 1000 cc. Filter.

For use, this gargle is diluted with 10 volumes of water.

COMPOUND SALICYLIC ACID GARGLE
(V.C.N.Y.)

Salicylic Acid	100 Gm.
Alcohol	500 cc.
Glycerin	100 cc.
Methyl Salicylate	15 cc.
Oil of Clove	15 cc.
Distilled Water, a sufficient quantity,	
To make	1000 cc.

Dissolve the salicylic acid and the flavors in the alcohol. Add the glycerin and finally sufficient distilled water to make the product measure 1000 cc.

For use, 15 to 20 drops are diluted with $\frac{1}{4}$ tumblerful of hot water.

SALT, SODA AND BORAX GARGLE
(U.C.H.)

Sodium Chloride	333 Gm.
Sodium Bicarbonate	333 Gm.
Sodium Borate	334 Gm.
To make	1000 Gm.

Mix the powders intimately.

For use, dissolve 1 teaspoonful in a glass of hot water.

TANNIC ACID AND ALUM GARGLE
(V.C.N.Y.)

Tannic Acid	130 Gm.
Alum, in fine powder	130 Gm.
Glycerin	130 cc.
Distilled Water, a sufficient quantity,	
To make	1000 cc.

Mix the alum and tannic acid thoroughly with the glycerin, and add sufficient distilled water to make the product measure 1000 cc. Agitate until solution is effected.

For use, this gargle is diluted with 6 volumes of water.

WADSWORTH'S GARGLE
Wadsworth's Solution
(P.F.)

Sodium Chloride	8	Gm.
Sodium Bicarbonate	2.40	Gm.
Glycerin	420	cc.
Alcohol	300	cc.
Menthol	0.24	Gm.
Thymol	0.24	Gm.
Methyl Salicylate	0.70	cc.
Oil of Cinnamon	0.50	cc.
Oil of Eucalyptus	1.30	cc.
Tincture of Cudbear	16	cc.
Tincture of Krameria, R.B.	8	cc.
Purified Talc	20	Gm.
Distilled Water, a sufficient quantity,		
To make	1000	cc.

Dissolve the sodium salts in a mixture of the glycerin and 200 cc. of distilled water, and the other ingredients in the alcohol. Pour the aqueous solution into the alcoholic solution, add the talc and allow the mixture to stand with occasional agitation during 48 hours. Then filter, passing sufficient distilled water through the filter to make the product measure 1000 cc.

GELATINS

CHONDRUS JELLY
Gelatum Chondri
Irish Moss Gel
(N.F. IV)

Chondrus	100 Gm.
Water, a sufficient quantity.	

Wash the chondrus with cold water, then place it in a suitable vessel, add 5000 cc. of hot distilled water, and heat it on a water bath for 15 minutes, stirring frequently. Strain the decoction, while hot, through a strong muslin strainer; return the strained, mucilaginous liquid to the water bath, evaporate it to a semi-fluid consistency, then transfer it to shallow, flat-bottomed trays and evaporate it at a temperature not exceeding 90° C. so that the product may be detached in scales.

GELATIN OF ZINC OXIDE AND ICHTHAMMOL

Unna's Paste with Ichthammol

(R.B. I)

Gelatin.	150 Gm.
Zinc Oxide	100 Gm.
Glycerin	375 Gm.
Ichthammol.	20 Gm.
Distilled Water	355 cc.
To make	1000 Gm.

Soften the gelatin by soaking it in the distilled water, then add the glycerin, zinc oxide and ichthammol, previously rubbed together to a smooth paste. Heat on a water bath till the gelatin is dissolved and the product is of uniform consistence. Pour into a flat dish to solidify.

GLYCEROGELATINS

FIRM ZINC GLYCEROGELATIN

Glycerogelatinum Zinci Durum

(N.F. V)

Glycerinated Gelatin.	300 Gm.
Glycerin	250 Gm.
Distilled Water	350 cc.
Zinc Oxide, in fine powder	100 Gm.
To make	1000 Gm.

Mix the zinc oxide thoroughly with the glycerin, add the water, and incorporate this mixture with the glycerinated gelatin, previously melted on a water bath. Continue the heat, with stirring, until a homogeneous mixture is obtained, pour it into chilled molds, and allow it to congeal.

SOFT ZINC GLYCEROGELATIN

Glycerogelatinum Zinci Molle

(N.F. V)

Glycerinated Gelatin.	200 Gm.
Glycerin	350 Gm.
Distilled Water	350 cc.
Zinc Oxide, in fine powder	100 Gm.
To make	1000 Gm.

Mix the zinc oxide thoroughly with the glycerin, add the water, and incorporate this mixture with the glycerinated gelatin, previously melted on a water bath. Continue the heat, with stirring, until a homogeneous mixture is obtained, pour it into chilled molds, and allow it to congeal.

GLYCERITES

BOROGLYCERITE OF STARCH
(R.B. I)

Boric Acid	10 Gm.
Starch	10 Gm.
Distilled Water	20 cc.
Glycerin	60 Gm.
To make	100 Gm.

Triturate the starch with the distilled water and add the boric acid, previously mixed with the glycerin. Heat the mixture to a temperature not exceeding 140° C. until a gelatinous mass is obtained.

GLYCERITE OF BORAX
Glyceritum Sodii Boratis
(B.P.)

Sodium Borate	165 Gm.
Glycerin, a sufficient quantity,	
To make	1000 cc.

Dissolve.

GLYCERITE OF GUAIAC
Glyceritum Guaiaci
(N.F. IV)

Guaiac, in powder	85	Gm.
Potassium Hydroxide	3.25	Gm.
Glycerin	600	cc.
Distilled Water, a sufficient quantity		
To make	1000	cc.

Dissolve the potassium hydroxide in 300 cc. of distilled water, add the powdered guaiac, and macerate the mixture during 24 hours with occasional agitation. Finally filter, and add the glycerin and sufficient distilled water to make the product measure 1000 cc.

AVERAGE DOSE—Metric, 2 cc.—Apothecaries, 30 minims.

GLYCERITE OF IODINE
Glycerin of Iodine
Morton's Fluid
(B.P.C. 1923)

Iodine . . . . 22.8 Gm.
Potassium Iodide . . . . 68.6 Gm.
Distilled Water 50   cc.
Glycerin, a sufficient quantity,

To make 1000   cc.

Dissolve the potassium iodide in the distilled water, add the iodine and, when dissolved, sufficient glycerin to make the product measure 1000 cc.

STRONGER GLYCERITE OF IODINE AND ZINC IODIDE
Talbot's Solution

Zinc Iodide . . . . 36.7 Gm.
Iodine . . . . 45.8 Gm.
Glycerin 370   cc.
Distilled Water, a sufficient quantity,

To make 1000   Gm.

Dissolve the zinc iodide in 70 cc. of distilled water, add the iodine, and agitate the mixture until solution is effected. Finally add the glycerin and sufficient distilled water to make the product weigh 1000 Gm. and mix thoroughly.

NOTE—Keep the glycerite in glass-stoppered or rubber-stoppered bottles. This preparation is not to be confused with the Glycerite of Iodine and Zinc Iodide of the N.F. which is a weaker preparation.

GLYCERITE OF LEAD SUBACETATE
Glycerinum Plumbi Subacetatis
(B.P.C. 1934)

Solution of Lead Subacetate . . . . 500 cc.
Glycerin . . . . 500 cc.
Distilled Water, recently boiled, a sufficient quantity

Evaporate the solution of lead subacetate to dryness on a water bath, add the glycerin and warm gently until the residue is dissolved; cool, add distilled water until the specific gravity of the mixture is about 1.48, and filter if necessary.

GLYCERITE OF PANCREATIN
Glycerinum Pancreatini
Glycerin of Pancreatin
(B.P.C. 1934)

Pancreatin	100 Gm.
Glycerin	500 cc.
Aromatic Elixir	50 cc.
Distilled Water, a sufficient quantity,	
To make	1000 cc.

Macerate the pancreatin in 300 cc. of distilled water for 24 hours, add the glycerin, and macerate for 7 days. Add the aromatic elixir and sufficient distilled water to make the product measure 1000 cc. and filter.

AVERAGE DOSE—Metric, 2 to 4 cc.—Apothecaries, ½ to 1 fluidrachm.

GLYCERITE OF STRONG PROTEIN SILVER
(R.B. I)

Strong Protein Silver.	100 Gm.
Distilled Water	100 cc.
Glycerin, a sufficient quantity,	
To make	1000 cc.

Dissolve the strong protein silver in the distilled water, and add sufficient glycerin to make the product measure 1000 cc.

INFUSIONS

COMPOUND INFUSION OF BUCHU AND METHENAMINE
(R.B. II)

Methenamine	60 Gm.
Potassium Acetate	150 Gm.
Infusion of Buchu*.	500 cc.
Infusion of Uva Ursi,* a sufficient quantity,	
To make	1000 cc.

Dissolve the methenamine and potassium acetate in the mixed infusions.

AVERAGE DOSE—Metric, 8 cc.—Apothecaries, 2 fluidrachms.

FRESH INFUSION OF CALUMBA
Infusum Calumbæ Recens
(B.P. 1932)

Calumba, in coarse powder	50 Gm.
Distilled Water, cold	1000 cc.

* Prepared according to the general formula for Infusions (see U.S.P. XII, page 218).

Infuse in a covered vessel for half an hour and strain.

AVERAGE DOSE—Metric, 15 to 30 cc.—Apothecaries, ½ to 1 fluidounce.

NOTE—This infusion should be freshly prepared.

INFUSION OF CINCHONA
Infusum Cinchonæ
(N.F. IV)

Cinchona, in No. 40 powder.	60 Gm.
Aromatic Sulfuric Acid	10 cc.
Distilled Water, a sufficient quantity,	
To make	1000 cc.

Mix the acid with 500 cc. of distilled water and moisten the powder with 30 cc. of the mixture; pack it firmly in a conical glass percolator, and pour upon it gradually, first the remainder of the mixture, and afterwards distilled water, until the percolate measures 1000 cc.

AVERAGE DOSE—Metric, 50 cc.—Apothecaries, 1½ fluidounces.

COMPOUND INFUSION OF DIGITALIS
(N.Y.H.F.)

Potassium Acetate	75 Gm.
Infusion of Digitalis, a sufficient quantity,	
To make	1000 cc.

Dissolve.

AVERAGE DOSE—Metric, 4 cc.—Apothecaries, 1 fluidrachm.

INFUSION OF LINSEED
Infusum Lini
Linseed Tea
(B.P.C. 1934)

Linseed.	35 Gm.
Glycyrrhiza, in coarse powder	10 Gm.
Distilled Water, boiling.	1000 cc.

Infuse in a covered vessel for 15 minutes and strain.

AVERAGE DOSE—Metric, 30 to 120 cc.—Apothecaries, 1 to 4 fluidounces.

NOTE—This infusion should be freshly prepared.

FRESH COMPOUND INFUSION OF BITTER ORANGE PEEL
Infusum Aurantii Compositum Recens
(B.P.C. 1934)

Bitter Orange Peel, in coarse powder	25 Gm.
Lemon Peel, in coarse powder	10 Gm.
Clove, bruised	5 Gm.
Distilled Water, boiling	1000 cc.

Infuse in a covered vessel for 15 minutes and strain.

AVERAGE DOSE—Metric, 15 to 30 cc.—Apothecaries, ½ to 1 fluidounce.

NOTE—This infusion should be freshly prepared.

INFUSION OF QUASSIA
Infusum Quassiæ
(B.P. 1932)

Quassia, rasped	10 Gm.
Distilled Water, cold	1000 cc.

Infuse in a covered vessel for 15 minutes and strain.

AVERAGE DOSE—Metric, 15 to 30 cc.—Apothecaries, ½ to 1 fluidounce.

NOTE—This infusion should be freshly prepared.

COMPOUND INFUSION OF ROSE
Infusum Rosæ Compositum
(N.F. V)

Rose	13 Gm.
Diluted Sulfuric Acid	9 cc.
Sucrose	40 Gm.
Distilled Water, boiling	1000 cc.

Pour the boiling distilled water upon the rose in a glass or porcelain vessel, add the acid, cover the vessel, and digest the drug for 1 hour. Dissolve the sucrose in the liquid and strain the infusion.

AVERAGE DOSE—Metric, 100 cc.—Apothecaries, 3 fluidounces.

INFUSION OF WILD CHERRY
Infusum Pruni Virginianæ
(N.F. IV)

Wild Cherry, in No. 20 powder	40 Gm.
Glycerin	50 cc.
Distilled Water, cold, a sufficient quantity, To make	1000 cc.

Macerate the wild cherry in 900 cc. of cold distilled water in a cylindrical percolator for 1 hour, and then draw off and collect the percolate in a receiving bottle containing the glycerin.   When the liquid has passed below the surface of the drug, press it down firmly and pour on sufficient distilled water to make the infusion measure 1000 cc., and mix well.

AVERAGE DOSE—Metric, 60 cc.—Apothecaries, 2 fluidounces.

NOTE—This infusion should be freshly prepared.

INHALANTS

BENZOIN INHALANT
(N.Y.H.F.)

Oil of Dwarf Pine Needles,
Compound Tincture of Benzoin, of each, an equal volume.
  Mix.

For use, add 4 cc. or 1 fluidrachm to 1 quart of boiling water for vapor inhalation.

COMPOUND BENZOIN INHALANT
Inhalatio Benzoini Composita
(N.Y.P.G.H.)

Menthol	30 Gm.
Oil of Eucalyptus	30 cc.
Chloroform	20 cc.
Compound Tincture of Benzoin, a sufficient quantity,	
To make	1000 cc.

Dissolve the menthol in the oil of eucalyptus and chloroform, then add sufficient compound tincture of benzoin to make the product measure 1000 cc.

For use, add 4 cc. or 1 fluidrachm to 1 quart of boiling water for vapor inhalation.

COMPOUND BENZOIN AND CREOSOTE INHALANT
(R.B. II)

Camphor	20 Gm.
Menthol	20 Gm.
Oil of Eucalyptus	80 cc.
Creosote	40 cc.
Compound Tincture of Benzoin, a sufficient quantity,	
To make	1000 cc.

Dissolve the camphor and the menthol in 500 cc. of the tincture and add the oil of eucalyptus and creosote.   Finally add sufficient compound tincture of benzoin to make the product measure 1000 cc.

For use, add 4 cc. or 1 fluidrachm to 1 quart of boiling water for vapor inhalation.

COMPOUND CREOSOTE INHALANT
(B.N.Y.)

Chloroform,
Alcohol,
Creosote, of each, an equal volume.

Mix.

For use, 20 drops inhaled from a sponge every 5 hours.

CREOSOTE AND PHENOL INHALANT
(R.B. II)

Creosote . . . .   60 cc.
Liquefied Phenol . . . .   60 cc.
Alcohol, a sufficient quantity,

To make . . . .   1000 cc.

Mix.

For use, add 4 cc. or 1 fluidrachm to 1 quart of boiling water for vapor inhalation.

INHALANT FLUID
(R.B. I)

Oil of Eucalyptus. . . . .   75 cc.
Oil of Dwarf Pine Needles . . . .   75 cc.
Methyl Salicylate . . . .   75 cc.
Compound Tincture of Benzoin, a sufficient quantity,

To make . . . .   1000 cc.

Mix.

For use, add 4 cc. or 1 fluidrachm to 1 quart of boiling water for vapor inhalation.

VAPOR INHALANT
(U.C.H.)

Menthol . . . .   66 Gm.
Camphor   . . . .   100 Gm.
Oil of Cinnamon   . . . .   33 cc.
Oil of Dwarf Pine Needles . . . .   100 cc.
Eucalyptol . . . .   500 cc.
Alcohol, a sufficient quantity,

To make . . . .   1000 cc.

Dissolve all the ingredients in the alcohol.

For use, add 4 cc. or 1 fluidrachm to 1 quart of boiling water for vapor inhalation.

JELLIES

GLYCERITE OF BOROGLYCERIN JELLY

Glycerin Jelly

(R.B. I)

Gelatin	2 Gm.
Distilled Water	47 cc.
Glycerin	5 Gm.
Glycerite of Boroglycerin	46 Gm.
To make	100 Gm.

Soak the gelatin in the distilled water for 12 hours, warm to solution with the aid of gentle heat. Add the glycerin and glycerite of boroglycerin and pour into a wide-mouthed glass jar to cool.

ZINC AND MAGNESIA JELLY

(R.B. II)

Zinc Oxide	100 Gm.
Magnesia Magma	100 Gm.
Glycerin Lubricant, R.B.	800 Gm.
To make	1000 Gm.

Triturate the zinc oxide with the magnesia magma and to this add gradually, with constant trituration, the glycerin lubricant.

LINIMENTS

AMMONIA AND CAMPHOR LINIMENT

Linimentum Ammoniæ cum Camphora

(B.P.C.)

Diluted Solution of Ammonia	250 cc.
Camphor Liniment	250 cc.
Olive Oil, a sufficient quantity,	
To make	1000 cc.

Mix by agitation.

AMMONIUM IODIDE LINIMENT

Linimentum Ammonii Iodidi

(N.F. IV)

Iodine	4 Gm.
Oil of Rosemary	15 cc.
Oil of Lavender	15 cc.
Camphor	32 Gm.
Diluted Solution of Ammonia	110 cc.
Alcohol, a sufficient quantity,	
To make	1000 cc.

Dissolve the iodine, the oils, and the camphor in 750 cc. of alcohol, then add the diluted solution of ammonia, and finally sufficient alcohol to make the product measure 1000 cc.

If a precipitate forms, filter the liniment before dispensing it.

ANODYNE LINIMENT
Linimentum Anodynum
(B.N.Y.)

Chloral Hydrate	16 Gm.
Camphor	16 Gm.
Chloroform	16 cc.
Ethyl Oxide	16 cc.
Oil of Sassafras	8 cc.
Tincture of Opium	8 cc.
Camphor and Soap Liniment, a sufficient quantity,	
To make	1000 cc.

Dissolve the chloral hydrate and camphor in a mixture of the chloroform, ethyl oxide and oil of sassafras. To this add the tincture of opium and sufficient camphor and soap liniment to make the product measure 1000 cc.

LINIMENT OF ARNICA
Arnica Opodeldoc
(B.P.C. 1934)

Hard Soap	200 Gm.
Tincture of Arnica	250 cc.
Camphor	50 Gm.
Alcohol, a sufficient quantity,	
To make	1000 cc.

Dissolve the hard soap in a mixture of the tincture of arnica and 500 cc. of alcohol on a water bath, dissolve the camphor in the solution and add sufficient alcohol to make the product measure 1000 cc. Pour into suitable containers and allow to solidify.

BELLADONNA AND CHLOROFORM LINIMENT
(N.Y.H.F.)

Chloroform	50 cc.
Tincture of Aconite	150 cc.
Fluidextract of Belladonna Root	100 cc.
Spirit of Camphor	200 cc.
Camphor and Soap Liniment, a sufficient quantity,	
To make	1000 cc.

Mix by agitation.

COMPOUND BELLADONNA LINIMENT
(V.C.N.Y.)

Tincture of Belladonna	265 cc.
Tincture of Aconite.	130 cc.
Chloroform	130 cc.
Camphor and Soap Liniment, a sufficient quantity,	
To make	1000 cc.

Mix by agitation.

PUSEY'S CALAMINE AND ZINC OXIDE LINIMENT
I

Prepared Calamine	60	Gm.
Zinc Oxide	60	Gm.
Tragacanth, in fine powder	2.5	Gm.
Glycerin	1.5	cc.
Liquefied Phenol	1.7	cc.
Olive Oil	240	cc.
Oil of Bergamot	3	cc.
Distilled Water, a sufficient quantity,		
To make	1000	cc.

Place the tragacanth and olive oil in a dry bottle and shake. Add 120 cc. of distilled water, little by little, shaking after each addition, until a satisfactory emulsion is made. Triturate the prepared calamine and zinc oxide in a mortar with the glycerin, adding distilled water slowly to form a smooth paste. Add this to the emulsion and shake until a uniform mixture results. Add the liquefied phenol and oil of bergamot and then sufficient distilled water to make the product measure 1000 cc. Mix thoroughly by shaking.

II
(Improved Formula)

Prepared Calamine.	100 Gm.
Zinc Oxide	100 Gm.
Petrolatum Liniment, Pusey, R.B., a sufficient quantity,	
To make	1000 cc.

Triturate the prepared calamine and zinc oxide, incorporating gradually sufficient petrolatum liniment to make the product measure 1000 cc. and triturate until uniform.

CAMPHOR AND CHLORAL LINIMENT
(B.N.Y.)

Camphor	45 Gm.
Chloral Hydrate	45 Gm.
Menthol	45 Gm.
Oil of Cajuput	170 cc.
Alcohol, a sufficient quantity,	
To make	1000 cc.

Dissolve the solid ingredients in 700 cc. of alcohol, add the oil of cajuput, and then enough alcohol to make 1000 cc.

CAMPHOR AND TURPENTINE LINIMENT
Linimentum Camphoræ et Olei Terebinthinæ
(R.B. II)

Spirit of Camphor,
Oil of Turpentine,
Olive Oil, of each, an equal volume.

Mix.

Dispense with a "shake well" label.

CAPSICUM LINIMENT
Linimentum Capsici
(B.P.C. 1934)

Stronger Tincture of Capsicum, R.B.	350	cc.
Oleic Acid	125	cc.
Oil of Lavender	6.2	cc.
Alcohol, a sufficient quantity,		
To make	1000	cc.

Mix the stronger tincture of capsicum with 500 cc. of alcohol, add the oleic acid and oil of lavender, and sufficient alcohol to make the product measure 1000 cc.

BALSAMIC CAPSICUM LINIMENT
Linimentum Capsici Balsamicum
(Lux. F.)

Diluted Solution of Ammonia	150 cc.
Oleo-Balsamic Mixture, R.B.	150 cc.
Spirit of Camphor	150 cc.
Camphor and Soap Liniment	150 cc.
Tincture of Capsicum	100 cc.
Tincture of Caramel, R.B.	15 cc.
Alcohol, a sufficient quantity,	
To make	1000 cc.

Mix, and filter if necessary.

COMPOUND CAPSICUM LINIMENT
Linimentum Capsici Compositum
(Ph. Aust.)

Capsicum, in coarse powder	100 Gm.
Black Pepper, in coarse powder	100 Gm.
Soft Soap	25 Gm.
Camphor	25 Gm.
Eugenol	5 cc.
Oil of Rosemary	5 cc.
Cinnamic Aldehyde	1 cc.
Diluted Solution of Ammonia	208 cc.
Alcohol	912 cc.
Distilled Water	58 cc.
To make about	1000 cc.

Macerate the first four ingredients in the mixed alcohol and distilled water during 8 days, then express and filter, and add the other ingredients.

CAPSICUM AND AMMONIA LINIMENT
(R.B. II)

Diluted Solution of Ammonia	265 cc.
Tincture of Capsicum.	265 cc.
Camphor and Soap Liniment, a sufficient quantity,	
To make	1000 cc.

Add the diluted solution of ammonia to the tincture of capsicum which has been previously mixed with 450 cc. of camphor and soap liniment. Finally add sufficient camphor and soap liniment to make the product measure 1000 cc.

COMPOUND LINIMENT OF CAPSICUM AND CAMPHOR

Tincture of Capsicum	150 cc.
Alcohol	200 cc.
Spirit of Camphor	100 cc.
Spirit of Ether.	100 cc.
Diluted Solution of Ammonia	20 cc.
Oil of Turpentine	10 cc.
Sodium Chloride	20 Gm.
Ammonium Chloride	50 Gm.
Water, a sufficient quantity,	
To make	1000 cc.

Mix the tincture and spirits with the alcohol and oil of turpentine; dissolve the salts in the water and diluted solution of ammonia, and gradually mix the two solutions.

NOTE—Dispense with a "shake well" label

LINIMENT OF CHLOROFORM, MENTHOL AND BELLADONNA

Menthol	8 Gm.
Fluidextract of Belladonna Root	64 cc.
Chloroform Liniment, a sufficient quantity,	
To make	1000 cc.

Dissolve the menthol in the mixture of the fluidextract and chloroform liniment.

NOTE—Dispense with a "shake well" label.

GIBSON'S LINIMENT
(R.B. I)

Oil of Anise	8 cc.
Oil of Cedar Leaf	8 cc.
Oil of Sassafras	8 cc.
Oil of Hemlock Spruce	8 cc.
Chloroform	45 cc.
Tincture of Capsicum	60 cc.
Spirit of Camphor	60 cc.
Stronger Solution of Ammonia	20 cc.
Alcohol, a sufficient quantity,	
To make	1000 cc.

Mix.

MENTHOL LINIMENT
Linimentum Mentholis
I
(B.P.C.)

Menthol	200 Gm.
Chloroform	250 cc.
Olive Oil or Peanut Oil, a sufficient quantity,	
To make	1000 cc.

Dissolve the menthol in the chloroform and add sufficient olive oil to make the product measure 1000 cc.

II
(Liebreich)

Menthol	50 Gm.
Olive Oil or Peanut Oil	450 cc.
Solution of Calcium Hydroxide, a sufficient quantity,	
To make	1000 cc.

Triturate the finely powdered menthol with the olive oil. Then add sufficient solution of calcium hydroxide, with vigorous agitation, to make the product measure 1000 cc.

COMPOUND METHYL SALICYLATE LINIMENT

I

Analgesic Liniment
(Aust. Ph. F.)

Menthol	45 Gm.
Olive Oil or Peanut Oil	300 cc.
Oil of Camphor	250 cc.
Methyl Salicylate, a sufficient quantity,	
To make	1000 cc.

Mix the oil of camphor and 200 cc. of methyl salicylate and in this dissolve the menthol. Add the olive oil and sufficient methyl salicylate to make the product measure 1000 cc.

II

(G.H.N.Y.)

Ichthammol	100 Gm.
Methyl Salicylate	100 cc.
Camphor and Soap Liniment, a sufficient quantity,	
To make	1000 cc.

Triturate the ichthammol with a solution of the methyl salicylate in 750 cc. of camphor and soap liniment, then add sufficient camphor and soap liniment to make the product measure 1000 cc.

COMPOUND LINIMENT OF MUSTARD

Linimentum Sinapis Compositum

(N.F. V)

Oil of Mustard	30 cc.
Fluidextract of Mezereum, R.B.	200 cc.
Camphor	60 Gm.
Menthol	20 Gm.
Castor Oil	150 cc.
Alcohol, a sufficient quantity,	
To make	1000 cc.

Dissolve the camphor and menthol in 500 cc. of alcohol, add the fluidextract of mezereum, then the oil of mustard and castor oil, and finally sufficient alcohol to make the product measure 1000 cc. Mix thoroughly.

PUSEY'S PETROLATUM LINIMENT

Heavy Liquid Petrolatum	132	cc.
Oil of Bergamot	2.5	cc.
Oil of Lavender	2.5	cc.
Sodium Benzoate	4	Gm.
Tragacanth, in fine powder	15	Gm.
Distilled Water, a sufficient quantity,		
To make	1000	cc.

Triturate the liquid petrolatum with the tragacanth until smooth, add at once 320 cc. of distilled water, and make an emulsion. Dissolve the sodium benzoate in 100 cc. of distilled water and add gradually to the emulsion. Add the oils, and lastly sufficient distilled water to make the product measure 1000 cc.

LINIMENT OF ZINC OXIDE
Linimentum Zincicum Spissum, Zinkliniment
(Ph. Svec.)

Salicylic Acid, No. 40 powder . . . .   1 Gm.
Zinc Oxide, No. 40 powder . . . .   200 Gm.
Wool Fat . . . .   100 Gm.
Olive Oil or Peanut Oil . . . .   300 Gm.
Solution of Calcium Hydroxide, a sufficient quantity,
                    To make . . . .   1000 Gm.

Melt the wool fat with the aid of gentle heat and mix it with the olive oil.   Mix the salicylic acid with the zinc oxide and gradually mix with it the oily mixture; gradually add with constant trituration the solution of calcium hydroxide, and continue the trituration until the product is uniformly mixed.

LIQUID PARENOL
Parenol Liquidum
(B.P.C.)

Light Liquid Petrolatum . . . .   700 cc.
White Wax . . . .   50 Gm.
Distilled Water, a sufficient quantity,
                    To make . . . .   1000 cc.

Melt the wax in the liquid petrolatum, pour the mixture into a warm mortar and add gradually sufficient distilled water, previously warmed, to make the product measure 1000 cc.

Dispense with a "shake well" label.

This is a neutral liniment.   It does not become rancid, and besides being useful in the treatment of skin diseases and as a vehicle for injections, it is also a lubricant for catheters, etc.

LOTIONS

ALKALINE LOTION
Lotio Alkalina
(B.P.C. 1923)

Sodium Bicarbonate . . . .   10 Gm.
Sodium Borate . . . .   10 Gm.
Water, a sufficient quantity,
                    To make . . . .   1000 cc.

Dissolve.

AMMONIUM CHLORIDE LOTION
Lotio Ammonii Chloridi

Lotio Evaporans
(B.P.C.)

Ammonium Chloride	30 Gm.
Alcohol	125 cc.
Water, a sufficient quantity,	
To make	1000 cc.

Dissolve, and filter if necessary.

ANALGESIC LOTION
Lotion of Ethylaminobenzoate

Ethylaminobenzoate	25 Gm.
Menthol	2 Gm.
Lotion of Calamine and Phenol, a sufficient quantity,	
To make	1000 cc.

Triturate together the ethylaminobenzoate and menthol and gradually add the calamine and phenol lotion.

NOTE—Dispense with a "shake well" label.

ANTIPRURITIC LOTION
(P.F.)

Menthol	0.35	Gm.
Liquefied Phenol	12	cc.
Bismuth Subnitrate	90	Gm.
Zinc Oxide	90	Gm.
Bitter Almond Water	180	cc.
Deodorizing Cleansing Solution, R.B., No. I	360	cc.
Rose Water, a sufficient quantity,		
To make	1000	cc.

Triturate intimately the first four ingredients, preferably dissolving the menthol in a small quantity of alcohol. Then add the bitter almond water, cleansing solution, and sufficient rose water to make the product measure 1000 cc.

ASTRINGENT LOTION
Lotio Adstringens
(N.Y.P.G.H.)

Alum	2 Gm.
Zinc Sulfate	2 Gm.
Liquefied Phenol	2 cc.
Glycerin	135 cc.
Water, a sufficient quantity,	
To make	1000 cc.

Dissolve the alum and the zinc sulfate in 500 cc. of the water and add the glycerin in which the liquefied phenol has been dissolved. Lastly add sufficient water to make the product measure 1000 cc., and filter.

LOTION OF BENZYL BENZOATE
(Phar. Jour.)

Benzyl Benzoate	333 cc.
Oleic Acid	166 cc.
Potassium Hydroxide, approximately	33 Gm.
Alcohol, a sufficient quantity,	
To make	1000 cc.

Dissolve the potassium hydroxide in 45 cc. of alcohol. Add to the oleic acid and adjust with more of such alkaline solution if necessary until neutral in reaction, using 2 drops of phenolphthalein T.S. as the indicator. Not more than a faint pink color shall be produced. Lastly add the benzyl benzoate and sufficient alcohol to make the product measure 1000 cc.

BISMUTH LOTION
Lotio Bismuthi
(R.B. II)

Bismuth Subnitrate.	20 Gm.
Tragacanth, in fine powder	2 Gm.
Glycerin	250 cc.
Water, a sufficient quantity,	
To make	1000 cc.

Triturate the bismuth subnitrate and tragacanth with the glycerin. Add gradually sufficient water to make the product measure 1000 cc. and mix thoroughly.

COMPOUND BISMUTH LOTION
Lotio Bismuthi Composita
(Startin)

Bismuth Subnitrate.	250 Gm.
Zinc Oxide	250 Gm.
Spirit of Camphor	250 cc.
Glycerin	250 cc.
Water, a sufficient quantity,	
To make	1000 cc.

Triturate the solids with the glycerin. Add the spirit of camphor with continued trituration and then add sufficient water to make the product measure 1000 cc.

BOECK'S LOTION

Boeck's Paste, Lotion of Lead, Talc, Starch and Tar
(R.B. I)

Solution of Lead Subacetate.	20 cc.
Solution of Coal Tar	150 cc.
Starch	200 Gm.
Purified Talc	200 Gm.
Glycerin	100 cc.
Mucilage of Acacia.	15 cc.
Water, a sufficient quantity,	
To make	1000 cc.

Triturate the purified talc and starch with the solution of coal tar and the glycerin. Add the solution of lead subacetate, mix well, then add the mucilage of acacia and sufficient water to make the product measure 1000 cc.

This preparation develops a compact sediment upon standing. Vigorous agitation will re-establish the suspension.

PUSEY'S BORIC ACID LOTION
(R.B. II)

Oil of Rose	0.05	cc.
Oil of Lavender	0.10	cc.
Oil of Bergamot	0.20	cc.
Tragacanth, in fine powder	5	Gm.
Boric Acid	15	Gm.
Glycerin	15	cc.
Water, a sufficient quantity,		
To make	1000	cc.

Mix the tragacanth with the glycerin and add 500 cc. of water. Dissolve the boric acid in this liquid and add the oils and sufficient distilled water to make the product measure 1000 cc.

CALAMINE AND CHALK LOTION
(R.B. I)

Prepared Calamine.	50 Gm.
Prepared Chalk	50 Gm.
Glycerin	150 cc.
Solution of Calcium Hydroxide, a sufficient quantity,	
To make	1000 cc.

Triturate the prepared chalk and prepared calamine until smooth and add gradually the solution of calcium hydroxide and the glycerin.

CALAMINE AND ZINC OXIDE LOTION

Bulkley's Calamine and Zinc Oxide Lotion

Prepared Calamine.	32 Gm.
Zinc Oxide	64 Gm.
Glycerin	75 cc.
Solution of Calcium Hydroxide.	120 cc.
Water, or Rose Water, a sufficient quantity,	
To make	1000 cc.

Triturate the solids with the glycerin, add the solution of calcium hydroxide and sufficient water, or rose water, to make the product measure 1000 cc.

CALAMINE, ZINC OXIDE AND PHENOL LOTION

Bulkley's Phenolated Calamine Lotion

Liquefied Phenol.	10 cc.
Calamine and Zinc Oxide Lotion, R.B., a sufficient quantity,	
To make	1000 cc.

Mix.

Note—This preparation is not to be confused with Phenolated Lotion of Calamine, N.F. VII.

CALAMINE, ZINC OXIDE AND OIL LOTION
(R.B. II)

Prepared Calamine.	125 Gm.
Zinc Oxide	125 Gm.
Solution of Calcium Hydroxide.	500 cc.
Olive Oil or Peanut Oil	165 cc.
Tragacanth, in fine powder	6 Gm.
Water or Rose Water, a sufficient quantity,	
To make	1000 cc.

Emulsify the olive oil with the solution of calcium hydroxide by shaking thoroughly. Thoroughly triturate the prepared calamine, zinc oxide, and tragacanth together, add the emulsified mixture, and then sufficient water or rose water to make the product measure 1000 cc.

CAMPHOR, MENTHOL, BORIC ACID AND SODIUM BICARBONATE LOTION
(R.B. II)

Camphor	7.5	Gm.
Menthol	15	Gm.
Boric Acid	15	Gm.
Sodium Bicarbonate	15	Gm.
Alcohol.	250	cc.
Water, a sufficient quantity,		
To make	1000	cc.

Dissolve the camphor and menthol in the alcohol, and the boric acid and sodium bicarbonate in 700 cc. of water, pour the alcoholic solution gradually into the aqueous solution, and after the mixture has been permitted to stand for 24 hours, filter. Add sufficient water through the filter to make the product measure 1000 cc.

CHLORAL AND CAMPHOR LOTION
(R.B. I)

Chloral Hydrate	320 Gm.
Spirit of Camphor, a sufficient quantity,	
To make	1000 cc.

Dissolve.

COAL TAR LOTION
(R.B. I)

Coal Tar	500 Gm.
Carbon Tetrachloride, a sufficient quantity,	
To make	1000 cc.

Dissolve the coal tar in the carbon tetrachloride and filter if necessary.

ALKALINE COAL TAR LOTION
Lotio Picis Carbonis Alkalina
(B.P.C. 1934)

Solution of Coal Tar	5 cc.
Sodium Bicarbonate	12.5 Gm.
Water, a sufficient quantity,	
To make	1000 cc.

Dissolve the sodium bicarbonate in 500 cc. of water, and add the solution of coal tar and sufficient water to make the product measure 1000 cc.

COOLING LOTION
Lotio Refrigerans
(R.B. I)

Potassium Nitrate	200 Gm.
Ammonium Chloride	200 Gm.
Water, a sufficient quantity,	
To make	1000 cc.

Dissolve and filter. This solution is to be used immediately after compounding.

COMPOUND JUNIPER TAR LOTION
(V.C.N.Y.)

Juniper Tar	195	cc.
Castor Oil	150	cc.
Salicylic Acid	32.5	Gm.
Alcohol, a sufficient quantity,		
To make	1000	cc.

Dissolve the salicylic acid in 500 cc. of alcohol, add the castor oil and juniper tar, and finally sufficient alcohol to make the product measure 1000 cc.

KUMMERFELD'S LOTION
Aqua Cosmetica
Kummerfeld's Cosmetic Water

I

Spirit of Camphor	100	cc.
Alcohol	100	cc.
Tragacanth, ribbon	15	Gm.
Precipitated Sulfur	60	Gm.
Water, a sufficient quantity,		
To make	1000	cc.

Mix the spirit of camphor with the alcohol. Macerate the tragacanth in 500 cc. of distilled water until thoroughly softened and suspend the sulfur in the product by trituration. Mix the two liquids, and finally add sufficient water to make the product measure 1000 cc.

II
(Hager)

Precipitated Sulfur	40	Gm.
Camphor	3.33	Gm.
Acacia, in fine powder	6.66	Gm.
Solution of Calcium Hydroxide	500	cc.
Water or Rose Water, a sufficient quantity,		
To make	1000	cc.

Triturate the solid ingredients until intimately mixed, using a few drops of alcohol to insure the pulverization of the camphor, and incorporate with the solution of calcium hydroxide. Add sufficient rose water to make the product measure 1000 cc.

LEAD AND ZINC LOTION
(B.N.Y.)

Zinc Oxide	75	Gm.
Solution of Lead Subacetate	100	cc.
Glycerin	125	cc.
Solution of Calcium Hydroxide, a sufficient quantity,		
To make	1000	cc.

Triturate the zinc oxide with the glycerin to a smooth paste, add the solution of lead subacetate, and finally sufficient solution of calcium hydroxide to make the product measure 1000 cc.

COMPOUND LIME LOTION
(R.B. I)

Zinc Oxide . . . . 60 Gm.
Starch . . . . 60 Gm.
Solution of Calcium Hydroxide. . . . . 500 cc.
Water or Rose Water, a sufficient quantity,

              To make . . . . 1000 cc.

Triturate the starch with the solution of calcium hydroxide and heat until gelatinized.   Rub the zinc oxide to a smooth mixture with this liquid and, when cool, add sufficient water or rose water to make the product measure 1000 cc.

EMULSIFIED LINSEED OIL LOTION WITH PHENOL
(B.N.Y.)

Potassium Hydroxide . . . . 7 Gm.
Phenol . . . . 133 Gm.
Water . . . . 140 cc.
Linseed Oil, a sufficient quantity,

              To make . . . . 1000 cc.

Dissolve the phenol in 500 cc. of warm linseed oil, cool and add sufficient linseed oil to make 860 cc.   Add the potassium hydroxide dissolved in the water and agitate vigorously.

NOTE—To be dispensed with a "shake well" label.

MACNAIR'S LOTION

Ferric Chloride . . . . 25 Gm.
Sodium Chloride. . . . . 25 Gm.
Glycerin . . . . 200 cc.
Water, a sufficient quantity,

              To make . . . . 1000 cc.

Dissolve the salts in the mixed liquids.

MAGNESIA AND ZINC LOTION
Lotio Magnesiæ et Zinci
(V.C.N.Y.)

Magnesium Carbonate . . . . 35 Gm.
Zinc Oxide . . . . 35 Gm.
Water, or Rose Water, a sufficient quantity,

              To make . . . . 1000 cc.

Mix the powders and triturate thoroughly with the water or rose water, added gradually until the product measures 1000 cc.

LOTION OF MAGNESIUM CARBONATE AND ZINC OXIDE WITH PHENOL

I

Phenol	8 Gm.
Zinc Oxide	40 Gm.
Light Magnesium Carbonate	125 Gm.
Expressed Almond Oil or Persic Oil	125 cc.
Glycerin	40 cc.
Solution of Calcium Hydroxide	375 cc.
Water or Rose Water, a sufficient quantity,	
To make	1000 cc.

Mix the zinc oxide and magnesium carbonate with the expressed almond oil and glycerin to a smooth paste; gradually add the solution of calcium hydroxide with constant agitation, and lastly add the water or rose water and phenol, slowly and with constant agitation.

NOTE—Dispense with a "shake well" label.

II

Johnson's Lotion

Phenol	10 Gm.
Zinc Oxide	40 Gm.
Magnesium Carbonate	100 Gm.
Expressed Oil of Almond or Persic Oil	120 Gm.
Glycerin	40 cc.
Menthol	5 Gm.
Solution of Calcium Hydroxide, a sufficient quantity,	
To make	1000 cc.

Mix the zinc oxide and magnesium carbonate with the oil and gradually add the solution of calcium hydroxide, with constant agitation. Triturate the phenol with the menthol and add the glycerin, and add this mixture to the oil and the solution of calcium hydroxide mixture. Triturate until the product is uniformly mixed.

NOTE—Dispense with a "shake well" label.

MENTHOL AND AMMONIA LOTION
(R.B. I)

Menthol	20 Gm.
Alcohol	750 cc.
Strong Solution of Ammonia, a sufficient quantity,	
To make	1000 cc.

Dissolve the menthol in the alcohol, and add sufficient strong solution of ammonia to make the product measure 1000 cc.

OXGALL LOTION
(B.N.Y.)

Purified Ox Bile, R.B.	530 cc.
Glycerin	350 cc.
Salicylic Acid	5 Gm
Water, a sufficient quantity,	
To make	1000 cc.

Dissolve the salicylic acid in the glycerin, add the purified ox bile and sufficient water to make the product measure 1000 cc.

PATTON'S LOTION

Sodium Bicarbonate	20 Gm.
Sodium Sulfite	20 Gm.
Glycerin	40 cc.
Fluidextract of Grindelia	300 cc.
Water, a sufficient quantity,	
To make	1000 cc.

Dissolve the salts in 500 cc. of water, add the glycerin and the fluidextract of grindelia, mix well and add sufficient distilled water to make the product measure 1000 cc.

RESORCINOL LOTION
Lotio Resorcinolis
Elliott's Resorcin Lotion

Resorcinol	50 Gm.
Diluted Alcohol, a sufficient quantity,	
To make	1000 cc.

Dissolve.

NOTE—Andeer's Lotion differs from the above in that it contains twice the amount of resorcinol.

COMPOUND RESORCINOL LOTION
Lotio Resorcinolis Composita
Spiritus Resorcinolis, Spiritus Capillaris
(Aust. Ph. F.)

Resorcinol	25 Gm.
Castor Oil	25 cc.
Perfumed Spirit	200 cc.
Alcohol, a sufficient quantity,	
To make	1000 cc.

Dissolve the resorcinol in the perfumed spirit and add the castor oil and sufficient alcohol to make the product measure 1000 cc.

NOTE—This lotion may discolor the hair.

SALICYLIC ACID LOTION
(R.B. I)

Salicylic Acid	10 Gm.
Glycerin	40 cc.
Alcohol, a sufficient quantity,	
To make	1000 cc.

Dissolve the salicylic acid in 900 cc. of alcohol and add the glycerin and sufficient alcohol to make the product measure 1000 cc.

SODIUM BICARBONATE LOTION
(R.B. I)

Sodium Bicarbonate	90 Gm.
Perfume, as desired,	
Water, a sufficient quantity,	
To make	1000 cc.

Dissolve and filter.

SODIUM BICARBONATE, BORAX AND PHENOL LOTION
(R.B. I)

Sodium Bicarbonate	20 Gm.
Sodium Borate	8 Gm.
Liquefied Phenol.	11 cc.
Water or Rose Water, a sufficient quantity,	
To make	1000 cc.

Dissolve.

SODIUM THIOSULFATE LOTION
(R.B. I)

Sodium Thiosulfate.	120 Gm.
Glycerin	120 cc.
Water, a sufficient quantity,	
To make	1000 cc.

Dissolve the sodium thiosulfate in 500 cc. of water and add the glycerin and sufficient water to make the product measure 1000 cc.

STARCH LOTION
(U.C.H.)

Starch	200 Gm.
Zinc Oxide	200 Gm.
Glycerin	100 cc.
Solution of Calcium Hydroxide, a sufficient quantity,	
To make	1000 cc.

Triturate the starch and the zinc oxide together and gradually add the glycerin, triturating until a paste results; gradually add the solution of calcium hydroxide until a uniform mixture results and the product measures 1000 cc.

To be applied locally.

STAVESACRE LOTION
Lotio Staphisagriæ
Nursery Hair Lotion
(B.P.C. 1934)

Stavesacre, in coarse powder.	100	Gm.
Acetic Acid	50	cc.
Alcohol	100	cc.
Oil of Lemon	0.4	cc.
Oil of Lavender	0.2	cc.
Oil of Geranium	0.2	cc.
Glycerin	50	cc.
Water, a sufficient quantity,		
To make	1000	cc.

Boil the stavesacre with the acetic acid and 800 cc. of water for 10 minutes in a covered vessel and set aside until cold. Add the oils previously dissolved in the alcohol, filter, and add the glycerin and sufficient water to make the product measure 1000 cc.

SULFUR LOTION
Lotio Sulfuris
(B.P.C. 1934)

Precipitated Sulfur.	68 Gm.
Glycerin	31 cc.
Alcohol	125 cc.
Water or Rose Water	400 cc.
Solution of Calcium Hydroxide, a sufficient quantity,	
To make	1000 cc.

Triturate the precipitated sulfur with the alcohol, glycerin and rose water to form a smooth cream, and finally add sufficient solution of calcium hydroxide to make the product measure 1000 cc.

SULFUR AND CAMPHOR LOTION
Sulfur Face Lotion
(R.B. II)

Precipitated Sulfur.	64 Gm.
Camphor, in fine powder	4 Gm.
Acacia, in powder	8 Gm.
Water or Rose Water	500 cc.
Solution of Calcium Hydroxide, a sufficient quantity,	
To make	1000 cc.

Mix the camphor with the precipitated sulfur and acacia. Triturate the mixture with the rose water, and add sufficient solution of calcium hydroxide to make the product measure 1000 cc.

CAUTION—*Care should be exercised not to apply this lotion after the use of face powders containing bismuth or similar substances which react with sulfur.*

SULFURATED POTASH LOTION
(R.B. I)

Sulfurated Potash . . . .   200 Gm.
Water, a sufficient quantity,

            To make . . . .   1000 cc.

Dissolve the sulfurated potash in 800 cc. of water. Filter and wash the filter with sufficient water to make the product measure 1000 cc.

THYMOL, CAMPHOR AND AMMONIA LOTION
(R.B. I)

Thymol. . . . .   20 Gm.
Spirit of Camphor . . . .   800 cc.
Diluted Solution of Ammonia, a sufficient quantity,

            To make . . . .   1000 cc.

Dissolve the thymol in the spirit of camphor, and add sufficient diluted solution of ammonia to make the product measure 1000 cc.

TRIPLEX LOTION
(St. J. H.)

Prepared Calamine, in fine powder . . . .   20 Gm.
Zinc Oxide, in fine powder . . . .   20 Gm.
Solution of Lead Subacetate.   5 cc.
Liquefied Phenol . . . .   15 cc.
Glycerin . . . .   30 cc.
Water, a sufficient quantity,

            To make . . . .   1000 cc.

Triturate the prepared calamine and zinc oxide with the liquefied phenol and glycerin, add the solution of lead subacetate and sufficient water to make the product measure 1000 cc.

WHITE LOTION WITH SULFUR
Lotio Alba Composita

Compound White Lotion
(R.B. I)

Precipitated Sulfur. . . . .   40 Gm.
White Lotion, N.F., a sufficient quantity,

            To make . . . .   1000 cc.

Mix.

NOTE—This lotion should be freshly prepared. It generates gas upon standing and should be dispensed in an incompletely filled bottle.

CONCENTRATED WHITE LOTION
Lotio Alba Concentrata
(R.B. II)

Zinc Sulfate.	400 Gm.
Sulfurated Potash	220 Gm.
Glycerin	30 cc.
Rose Water	30 cc.
Water, a sufficient quantity,	
To make	1000 cc.

Dissolve the zinc sulfate in sufficient water to make 600 cc. and the sulfurated potash in sufficient water to make 340 cc. Filter each solution, using separate filters, and add the second solution slowly to the first. Add the rose water and glycerin and mix thoroughly by shaking.

NOTE—It is absolutely necessary that a good quality of sulfurated potash be used and that the lotion be freshly prepared.

WHITFIELD'S LOTION
(R.B. II)

Benzoic Acid	5 Gm.
Salicylic Acid	3 Gm.
Acetone.	25 cc.
Diluted Alcohol, a sufficient quantity,	
To make	100 cc.

Dissolve the acids in the acetone and add gradually sufficient diluted alcohol to make the product measure 100 cc.

MEDICATED EYE LOTIONS
ALUM AND BORIC ACID EYE LOTION

Alum.	4 Gm.
Boric Acid.	20 Gm.
Distilled Water, a sufficient quantity,	
To make	1000 cc.

Dissolve and filter.

AROMATIC EYE WASH
(N.Y.H.F.)

Camphor Water	333 cc.
Aromatic Alkaline Solution	333 cc.
Saturated Solution of Boric Acid	334 cc.
To make	1000 cc.

Mix.

NOTE—To be used with an eye cup.

ASTRINGENT EYE WASH
Collyrium Adstringens
(R.B. I)

Zinc Sulfate.	0.5 Gm.
Sodium Borate	32 Gm.
Boric Acid.	16 Gm.
Glycerin	50 cc.
Peppermint Water	75 cc.
Rose Water.	150 cc.
Camphor Water	150 cc.
Distilled Water, a sufficient quantity,	
To make	1000 cc.

Dissolve the zinc sulfate in the peppermint water, and the sodium borate and boric acid in the glycerin and rose water. Mix the two solutions, and add the camphor water and sufficient distilled water to make the product measure 1000 cc. Filter.

YELLOW ASTRINGENT EYE LOTION
Collyrium Adstringens Luteum
Horst's Eye Wash

(Ph. Aust. VIII)

Zinc Sulfate.	5 Gm.
Ammonium Chloride	2 Gm.
Camphor	2 Gm.
Crocus	1 Gm.
Alcohol	70 cc.
Distilled Water, a sufficient quantity,	
To make	1000 cc.

Dissolve the zinc sulfate and ammonium chloride in 900 cc. of distilled water and add the camphor previously dissolved in the alcohol. Lastly, add the crocus, agitate frequently during 24 hours and then filter, adding sufficient distilled water, through the filter, to make the product measure 1000 cc.

SOLUTION OF ATROPINE SULFATE (FOR EYE USE)
(E.H.P.)

Atropine Sulfate	8.3 Gm.
Distilled Water, a sufficient quantity,	
To make	1000 cc.

Dissolve.

NOTE—This solution is to be used for the eyes and must be used on the advice of a physician only. A dilute solution of atropine sulfate may be prepared by diluting this solution with an equal part of distilled water.

BORIC ACID AND BORAX EYE LOTION
(B.N.Y.)

Boric Acid	50 Gm.
Sodium Borate	50 Gm.
Camphor Water	250 cc.
Distilled water, a sufficient quantity,	
To make	1000 cc.

Dissolve and filter.

LANCASTER'S PREPARATION FOR EYE WASH

Boric Acid	2	Gm.
Sodium Borate	22	Gm.
Thymol	0.15	Gm.
Menthol	0.1	Gm.
Oil of Eucalyptus	0.4	cc.
Oil of Wintergreen	0.4	cc.

Triturate the powders intimately with the oils until uniform.

DOSE—One-half teaspoonful to 1 pint of boiling water. Cool and use with an eye cup.

MITTENDORF'S EYE WATER
(R.B. I)

Spirit of Camphor	25 cc.
Spirit of Lavender	25 cc.
Spirit of Rosemary*	25 cc.
Brandy	25 cc.

Mix and set aside for a few days. Filter.
For use this spirit is diluted with 9 volumes of water.

ROMERSHAUSEN'S EYE WATER

Romershausen's Augenwasser
(E.B. III)

Compound Tincture of Fennel, R.B..	165 cc.
Distilled Water, a sufficient quantity,	
To make	1000 cc.

Mix.

---

* Prepared according to the general formula for Spirits of Volatile Oils (see N.F. VII, page 387).

TANNIC ACID AND BORAX EYE LOTION
(N.Y.P.G.H.)

Tannic Acid.	20 Gm.
Sodium Borate	20 Gm.
Glycerin	120 cc.
Camphor Water, a sufficient quantity,	
To make	1000 cc.

Dissolve the sodium borate in the glycerin and add to 500 cc. of camphor water in which the tannic acid has been previously dissolved. Add sufficient camphor water to make the product measure 1000 cc., and filter.

WILLIAMS' EYE LOTION
(P.F.)

Sodium Borate.	16.5 Gm.
Camphor Water, a sufficient quantity,	
To make	1000 cc.

Dissolve and filter.

ZINC SULFATE AND BORIC ACID EYE LOTION
(B.N.Y.)

Zinc Sulfate.	2 Gm.
Boric Acid.	22 Gm.
Camphor Water	250 cc.
Distilled Water, a sufficient quantity,	
To make	1000 cc.

Dissolve and filter.

LUBRICANTS

CHONDRUS LUBRICANT
(N.F. V with Phenol)

Chondrus.	30 Gm.
Liquefied Phenol	2 cc.
Water, a sufficient quantity,	
To make	1000 cc.

Wash the chondrus with cold water, then place it in a double boiler and heat it with 800 cc. of water for half an hour. Strain through muslin. Add the liquefied phenol, and sufficient water to make the product measure 1000 cc.

This forms a thin lubricating liquid; if a thicker lubricant is desired, the strained liquid may be evaporated about one-third and the liquefied phenol added.

GLYCERIN LUBRICANT

Glyceritum Tragacanthæ Compositum
(R.B. I)

Tragacanth, in fine powder	15 Gm.
Liquefied Phenol	20 cc.
Alcohol	40 cc.
Distilled Water	600 cc.
Glycerin, a sufficient quantity,	
To make	1000 Gm.

Agitate the tragacanth in a wide-mouthed bottle with the alcohol, add the distilled water, and set aside overnight.   Then add the liquefied phenol and sufficient glycerin to make the product weigh 1000 Gm.

This preparation has the consistency of a thick liquid.   If intended for collapsible tubes, it should be made into a paste by increasing the quantity of tragacanth to 25 Gm.

LIQUID PARENOL

Parenol Liquidum
(B.P.C.)

See page 71.

LUND'S OILY LUBRICANT

Oleum Lubricans

Lubricating or Catheter Oil, Lund's Oil
(B.P.C.)

Phenol	50 Gm.
Castor Oil	200 cc.
Expressed Almond Oil or Persic Oil, a sufficient quantity,	
To make	1000 cc.

Dissolve the phenol in the mixed oils.

This oil is used to some extent to lubricate catheters.   Gum lubricants are generally preferred as they can be removed by water and do not attack the material of which the catheter is composed.

SURGEONS' LUBRICATING JELLY
(R.B. II)

Tragacanth, in selected ribbons	25	Gm.
Boric Acid	12.5	Gm.
Alcohol	40	Gm.
Glycerin	80	Gm.
Solution of Formaldehyde	4	cc.
Methyl Salicylate, 1% alcoholic solution	40	cc.
Water, a sufficient quantity,		
To make about	1000	Gm.

Macerate the tragacanth in the water, in which the boric acid has been dissolved. Strain through fine cheese-cloth. Add the alcohol, glycerin, solution of formaldehyde, methyl salicylate, and sufficient water to make the product weigh 1000 Gm.; mix thoroughly.

SURGICAL LUBRICANT FOR CATHETERS
(Ext. Ph.)

Starch	80 Gm.
Glycerin	700 cc.
Distilled Water	170 cc.
Boric Acid	50 Gm.
Liquefied Phenol	20 cc.

Heat to boiling the glycerin, distilled water and starch; add the boric acid and warm the mixture until dissolved. Cool, and add the liquefied phenol.

NOTE—This lubricant is non-greasy and can readily be removed with water.

MAGMAS

MAGMA OF FERRIC HYDROXIDE
Precipitated Ferric Hydroxide (Moist)
(N.F. IV)

Solution of Ferric Sulfate	330 cc.
Diluted Solution of Ammonia	460 cc.
Water, a sufficient quantity,	
To make	1000 Gm.

Add the solution of ferric sulfate, previously diluted with 3300 cc. of cold water, to the diluted solution of ammonia, previously diluted with 1600 cc. of cold water, stirring constantly. As soon as the precipitate has subsided, draw off the clear liquid by means of a siphon, then mix the precipitate intimately with about 3300 cc. of cold water. Again draw off the clear liquid after subsidence of the precipitate, and repeat this operation until a portion of the decanted liquid gives not more than a slight cloudiness with barium chloride T.S. Finally, transfer the precipitate to a wet strainer, and, after it has drained, mix it with sufficient cold water to make the product weigh 1000 Gm.

NOTE—This preparation is not to be confused with Magma of Ferric Hydroxide, U.S.P. XI, known as Arsenic Antidote which follows.

MAGMA OF FERRIC HYDROXIDE
Magma Ferri Hydroxidi
Ferri Hydroxidi cum Magnesii Oxido U.S.P. X, Arsenic Antidote
(U.S.P. XI)

Solution of Ferric Sulfate	40 cc.
Magnesium Oxide	10 Gm.
Distilled Water, a sufficient quantity,	

Mix the solution of ferric sulfate with 125 cc. of distilled water and keep the liquid in a large, well-stoppered bottle. Rub the magnesium oxide with cold distilled water to a smooth, thin mixture, transfer this to a bottle capable of holding 1000 cc., fill it with distilled water to about three-fourths of its capacity, and keep it tightly stoppered. When the preparation is needed, shake the magnesium oxide mixture until it is of a thin, creamy consistence, slowly add to it the diluted solution of ferric sulfate, and shake it until a uniformly smooth mixture results.

NOTE—In this process the 10 Gm. of magnesium oxide may be replaced by 300 cc. of magnesia magma, diluting it with sufficient distilled water to make the required volume.

The diluted solution of ferric sulfate and the magnesia mixture should be kept on hand in separate bottles ready for immediate use so that the antidote can be quickly prepared.

AVERAGE DOSE—Metric, 120 cc.—Apothecaries, 4 fluidounces.

MAGMA OF SULFURATED ZINC
Magma Zinci Sulfurati
Magma of Lotio Alba
(R.B. II)

Sulfurated Potash	240 Gm.
Zinc Sulfate.	313 Gm.
Distilled Water	430 cc.
Perfumed Spirit, as desired,	
Glycerin, a sufficient quantity,	
To make	1000 Gm.

Dissolve the sulfurated potash in 240 cc. of water and the zinc sulfate separately in 190 cc. of water. Add the first solution to the second, mix and set aside for the precipitate to settle. Decant the supernatant liquid and reject it. To the precipitate add the perfumed spirit, if desired, and sufficient glycerin to make the product weigh 1000 Gm.

MIXTURES

Mixtures are not always clear solutions when prepared. In such cases where the mixture is not clear, it is *advisable* to dispense the mixture with a "shake well" label attached.

A.C.E. MIXTURE
Anesthetic Mixture
(R.B. II)

Dehydrated Alcohol	167 cc.
Chloroform	333 cc.
Ether.	500 cc.
To make	1000 cc.

Mix.

NOTE—This mixture must be freshly prepared and must be placed in a well-stoppered container protected from air.

MIXTURE OF ACETYLSALICYLIC ACID
Mistura Acidi Acetylsalicylici
(B.P.C. 1934)

Acetylsalicylic Acid, in fine powder	34.3 Gm.
Tragacanth, in fine powder	3.4 Gm.
Acacia, in fine powder	4.6 Gm.
Starch, in fine powder	4.6 Gm.
Sucrose, in fine powder.	10.3 Gm.
Chloroform Water, a sufficient quantity,	
To make	1000 cc.

Mix the powders and add gradually, with constant trituration, sufficient chloroform water to make the product measure 1000 cc.

AVERAGE DOSE—Metric, 15 to 30 cc.—Apothecaries, ½ to 1 fluidounce.

NOTE—This mixture should be freshly prepared.

AMMONIUM CARBONATE MIXTURE
(N.Y.H.F.)

Ammonium Carbonate, in hard translucent pieces	8 Gm.
Spirit of Camphor	50 cc.
Spirit of Ethyl Nitrite.	160 cc.
Distilled Water	35 cc.
Syrup of Tolu Balsam, a sufficient quantity,	
To make	1000 cc.

Powder the ammonium carbonate and dissolve in the distilled water.   Add 500 cc. of syrup of tolu balsam.   To this add the spirits, and finally sufficient syrup of tolu balsam to make the product measure 1000 cc.

AVERAGE DOSE—Metric, 4 cc.—Apothecaries, 1 fluidrachm.

NOTE—This mixture should be freshly prepared.

AMMONIUM CARBONATE AND CAMPHOR MIXTURE
Mistura Ammonii Carbonatis et Camphoræ
(B.N.Y.)

Ammonium Carbonate, in hard translucent pieces	15 Gm.
Spirit of Camphor	300 cc.
Spirit of Ethyl Nitrite.	150 cc.
Aromatic Elixir, a sufficient quantity,	
To make	1000 cc.

Powder the ammonium carbonate and dissolve in 500 cc. of the aromatic elixir, and add the spirit of camphor and spirit of ethyl nitrite. Finally add sufficient aromatic elixir to make the product measure 1000 cc.

AVERAGE DOSE—Metric, 4 cc.—Apothecaries, 1 fluidrachm.

NOTE—This mixture should be freshly prepared.

AMMONIUM CHLORIDE MIXTURE
Mistura Ammonii Chloridi
Mistura Solvens Simplex

I
(N.F. IV)

Ammonium Chloride	25 Gm.
Extract of Glycyrrhiza	65 Gm.
Distilled Water, a sufficient quantity,	
To make	1000 cc.

Dissolve.

AVERAGE DOSE—Metric, 8 cc.—Apothecaries, 2 fluidrachms.

II
(V.C.N.Y)

Ammonium Chloride	40 Gm.
Spirit of Chloroform	23 cc.
Syrup of Tolu Balsam.	250 cc.
Syrup.	250 cc.
Distilled Water, a sufficient quantity,	
To make	1000 cc.

Dissolve the ammonium chloride in 400 cc. of distilled water, add the syrup of tolu balsam, syrup and spirit of chloroform. Finally add sufficient distilled water to make the product measure 1000 cc.

AVERAGE DOSE—Metric, 8 cc.—Apothecaries, 2 fluidrachms.

AMMONIUM CHLORIDE AND POTASSIUM IODIDE MIXTURE
(B.N.Y.)

Potassium Iodide	15 Gm.
Ammonium Chloride	30 Gm.
Fluidextract of Glycyrrhiza	150 cc.
Distilled Water, a sufficient quantity,	
To make	1000 cc.

Dissolve the potassium iodide and ammonium chloride in 500 cc. of distilled water, add the fluidextract of glycyrrhiza and finally sufficient distilled water to make the product measure 1000 cc.

AVERAGE DOSE—Metric, 4 cc.—Apothecaries, 1 fluidrachm.

AMMONIUM CHLORIDE AND IPECAC MIXTURE
I
(B.N.Y.)

Ammonium Chloride	15 Gm.
Camphorated Tincture of Opium	100 cc.
Syrup of Ipecac	100 cc.
Syrup of Wild Cherry	250 cc.
Syrup of Tolu Balsam, a sufficient quantity,	
To make	1000 cc.

Dissolve the ammonium chloride in the syrups of ipecac and wild cherry, and add the camphorated tincture of opium. Finally add sufficient syrup of tolu balsam to make the product measure 1000 cc.

AVERAGE DOSE—Metric, 4 cc.—Apothecaries, 1 fluidrachm.

II
(N.Y.H.F.)

Ammonium Chloride	75 Gm.
Fluidextract of Ipecac	25 cc.
Syrup of Tolu Balsam, a sufficient quantity,	
To make	1000 cc.

Dissolve the ammonium chloride in 750 cc. of syrup of tolu balsam and add the fluidextract of ipecac, and finally add sufficient syrup of tolu balsam to make the product measure 1000 cc.

AVERAGE DOSE—Metric, 4 cc.—Apothecaries, 1 fluidrachm.

MIXTURE OF AMMONIUM IODIDE AND BROMIDE WITH LOBELIA
(B.N.Y.)

Ammonium Iodide	30 Gm.
Ammonium Bromide	50 Gm.
Syrup of Tolu Balsam	325 cc.
Tincture of Lobelia, a sufficient quantity,	
To make	1000 cc.

Dissolve the ammonium bromide and ammonium iodide in 500 cc. of the tincture of lobelia, add the syrup of tolu balsam and sufficient tincture of lobelia to make the product measure 1000 cc.

AVERAGE DOSE—Metric, 2 cc.—Apothecaries, 30 minims.

NOTE—This mixture must be freshly prepared.

ANTACID MIXTURE
(N.Y.H.F.)

Magnesium Sulfate.	125 Gm.
Magnesium Carbonate	65 Gm.
Aromatic Spirit of Ammonia.	60 cc.
Distilled Water, a sufficient quantity,	
To make	1000 cc.

Dissolve the magnesium sulfate in 500 cc. of distilled water. Triturate the magnesium carbonate with this solution until a smooth mixture is obtained. Add the aromatic spirit of ammonia and finally sufficient distilled water to make the product measure 1000 cc.

Average dose—Metric, 4 cc.—Apothecaries, 1 fluidrachm.

ANTIMONIAL MIXTURE
(V.C.N.Y.)

Tincture of Antimony.	150 cc.
Tincture of Ipecac	150 cc.
Spirit of Ethyl Nitrite.	150 cc.
Solution of Ammonium Acetate, a sufficient quantity,	
To make	1000 cc.

Mix the tincture of antimony, tincture of ipecac and spirit of ethyl nitrite. Add sufficient solution of ammonium acetate to make the product measure 1000 cc.

Average dose—Metric, 4 cc.—Apothecaries, 1 fluidrachm.

ANTIPYRINE, BROMIDE AND CAFFEINE MIXTURE
A.B.C. Headache Mixture
(R.B. I)

Ammonium Bromide	25 Gm.
Antipyrine.	25 Gm.
Citrated Caffeine	12.5 Gm.
Chloroform Water, a sufficient quantity,	
To make	1000 cc.

Dissolve, and filter if necessary.

Average dose—Metric, 4 cc.—Apothecaries, 1 fluidrachm.

MIXTURE OF ANTIPYRINE AND GLYCYRRHIZA
(B.N.Y.)

Antipyrine.	30 Gm.
Fluidextract of Glycyrrhiza	30 cc.
Syrup.	500 cc.
Distilled Water, a sufficient quantity,	
To make	1000 cc.

Dissolve the antipyrine in 250 cc. of distilled water and add the fluidextract of glycyrrhiza, syrup and sufficient distilled water to make the product measure 1000 cc.

Average dose—Metric, 4 cc.—Apothecaries, 1 fluidrachm.

MIXTURE OF ANTIPYRINE AND SODIUM BROMIDE WITH BELLADONNA
(N.Y.H.F.)

Antipyrine	25 Gm.
Tincture of Belladonna	50 cc.
Sodium Bromide.	33 Gm.
Syrup of Tolu Balsam.	325 cc.
Distilled Water, a sufficient quantity,	
To make	1000 cc.

Dissolve the antipyrine and sodium bromide in 500 cc. of distilled water, add the syrup of tolu balsam, tincture of belladonna, and sufficient distilled water to make the product measure 1000 cc.

AVERAGE DOSE—Metric, 4 cc.—Apothecaries, 1 fluidrachm.

MIXTURE OF ANTIPYRINE, SODIUM BROMIDE AND VALERIAN WITH CHLOROFORM
(V.C.N.Y.)

Antipyrine	50 Gm.
Sodium Bromide.	115 Gm.
Spirit of Chloroform	75 cc.
Tincture of Valerian	500 cc.
Distilled Water, a sufficient quantity,	
To make	1000 cc.

Dissolve the antipyrine and sodium bromide in 300 cc. of distilled water. Add the spirit of chloroform and tincture of valerian and sufficient distilled water to make the product measure 1000 cc.

AVERAGE DOSE—Metric, 4 cc.—Apothecaries, 1 fluidrachm.

ASTRINGENT MIXTURE
(V.C.N.Y.)

Tincture of Kino	333 cc.
Tincture of Krameria, R.B.	333 cc.
Tincture of Gambir, R.B.	334 cc.
To make	1000 cc.

Mix.

AVERAGE DOSE—Metric, 4 cc.—Apothecaries, 1 fluidrachm.

BELLADONNA, BROMIDE AND CHLOROFORM MIXTURE
(Phillip)

Sodium Bromide.	300 Gm.
Tincture of Belladonna	200 cc.
Spirit of Chloroform	200 cc.
Peppermint Water, a sufficient quantity,	
To make	1000 cc.

Dissolve the sodium bromide in 500 cc. of peppermint water, add the tincture of belladonna and spirit of chloroform, and sufficient peppermint water to make the product measure 1000 cc.

AVERAGE DOSE—Metric, 4 cc.—Apothecaries, 1 fluidrachm.

MIXTURE OF BISMUTH AND CAMPHORATED OPIUM
(E.H.P.)

Bismuth Subcarbonate	81 Gm.
Camphorated Tincture of Opium	250 cc.
Chalk Mixture, a sufficient quantity,	
To make	1000 cc.

Mix the bismuth subcarbonate with the chalk mixture and add the camphorated tincture of opium, and mix well.

AVERAGE DOSE—Metric, 8 cc.—Apothecaries, 2 fluidrachms.

NOTE—This mixture should be dispensed with a "shake well" label.   To be dispensed on prescription only.

BISMUTH, RESORCINOL, CARDAMOM AND PEPSIN MIXTURE
(R.B. I)

Resorcinol	16 Gm.
Bismuth Subnitrate	40 Gm.
Bismuth Subgallate.	40 Gm.
Compound Tincture of Cardamom	250 cc.
Elixir of Pepsin and Rennin	500 cc.
Cinnamon Water, a sufficient quantity,	
To make	1000 cc.

Dissolve the resorcinol in the compound tincture of cardamom, add the salts and elixir and sufficient cinnamon water to make the product measure 1000 cc.

AVERAGE DOSE—Metric, 4 cc.—Apothecaries, 1 fluidrachm.

BLACK MIXTURE
I
(N.Y.P.G.H.)

Sodium Bromide.	250 Gm.
Pepsin	15 Gm.
Activated Charcoal, in fine powder	75 Gm.
Glycerin	200 cc.
Peppermint Water, a sufficient quantity,	
To make	1000 cc.

Dissolve the sodium bromide and pepsin in 500 cc. of peppermint water and add gradually to the mixture of the activated charcoal triturated with the glycerin. Add sufficient peppermint water to make the product measure 1000 cc.

AVERAGE DOSE—Metric, 4 cc.—Apothecaries 1 fluidrachm.

NOTE—Do not confuse this mixture with Hammond's mixture of the R.B. or Lotio Nigra of the N.F.

II
Hammond's Mixture
(Can. Ph. J.)

Pepsin	57 Gm.
Activated Charcoal	65 Gm.
Potassium Bromide	259 Gm.
Distilled Water, a sufficient quantity,	
To make	1000 cc.

Mix the activated charcoal with a portion of the distilled water; dissolve the pepsin and potassium bromide in the remainder of the distilled water, and mix the two solutions.

AVERAGE DOSE—Metric, 4 cc.—Apothecaries, 1 fluidrachm.

NOTE—This mixture should be dispensed with a "shake well" label. Do not confuse this mixture with Black Mixture, I of the R.B.

BORIC ACID AND HYOSCYAMUS MIXTURE
(V.C.N.Y.)

Boric Acid	230 Gm.
Tincture of Hyoscyamus	450 cc.
Distilled Water, a sufficient quantity,	
To make	1000 cc.

Triturate the boric acid with the tincture of hyoscyamus and add gradually sufficient distilled water to make the product measure 1000 cc.

Dispense with a "shake well" label.

AVERAGE DOSE—Metric, 2 cc.—Apothecaries, 30 minims.

ALKALINE MIXTURE OF BROMIDES
Mistura Bromidorum Alkalina
(N.Y.H.F.)

Sodium Bromide	20 Gm.
Potassium Bromide	20 Gm.
Ammonium Bromide	20 Gm.
Tincture of Capsicum	20 cc.
Aromatic Spirit of Ammonia	125 cc.
Syrup of Ginger	125 cc.
Distilled Water, a sufficient quantity,	
To make	1000 cc.

Dissolve the bromides in 500 cc. of distilled water, add the syrup of ginger, tincture of capsicum and aromatic spirit of ammonia, and finally sufficient distilled water to make the product measure 1000 cc.

AVERAGE DOSE—Metric, 15 cc.—Apothecaries, 4 fluidrachms.

TRIPLE BROMIDE MIXTURE
I
(Hager)

Potassium Bromide	40 Gm.
Sodium Bromide.	20 Gm.
Ammonium Bromide	20 Gm.
Compound Tincture of Cardamom	100 cc.
Syrup of Orange.	200 cc.
Distilled Water, a sufficient quantity,	
To make	1000 cc.

Dissolve the bromides in 500 cc. of distilled water, add the compound tincture of cardamom and syrup of orange, filter and add sufficient distilled water through the filter to make the product measure 1000 cc.

AVERAGE DOSE—Metric, 12 cc.—Apothecaries, 3 fluidrachms.

II
(B.N.Y.)

Potassium Bromide.	75 Gm.
Sodium Bromide.	120 Gm.
Ammonium Bromide	150 Gm.
Distilled Water, a sufficient quantity,	
To make	1000 cc.

Dissolve and filter if necessary.

AVERAGE DOSE—Metric, 4 cc.—Apothecaries, 1 fluidrachm.

BROMIDE AND HYOSCYAMUS MIXTURE
(V.C.N.Y.)

Potassium Bromide	242 Gm.
Tincture of Hyoscyamus	500 cc.
Peppermint Water, a sufficient quantity,	
To make	1000 cc.

Dissolve the potassium bromide in 300 cc. of peppermint water, add the tincture of hyoscyamus, and sufficient peppermint water to make the product measure 1000 cc.

AVERAGE DOSE—Metric, 4 cc.—Apothecaries, 1 fluidrachm.

MIXTURE OF BROMIDE AND VALERIAN
(R.B. II)

Sodium Bromide	125 Gm.
Ammoniated Tincture of Valerian	250 cc.
Fluidextract of Glycyrrhiza	20 cc.
Syrup.	380 cc.
Distilled Water, a sufficient quantity,	
To make	1000 cc.

Dissolve the sodium bromide in 250 cc. of the distilled water, add the syrup, fluid-extract of glycyrrhiza, ammoniated tincture of valerian, and sufficient distilled water to make the product measure 1000 cc.

AVERAGE DOSE—Metric, 4 cc.—Apothecaries, 1 fluidrachm.

BROWN MIXTURE WITH AMMONIUM CHLORIDE
(R.B. I)

Ammonium Chloride	50 Gm.
Compound Mixture of Opium and Glycyrrhiza, a sufficient quantity,	
To make	1000 cc.

Dissolve.

Dispense with a "shake well" label.

AVERAGE DOSE—Metric, 4 cc.—Apothecaries, 1 fluidrachm.

COMPOUND BUCHU MIXTURE
(V.C.N.Y.)

Fluidextract of Buchu	80 cc.
Potassium Citrate	45 Gm.
Spirit of Ethyl Nitrite.	130 cc.
Distilled Water, a sufficient quantity,	
To make	1000 cc.

Dissolve the potassium citrate in 500 cc. of distilled water. Add the fluidextract of buchu, spirit of ethyl nitrite, and finally sufficient distilled water to make the product measure 1000 cc.

AVERAGE DOSE—Metric, 15 cc.—Apothecaries, 4 fluidrachms.

NOTE—This mixture must be freshly prepared.

AROMATIC CAMPHOR MIXTURE
Mistura Camphoræ Aromatica
Parrish's Camphor Mixture
(N.F. IV)

Compound Tincture of Lavender.	250 cc.
Sucrose.	35 Gm.
Camphor Water, a sufficient quantity,	
To make	1000 cc.

Mix the compound tincture of lavender with 500 cc. of camphor water, dissolve the sucrose in the mixture, and add sufficient camphor water to make the product measure 1000 cc.

AVERAGE DOSE—Metric, 8 cc.—Apothecaries, 2 fluidrachms.

COMPOUND MIXTURE OF CAPSICUM
(N.Y.H.F.)

Tincture of Capsicum.	10 cc.
Fluidextract of Ginger	12 cc.
Chloroform	20 cc.
Whisky, a sufficient quantity,	
To make	1000 cc.

Mix the chloroform with the tincture and fluidextract, and add sufficient whisky to make the product measure 1000 cc.

AVERAGE DOSE—Metric, 15 cc.—Apothecaries, 4 fluidrachms.

ACID CARDAMOM MIXTURE
(R.B. II)

Diluted Sulfuric Acid.	60 cc.
Compound Tincture of Cardamom	120 cc.
Sucrose.	240 Gm.
Spearmint Water, a sufficient quantity,	
To make	1000 cc.

Dissolve the sucrose in 500 cc. of spearmint water. Add the other ingredients and sufficient spearmint water to make the product measure 1000 cc.

AVERAGE DOSE—Metric, 8 cc.—Apothecaries, 2 fluidrachms.

CASCARA AND BELLADONNA MIXTURE
(R.B. II)

Fluidextract of Cascara Sagrada	300 cc.
Fluidextract of Glycyrrhiza	300 cc.
Tincture of Belladonna	30 cc.
Chloroform Water, a sufficient quantity,	
To make	1000 cc.

Mix.

AVERAGE DOSE—Metric, 8 cc.—Apothecaries, 2 fluidrachms.

AROMATIC CHALK MIXTURE
(R.B. II)

Magnesium Carbonate	30 Gm.
Aromatic Chalk Powder	150 Gm.
Aromatic Tincture of Rhubarb.	150 cc.
Peppermint Water, a sufficient quantity,	
To make	1000 cc.

Triturate the magnesium carbonate and aromatic chalk powder with 500 cc. of the peppermint water. Add the aromatic tincture of rhubarb and sufficient peppermint water to make the product measure 1000 cc.

AVERAGE DOSE—Metric, 15 cc.—Apothecaries, 4 fluidrachms.

MIXTURE OF CODEINE AND IPECAC
(N.Y.H.F.)

Codeine Phosphate	2 Gm.
Fluidextract of Ipecac	25 cc.
Syrup of Tolu Balsam, a sufficient quantity,	
To make	1000 cc.

Dissolve the codeine phosphate in a small amount of water; add to part of the syrup of tolu balsam, and finally add the fluidextract of ipecac and sufficient syrup of tolu balsam to make the product measure 1000 cc.

AVERAGE DOSE—Metric, 4 cc.—Apothecaries, 1 fluidrachm.

NOTE—To be dispensed on prescription only.

COLCHICUM, POTASSIUM IODIDE AND SARSAPARILLA MIXTURE
(V.C.N.Y.)

Strong Tincture of Colchicum Corm	150 cc.
Potassium Iodide	80 Gm.
Compound Syrup of Sarsaparilla	500 cc.
Distilled Water, a sufficient quantity,	
To make	1000 cc.

Dissolve the potassium iodide in 300 cc. of distilled water. Add the strong tincture of colchicum corm, compound syrup of sarsaparilla, and sufficient distilled water to make the product measure 1000 cc.

AVERAGE DOSE—Metric, 8 cc.—Apothecaries, 2 fluidrachms.

COLCHICUM AND POTASSIUM ACETATE MIXTURE
(B.N.Y.)

Potassium Acetate	150 Gm.
Tincture of Colchicum Seed	150 cc.
Distilled Water, a sufficient quantity,	
To make	1000 cc.

Dissolve the potassium acetate in 500 cc. of distilled water, add the tincture of colchicum seed and sufficient distilled water to make the product measure 1000 cc.

AVERAGE DOSE—Metric, 4 cc.—Apothecaries, 1 fluidrachm.

CREOSOTE MIXTURE
Mistura Creosoti
(B.P.C.)

Creosote	2 cc.
Syrup	60 cc.
Spirit of Juniper*	2 cc.
Distilled Water, a sufficient quantity,	
To make	1000 cc.

Shake the creosote and spirit of juniper with 900 cc. of distilled water. Add the syrup and sufficient distilled water to make the product measure 1000 cc.

AVERAGE DOSE—Metric, 15 cc.—Apothecaries, 4 fluidrachms.

CREOSOTE AND ALMOND OIL MIXTURE
(B.P.C.)

Creosote	4 Gm.
Expressed Almond Oil or Persic Oil	60 cc.
Syrup of Orange	120 cc.
Acacia, in fine powder	25 Gm.
Distilled Water, a sufficient quantity,	
To make	1000 cc.

Mix the creosote and the oil with the acacia; add at once 50 cc. of distilled water and triturate until an emulsion is formed. To this emulsion add the syrup and sufficient distilled water to make the product measure 1000 cc.

AVERAGE DOSE—Metric, 4 cc.—Apothecaries, 1 fluidrachm.

CREOSOTE AND COD LIVER OIL MIXTURE
(N.Y.H.F.)

Creosote	12.5 cc.
Cod Liver Oil	250 cc.
Extract of Malt, a sufficient quantity,	
To make	1000 cc.

* Prepared according to the general formula for Spirits of Volatile Oils (see N.F. VII, page 387).

Mix thoroughly by trituration or put through an homogenizer.

AVERAGE DOSE—Metric, 15 cc.—Apothecaries, 4 fluidrachms.

CREOSOTE AND GENTIAN MIXTURE
(V.C.N.Y.)

Creosote	15 cc.
Compound Tincture of Gentian, a sufficient quantity,	
To make	1000 cc.

Mix.

AVERAGE DOSE—Metric, 4 to 8 cc.—Apothecaries, 1 to 2 fluidrachms.

DIGITALIS MIXTURE
(V.C.N.Y.)

Tincture of Digitalis	150 cc.
Aromatic Elixir, a sufficient quantity,	
To make	1000 cc.

Mix.

AVERAGE DOSE—Metric, 4 cc.—Apothecaries, 1 fluidrachm.

COMPOUND DIGITALIS MIXTURE
(V.C.N.Y.)

Tincture of Digitalis	75 cc.
Tincture of Nux Vomica.	75 cc.
Compound Tincture of Cinchona, a sufficient quantity,	
To make	1000 cc.

Mix the tincture of digitalis and the tincture of nux vomica, then add sufficient compound tincture of cinchona to make the product measure 1000 cc.

AVERAGE DOSE—Metric, 4 cc.—Apothecaries, 1 fluidrachm.

A.B.C. DIURETIC MIXTURE
Potassium Acetate, Bicarbonate and Citrate Mixture
(B.N.Y.)

Potassium Acetate	30 Gm.
Potassium Bicarbonate	30 Gm.
Potassium Citrate	30 Gm.
Distilled Water, a sufficient quantity,	
To make	1000 cc.

Dissolve and filter if necessary.

AVERAGE DOSE—Metric, 15 cc.—Apothecaries, 4 fluidrachms.

A.B.C. DIURETIC MIXTURE WITH TRITICUM
Potassium Acetate, Bicarbonate and Citrate Mixture with Triticum
(B.N.Y.)

Potassium Acetate	60 Gm.
Potassium Bicarbonate	60 Gm.
Potassium Citrate	60 Gm.
Fluidextract of Triticum	125 cc.
Distilled Water, a sufficient quantity,	
To make	1000 cc.

Dissolve the salts in 500 cc. of distilled water, add the fluidextract of triticum and sufficient distilled water to make the product measure 1000 cc.

AVERAGE DOSE—Metric, 4 cc.—Apothecaries, 1 fluidrachm.

EXPECTORANT MIXTURE
I
(N.Y.P.G.H.)

Ammonium Carbonate	18 Gm.
Potassium Iodide	60 Gm.
Tincture of Belladonna	18 cc.
Compound Spirit of Ether.	180 cc.
Syrup of Wild Cherry.	150 cc.
Distilled Water, a sufficient quantity,	
To make	1000 cc.

Dissolve the ammonium carbonate and potassium iodide in 500 cc. of distilled water. Add the tincture of belladonna, compound spirit of ether, syrup of wild cherry, and sufficient distilled water to make the product measure 1000 cc.

Dispense with a "shake well" label.

AVERAGE DOSE—Metric, 4 cc.—Apothecaries, 1 fluidrachm.

II
Lobelia Expectorant Mixture
(R.B. I)

Potassium Iodide	60 Gm.
Tincture of Lobelia.	250 cc.
Syrup of Wild Cherry	125 cc.
Distilled Water, a sufficient quantity,	
To make	1000 cc.

Dissolve the potassium iodide in 500 cc. of distilled water, add the tincture of lobelia, syrup of wild cherry, and sufficient distilled water to make the product measure 1000 cc.

AVERAGE DOSE—Metric, 4 cc.—Apothecaries, 1 fluidrachm.

III
(R.B. I)

Anisated Spirit of Ammonia	75 cc.
Potassium Iodide	18 Gm.
Syrup of Tolu Balsam	250 cc.
Distilled Water, a sufficient quantity,	
To make	1000 cc.

Dissolve the potassium iodide in 500 cc. of distilled water, add the anisated spirit of ammonia and the syrup of tolu balsam. Finally add sufficient distilled water to make the product measure 1000 cc.

AVERAGE DOSE—Metric, 4 cc.—Apothecaries, 1 fluidrachm.

FRELEIGH'S MIXTURE

English Tonic
(R.B. I)

Spirit of Phosphorus, R.B.	22.5 cc.
Tincture of Calumba	53.5 cc.
Tincture of Gentian, R.B.	53.5 cc.
Tincture of Matricaria, R.B.	96.5 cc.
Tincture of Nux Vomica	96.5 cc.
Tincture of Ignatia, R.B.	96.5 cc.
Aromatic Tincture, R.B.	193.5 cc.
Tincture of Cinchona, R.B., a sufficient quantity,	
To make	1000 cc.

Mix, set aside for 48 hours and filter.

AVERAGE DOSE—Metric, 4 cc.—Apothecaries, 1 fluidrachm.

GRAY'S MIXTURE
(R.B. I)

Ammonium Chloride	60 Gm.
Diluted Hydrocyanic Acid	8 cc.
Chloroform	6 cc.
Syrup of Wild Cherry	500 cc.
Syrup of Lactucarium, R.B., a sufficient quantity,	
To make	1000 cc.

Dissolve the ammonium chloride in the syrup of wild cherry, add the chloroform and diluted hydrocyanic acid and sufficient syrup of lactucarium to make the product measure 1000 cc.

AVERAGE DOSE—Metric, 4 cc.—Apothecaries, 1 fluidrachm.

GRINDELIA MIXTURE
(v.c.n.y.)

Fluidextract of Grindelia . . . .   250 cc.
Compound Syrup of Sarsaparilla, a sufficient quantity,
           To make . . . .   1000 cc.

Mix.

AVERAGE DOSE—Metric, 4 cc.—Apothecaries, 1 fluidrachm.

MIXTURE OF GUAIAC
Mistura Guaiaci
(n.f. iv)

Tincture of Guaiac. . . . .   125 cc.
Honey . . . .   250 cc.
Cinnamon Water, a sufficient quantity,
           To make . . . .   1000 cc.

Place the honey in a mortar and add the tincture of guaiac gradually with brisk trituration. Then add sufficient cinnamon water, in portions, to make the product measure 1000 cc., mixing each portion thoroughly by trituration.

Dispense with a "shake well" label.

AVERAGE DOSE—Metric, 15 cc.—Apothecaries, 4 fluidrachms.

COMPOUND HYDRASTIS MIXTURE
(v.c.n.y.)

Fluidextract of Hydrastis . . . .   500 cc.
Fluidextract of Cascara Sagrada . . . .   150 cc.
Glycerin, a sufficient quantity,
           To make . . . .   1000 cc.

Mix the fluidextracts, and add gradually sufficient glycerin to make the product measure 1000 cc.

AVERAGE DOSE—Metric, 4 cc.—Apothecaries, 1 fluidrachm.

HYDROCHLORIC ACID AND GENTIAN MIXTURE
(n.y.h.f.)

Diluted Hydrochloric Acid . . . .   375 cc.
Compound Tincture of Gentian, a sufficient quantity,
           To make . . . .   1000 cc.

Mix.

AVERAGE DOSE—Metric, 4 cc., well diluted—Apothecaries, 1 fluidrachm, well diluted.

HYDROCHLORIC ACID AND PEPSIN MIXTURE
I
(V.C.N.Y.)

Diluted Hydrochloric Acid	300 cc.
Saccharated Pepsin	81 Gm.
Glycerin	75 cc.
Peppermint Water, a sufficient quantity,	
To make	1000 cc.

Dissolve the saccharated pepsin in a mixture of 300 cc. of peppermint water and the diluted hydrochloric acid. Add the glycerin and sufficient peppermint water to make the product measure 1000 cc. and filter if necessary.

AVERAGE DOSE—Metric, 4 cc.—Apothecaries, 1 fluidrachm.

II
(B.N.Y.)

Pepsin	18 Gm.
Diluted Hydrochloric Acid	37 cc.
Glycerin	325 cc.
Distilled Water, a sufficient quantity,	
To make	1000 cc.

Dissolve the pepsin in a mixture of the glycerin, diluted hydrochloric acid and 300 cc. of distilled water. Finally add sufficient distilled water to make the product measure 1000 cc.

AVERAGE DOSE—Metric, 8 cc.—Apothecaries, 2 fluidrachms.

ALKALINE HYOSCYAMUS MIXTURE
(B.N.Y.)

Potassium Bicarbonate	135 Gm.
Tincture of Hyoscyamus	30 cc.
Distilled Water, a sufficient quantity,	
To make	1000 cc.

Dissolve the potassium bicarbonate in 750 cc. of distilled water, add the tincture of hyoscyamus and sufficient distilled water to make the product measure 1000 cc.

AVERAGE DOSE—Metric, 15 cc.—Apothecaries, 4 fluidrachms.

MIXTURE OF HYOSCYAMUS AND POTASSIUM CITRATE
(B.N.Y.)

Potassium Citrate	150 Gm.
Tincture of Hyoscyamus	150 cc.
Distilled Water, a sufficient quantity,	
To make	1000 cc.

Dissolve the potassium citrate in 700 cc. of distilled water, add the tincture of hyoscyamus, and then sufficient distilled water to make the product measure 1000 cc.

AVERAGE DOSE—Metric, 4 cc.—Apothecaries, 1 fluidrachm.

H. X. B. MIXTURE

Lambert Treatment

(R.B. I)

Fluidextract of Hyoscyamus.   250 cc.
Fluidextract of Xanthoxylum . . . .   250 cc.
Fluidextract of Belladonna Leaf . . . .   75 cc.
Diluted Alcohol . . . .   425 cc.

To make . . . .   1000 cc.

Mix.

NOTE—This preparation is administered only when the patient can be kept under trained medical supervision.

AVERAGE DOSE—Metric, 0.5 cc.—Apothecaries, 8 minims.

IODIDE AND COLCHICUM MIXTURE

(N.Y.H.F.)

Potassium Iodide. . . . .   80 Gm.
Tincture of Colchicum Seed . . . .   250 cc.
Distilled Water, a sufficient quantity,

To make . . . .   1000 cc.

Dissolve the potassium iodide in 500 cc. of distilled water, add the tincture of colchicum seed and sufficient distilled water to make the product measure 1000 cc.

AVERAGE DOSE—Metric, 4 cc.—Apothecaries, 1 fluidrachm.

COMPOUND IRON MIXTURE

Mistura Ferri Composita

Griffith's Mixture

(N.F. IV)

Ferrous Sulfate, in clear crystals. . . . .   6 Gm.
Myrrh, in small pieces . . . .   18 Gm.
Sucrose. . . . .   18 Gm.
Potassium Carbonate. . . . .   8 Gm.
Spirit of Lavender . . . .   60 cc.
Water or Rose Water, a sufficient quantity,

To make . . . .   1000 cc.

Triturate the myrrh, sucrose and potassium carbonate in a mortar with 700 cc. of rose water, at first added very gradually, so that a uniform mixture results.   Add the spirit of lavender, then the ferrous sulfate previously dissolved in about 50 cc. of rose water, and lastly sufficient rose water to make the product measure 1000 cc.

AVERAGE DOSE—Metric, 15 cc.—Apothecaries, 4 fluidrachms.

NOTE—This mixture should be freshly prepared.

IRON CITRATE MIXTURE
Mistura Ferri Citratis
(Gray)

Iron and Ammonium Citrate	32 Gm.
Citric Acid.	5 Gm.
Tincture of Lemon.	8 cc.
Syrup.	750 cc.
Distilled Water, a sufficient quantity,	
To make	1000 cc.

Triturate the citric acid with the iron and ammonium citrate and dissolve in about 200 cc. of distilled water. Add the tincture of lemon and syrup and sufficient distilled water to make the product measure 1000 cc. Set aside for 24 hours and filter if necessary.

AVERAGE DOSE—Metric, 4 cc.—Apothecaries, 1 fluidrachm.

MIXTURE OF IRON AND AMMONIUM CHLORIDES
(G.H.N.Y.)

Tincture of Ferric Chloride	170 cc.
Ammonium Chloride	70 Gm.
Glycerin	350 cc.
Distilled Water, a sufficient quantity,	
To make	1000 cc.

Dissolve the ammonium chloride in 400 cc. of distilled water, add the glycerin, tincture of ferric chloride, and sufficient distilled water to make the product measure 1000 cc.

AVERAGE DOSE—Metric, 4 cc.—Apothecaries, 1 fluidrachm.

IRON, ARSENIC AND QUININE MIXTURE
(V.C.N.Y.)

Soluble Iron and Quinine Citrate	40 Gm.
Solution of Potassium Arsenite	22 cc.
Compound Tincture of Gentian, a sufficient quantity,	
To make	1000 cc.

Dissolve the soluble iron and quinine citrate in 750 cc. of compound tincture of gentian, add the solution of potassium arsenite, and sufficient compound tincture of gentian to make the product measure 1000 cc.

AVERAGE DOSE—Metric, 8 cc.—Apothecaries, 2 fluidrachms.

IRON AND POTASSIUM TARTRATE MIXTURE
(V.C.N.Y.)

Iron and Potassium Tartrate	80 Gm.
Glycerin	150 cc.
Distilled Water, a sufficient quantity,	
To make	1000 cc.

Dissolve the iron and potassium tartrate in 750 cc. of distilled water, add the glycerin, and sufficient distilled water to make the product measure 1000 cc.

AVERAGE DOSE—Metric, 8 cc.—Apothecaries, 2 fluidrachms.

MIXTURE OF IRON AND QUININE CITRATE
(P.F.)

Soluble Iron and Quinine Citrate . . . .   60 Gm.
Glycerin . . . .   650 cc.
Chloroform Water . . . .   120 cc.
Distilled Water, a sufficient quantity,
               To make . . . .   1000 cc.

Dissolve the soluble iron and quinine citrate in the chloroform water diluted with an equal quantity of distilled water.   Add the glycerin, and sufficient distilled water to make the product measure 1000 cc.

AVERAGE DOSE—Metric, 8 cc.—Apothecaries, 2 fluidrachms.

IRON AND STRYCHNINE MIXTURE
(V.C.N.Y.)

Soluble Ferric Pyrophosphate   160   Gm.
Strychnine Sulfate . . . .   0.5 Gm.
Fluidextract of Ginger   3   cc.
Glycerin   75   cc.
Distilled Water, a sufficient quantity,
               To make   1000   cc.

Dissolve the soluble ferric pyrophosphate in 500 cc. of distilled water and the strychnine sulfate in 100 cc. of distilled water.   Mix the solutions, add the glycerin, fluidextract of ginger, and sufficient distilled water to make the product measure 1000 cc.

AVERAGE DOSE—Metric, 4 cc.—Apothecaries, 1 fluidrachm.

The average dose contains 0.002 Gm. ($\frac{1}{30}$ grain) of strychnine sulfate.

COMPOUND IRON AND STRYCHNINE MIXTURE
(N.Y.H.F.)

Strychnine Sulfate . . . .   0.25 Gm.
Cinchonidine Sulfate   25   Gm.
Tincture of Ferric Chloride   162   cc.
Diluted Phosphoric Acid   400   cc.
Glycerin   125   cc.
Distilled Water, a sufficient quantity,
               To make   1000   cc.

Dissolve the strychnine sulfate and cinchonidine sulfate in the diluted phosphoric acid, and add the tincture of ferric chloride and glycerin.   Finally add sufficient distilled water to make the product measure 1000 cc.

AVERAGE DOSE—Metric, 4 cc.—Apothecaries, 1 fluidrachm.

The average dose contains 0.001 Gm. ($\frac{1}{60}$ grain) of strychnine sulfate.

COMPOUND MAGNESIUM SULFATE MIXTURE
Keith's Mixture
(R.B. I)

Heavy Magnesium Oxide	50 Gm.
Magnesium Sulfate	150 Gm.
Glycerin	180 cc.
Mucilage of Acacia	180 cc.
Peppermint Water, a sufficient quantity,	
To make	1000 cc.

Dissolve the magnesium sulfate in 500 cc. of peppermint water. Triturate the heavy magnesium oxide with the glycerin and the mucilage of acacia and add the solution of magnesium sulfate, and sufficient peppermint water to make the product measure 1000 cc.

Dispense with a "shake well" label.

AVERAGE DOSE—Metric, 4 to 8 cc.—Apothecaries, 1 to 2 fluidrachms.

LINSEED OIL MIXTURE
(B.N.Y.)

Linseed Oil	285 cc.
Methyl Salicylate	5 cc.
Oil of Cinnamon	5 cc.
Glycerin	15 cc.
Syrup	195 cc.
Mucilage of Chondrus, a sufficient quantity,	
To make	1000 cc.

Incorporate the mixed oils gradually with 200 cc. of mucilage of chondrus; add the glycerin and syrup and sufficient mucilage of chondrus to make the product measure 1000 cc.

AVERAGE DOSE—Metric, 15 cc.—Apothecaries, 4 fluidrachms.

COMPOUND MIXTURE OF LOBELIA AND HYOSCYAMUS
Compound Tincture of Lobelia and Hyoscyamus
(E.H.P.)

Tincture of Lobelia	75 cc.
Tincture of Hyoscyamus	75 cc.
Compound Spirit of Ether	75 cc.
Syrup of Tolu Balsam, a sufficient quantity,	
To make	1000 cc.

Mix the tinctures with the compound spirit of ether and gradually add sufficient syrup of tolu balsam to make the product measure 1000 cc.

AVERAGE DOSE—Metric, 4 cc.—Apothecaries, 1 fluidrachm.

MIXTURE OF OPIUM, RHUBARB AND GAMBIR
Loomis' Mixture
(P.F.)

Tincture of Opium	130 cc.
Compound Tincture of Rhubarb	60 cc.
Compound Tincture of Gambir.	100 cc.
Oil of Sassafras	10 cc.
Compound Tincture of Lavender, a sufficient quantity,	
To make	1000 cc.

Mix.

AVERAGE DOSE—Metric, 2 cc.—Apothecaries, 30 minims.

NOTE—To be dispensed on prescription only.

MAGNESIUM AND BISMUTH MIXTURE
White Mixture
(R.B. I)

Magnesium Carbonate	5 Gm.
Bismuth Subcarbonate	20 Gm.
Distilled Water, a sufficient quantity,	
To make	1000 cc.

Mix.

AVERAGE DOSE—Metric, 8 cc.—Apothecaries, 2 fluidrachms.

NOTE—This is a common American prescription and is not to be confused with the White Mixture of the British Pharmaceutical Codex, the formula for which is given below.

MAGNESIUM CARBONATE AND SULFATE MIXTURE
White Mixture
(B.P.C.)

Light Magnesium Carbonate	45 Gm.
Magnesium Sulfate.	275 Gm.
Peppermint Water, a sufficient quantity,	
To make	1000 cc.

Dissolve the magnesium sulfate in 800 cc. of peppermint water. Incorporate the light magnesium carbonate in this solution, and add sufficient peppermint water to make the product measure 1000 cc.

AVERAGE DOSE—Metric, 15 to 30 cc.—Apothecaries, ½ to 1 fluidounce.

NOTE—This mixture should be freshly prepared.

MERCURIC IODIDE MIXTURE
1-2-3 Mixture
(S.H.F.)

Mercury Bichloride	0.75 Gm.
Potassium Iodide	90 Gm.
Distilled Water	30 cc.
Compound Syrup of Sarsaparilla, a sufficient quantity,	
To make	1000 cc.

Dissolve the mercury bichloride in the distilled water, and the potassium iodide in 800 cc. of the compound syrup of sarsaparilla. Mix the two solutions, and add sufficient compound syrup of sarsaparilla to make the product measure 1000 cc.

AVERAGE DOSE—Metric, 4 cc.—Apothecaries, 1 fluidrachm.

NOTE—The preparation derives its synonym (1-2-3 Mixture) from the fact that the prescription is usually written in hospital clinics as follows:

Mercury Bichloride	1 grain
Potassium Iodide	2 drachms
Compound Syrup of Sarsaparilla	3 fluidounces

MIXTURE OF METHENAMINE AND AMMONIUM CHLORIDE
I
(Dauer, Med. Form.)

Methenamine	75 Gm.
Ammonium Chloride	125 Gm.
Peppermint Water, a sufficient quantity,	
To make	1000 cc.

Dissolve the methenamine and ammonium chloride in sufficient peppermint water to make 100 cc. and filter if necessary.

AVERAGE DOSE—Metric, 8 cc.—Apothecaries, 2 fluidrachms.

II
(R.B. II)

Methenamine	75 Gm.
Ammonium Chloride	150 Gm.
Fluidextract of Glycyrrhiza	65 cc.
Syrup	200 cc.
Distilled Water, a sufficient quantity,	
To make	1000 cc.

Dissolve the methenamine and ammonium chloride in 500 cc. of the distilled water. Add the syrup and fluidextract of glycyrrhiza, and finally sufficient distilled water to make the product measure 1000 cc.

AVERAGE DOSE—Metric, 4 to 8 cc.—Apothecaries, 1 to 2 fluidrachms.

METHENAMINE AND SODIUM BENZOATE MIXTURE
(N.Y.H.F.)

Methenamine	125 Gm.
Sodium Benzoate	125 Gm.
Distilled Water, a sufficient quantity,	
To make	1000 cc.

Dissolve.

AVERAGE DOSE—Metric, 4 cc.—Apothecaries, 1 fluidrachm.

MIXTURE OF OIL OF TAR
Mistura Olei Picis

Mistura Picis Liquidæ, Tar Mixture
(N.F. IV)

Rectified Oil of Tar	35 cc.
Extract of Glycyrrhiza	65 Gm.
Sucrose	250 Gm.
Chloroform	10 cc.
Oil of Peppermint	3 cc.
Alcohol	160 cc.
Distilled Water, a sufficient quantity,	
To make	1000 cc.

Add the extract of glycyrrhiza and sucrose to 500 cc. of distilled water, contained in a covered vessel, and heat the mixture with constant stirring until the extract and sucrose are dissolved. Cool, and add the rectified oil of tar, chloroform and oil of peppermint, previously dissolved in the alcohol, and lastly sufficient distilled water to make the product measure 1000 cc.

Dispense with a "shake well" label.

AVERAGE DOSE—Metric, 8 cc.—Apothecaries, 2 fluidrachms.

OLEO-BALSAMIC MIXTURE
Mistura Oleo-Balsamica

Hoffmann's Balsam
(N.F. V)

Oil of Lavender	4 cc.
Eugenol	4 cc.
Oil of Cinnamon	4 cc.
Oil of Thyme	4 cc.
Oil of Lemon	4 cc.
Oil of Myristica	4 cc.
Peruvian Balsam	16 cc.
Alcohol, a sufficient quantity,	
To make	1000 cc.

Dissolve the oils, eugenol and peruvian balsam in 900 cc. of alcohol, filter, and add sufficient alcohol through the filter to make the product measure 1000 cc.

MIXTURE OF OLEORESIN OF ASPIDIUM AND TURPENTINE
(B.N.Y.)

Oleoresin of Aspidium . . . . 134 Gm.
Rectified Oil of Turpentine . . . . 40 cc.
Acacia, in powder . . . . 174 Gm.
Chloroform . . . . 32 cc.
Distilled Water, a sufficient quantity,

To make . . . . 1000 cc.

Triturate the acacia with the oleoresin of aspidium and rectified oil of turpentine to a smooth cream. Add all at once 350 cc. of distilled water and mix thoroughly. Add the chloroform, and then sufficient distilled water to make the product measure 1000 cc.

AVERAGE DOSE—Caution! Single dose, once a day: Metric, 15 cc.—Apothecaries, 4 fluidrachms.

COMPOUND MIXTURE OF OPIUM AND CHALK
(E.H.P.)

Tincture of Opium . . . . 15 cc.
Tincture of Krameria . . . . 500 cc.
Chalk Mixture, a sufficient quantity,

To make . . . . 1000 cc.

Mix.

AVERAGE DOSE—Metric, 8 cc.—Apothecaries, 2 fluidrachms.

NOTE—This mixture should be dispensed with a "shake well" label. To be dispensed on prescription only.

MIXTURE OF OPIUM AND SASSAFRAS
Mistura Opii et Sassafras
Mistura Opii Alkalina, Godfrey's Cordial
(N.F. IV)

Tincture of Opium . . . . 35 cc.
Oil of Sassafras . . . . 1 cc.
Alcohol . . . . 50 cc.
Potassium Carbonate . . . . 8 Gm.
Syrup . . . . 325 cc.
Distilled Water, a sufficient quantity,

To make . . . . 1000 cc.

Mix the tincture of opium with the alcohol containing the oil of sassafras. Dissolve the potassium carbonate in 500 cc. of distilled water, mix this with the syrup, then add the mixture first prepared, and lastly sufficient distilled water to make the product measure 1000 cc. Allow the mixture to stand during 24 hours and then filter.

AVERAGE DOSE—Infants: Metric, 0.3 cc.—Apothecaries, 5 minims.

NOTE—To be dispensed on prescription only.

OSCHNER'S MIXTURE NO. 4

Potassium Iodide	10 Gm.
Sodium Iodide	10 Gm.
Tincture of Belladonna	20 cc.
Tincture of Hyoscyamus	20 cc.
Tincture of Lobelia	20 cc.
Fluidextract of Glycyrrhiza	310 cc.
Fluidextract of Grindelia	310 cc.
Syrup of Tolu Balsam, a sufficient quantity,	
To make	1000 cc.

Dissolve the potassium iodide and sodium iodide in the mixture of the syrup of tolu balsam and fluidextracts; gradually add the tinctures, and finally sufficient syrup of tolu balsam to make the product measure 1000 cc.

AVERAGE DOSE—Metric, 2 cc.—Apothecaries, 30 minims.

NOTE—This mixture should be freshly prepared and dispensed with a "shake well" label.

COMPOUND PEPSIN MIXTURE
(G.H.N.Y.)

Pepsin	22 Gm.
Diluted Hydrochloric Acid	70 cc.
Tincture of Nux Vomica	35 cc.
Elixir of Cinchona Alkaloids, a sufficient quantity,	
To make	1000 cc.

Dissolve the pepsin in 600 cc. of the elixir to which the diluted hydrochloric acid has been added in a glass mortar. Add the tincture of nux vomica, and finally sufficient elixir to make the product measure 1000 cc.

AVERAGE DOSE—Metric, 4 cc.—Apothecaries, 1 fluidrachm.

PEPSIN, BISMUTH AND NUX VOMICA MIXTURE
(N.Y.P.G.H.)

Bismuth Subnitrate	75 Gm.
Compound Tincture of Gentian	50 cc.
Tincture of Nux Vomica	75 cc.
Syrup of Ginger	250 cc.
Elixir of Pepsin and Rennin, a sufficient quantity,	
To make	1000 cc.

Triturate the bismuth subnitrate with the syrup of ginger, add the tinctures and sufficient elixir of pepsin and rennin to make the product measure 1000 cc.

Dispense with a "shake well" label.

AVERAGE DOSE—Metric, 4 cc.—Apothecaries, 1 fluidrachm.

PHENOLSULFONATE MIXTURE
Sulfocarbolate Mixture
(v.c.n.y.)

Sodium Phenolsulfonate	162 Gm.
Tincture of Nux Vomica	75 cc.
Tincture of Cubeb	150 cc.
Glycerin	225 cc.
Distilled Water, a sufficient quantity,	
To make	1000 cc.

Dissolve the sodium phenolsulfonate in 500 cc. of distilled water. Add the tinctures and glycerin, and sufficient distilled water to make the product measure 1000 cc.

Dispense with a "shake well" label.

AVERAGE DOSE—Metric, 4 cc.—Apothecaries, 1 fluidrachm.

PHOSPHORIC ACID MIXTURE
Mistura Acidi Phosphorici
(Starr)
(v.c.n.y.)

Diluted Phosphoric Acid	125 cc.
Tincture of Nux Vomica	62 cc.
Syrup of Hypophosphites, a sufficient quantity,	
To make	1000 cc.

Mix the tincture of nux vomica with 500 cc. of the syrup of hypophosphites and add the diluted phosphoric acid. Finally add sufficient syrup of hypophosphites to make the product measure 1000 cc.

AVERAGE DOSE—Metric, 4 cc.—Apothecaries, 1 fluidrachm.

P. I. N. S. MIXTURE
(r.b. i)

Camphorated Tincture of Opium	250 cc.
Syrup of Ipecac	250 cc.
Spirit of Ethyl Nitrite	250 cc.
Syrup of Squill	250 cc.
To make	1000 cc.

Mix.

AVERAGE DOSE—Metric, 2 cc.—Apothecaries, 30 minims.

NOTE—The letters P.I.N.S. are the first letters of the words paregoric, ipecac, nitre and squill in the colloquial formula. To be dispensed on prescription only.

POTASSIUM ACETATE MIXTURE
Mistura Potassii Acetatis
(v.c.n.y.)

Potassium Acetate	325 Gm.
Tincture of Hyoscyamus	225 cc.
Distilled Water, a sufficient quantity,	
To make	1000 cc.

Dissolve the potassium acetate in 500 cc. of distilled water.   Add the tincture of hyoscyamus, and sufficient distilled water to make the product measure 1000 cc.

Average dose—Metric, 4 cc.—Apothecaries, 1 fluidrachm.

COMPOUND MIXTURE OF POTASSIUM ACETATE
(e.h.p.)

Potassium Acetate	81 Gm.
Spirit of Ethyl Nitrite	162 cc.
Solution of Potassium Citrate, a sufficient quantity,	
To make	1000 cc.

Dissolve the potassium acetate in 100 cc. of the solution of potassium citrate, add the spirit of ethyl nitrite and lastly, sufficient solution of potassium citrate to make 1000 cc.

Average dose—Metric, 4 cc.—Apothecaries, 1 fluidrachm.

Note—This mixture must be freshly prepared.

MIXTURE OF POTASSIUM BICARBONATE AND COLCHICUM WITH CASCARA SAGRADA
(n.y.p.g.h.)

Potassium Bicarbonate	75	Gm.
Tincture of Colchicum Seed	22.5	cc.
Fluidextract of Cascara Sagrada	30	cc.
Syrup of Ginger	250	cc.
Distilled Water, a sufficient quantity,		
To make	1000	cc.

Dissolve the potassium bicarbonate in 500 cc. of distilled water, add the tincture, fluidextract and syrup, and finally sufficient distilled water to make the product measure 1000 cc.

Average dose—Metric, 4 cc.—Apothecaries, 1 fluidrachm.

POTASSIUM BROMIDE MIXTURE
(G.H.N.Y.)

Potassium Bromide. . . . .   70 Gm.
Ethereal Tincture of Valerian*. . . . .   85 cc.
Distilled Water, a sufficient quantity,

                  To make . . . .   1000 cc.

Dissolve the potassium bromide in the mixed liquids.

AVERAGE DOSE—Metric, 4 cc.—Apothecaries, 1 fluidrachm.

MIXTURE OF POTASSIUM CITRATE, AMMONIUM ACETATE AND SPIRIT OF ETHYL NITRITE
(L.H.F.)

Potassium Citrate . . . .   40 Gm.
Spirit of Ethyl Nitrite. . . . .   150 cc.
Syrup of Citric Acid . . . .   150 cc.
Solution of Ammonium Acetate . . . .   600 cc.
Distilled Water, a sufficient quantity,

                  To make . . . .   1000 cc.

Dissolve the potassium citrate in the solution of ammonium acetate, add the syrup of citric acid and spirit of ethyl nitrite. Then add sufficient distilled water to make the product measure 1000 cc.

AVERAGE DOSE—Metric, 4 cc.—Apothecaries, 1 fluidrachm.

NOTE—This preparation is intended for administration to children. This mixture should be freshly prepared.

POTASSIUM IODIDE, IPECAC AND OPIUM MIXTURE
(V.C.N.Y.)

Potassium Iodide . . . .   40 Gm.
Tincture of Opium . . . .   38 cc.
Tincture of Ipecac . . . .   115 cc.
Distilled Water, a sufficient quantity,

                  To make . . . .   1000 cc.

Dissolve the potassium iodide in 500 cc. of distilled water. Add the tincture of ipecac, tincture of opium, and sufficient distilled water to make the product measure 1000 cc.

AVERAGE DOSE—Metric, 8 cc.—Apothecaries, 2 fluidrachms.

NOTE—To be dispensed on prescription only.

* Prepared according to the general formula for Ethereal Tinctures (see N.F. VII, page 465).

POTASSIUM IODIDE AND SARSAPARILLA COMPOUND MIXTURE
(B.N.Y.)

Red Mercuric Iodide	0.5 Gm.
Potassium Iodide	125 Gm.
Compound Syrup of Sarsaparilla, a sufficient quantity,	
To make	1000 cc.

Dissolve the red mercuric iodide and the potassium iodide in a small volume of distilled water and then add the syrup.

AVERAGE DOSE—Metric, 4 cc.—Apothecaries, 1 fluidrachm.

QUININE MIXTURE
(B.N.Y.)

Quinine Sulfate	15 Gm.
Aromatic Elixir	500 cc.
Syrup, a sufficient quantity,	
To make	1000 cc.

Dissolve the quinine sulfate in the aromatic elixir and add sufficient syrup to make the product measure 1000 cc.

AVERAGE DOSE—Metric, 4 cc.—Apothecaries, 1 fluidrachm.

COMPOUND MIXTURE OF RHUBARB WITH CASCARA SAGRADA
(N.Y.H.F.)

Aromatic Fluidextract of Cascara Sagrada	250 cc.
Compound Mixture of Rhubarb, a sufficient quantity,	
To make	1000 cc.

Mix.

AVERAGE DOSE—Metric, 4 cc.—Apothecaries, 1 fluidrachm.

COMPOUND RHUBARB AND CASCARA MIXTURE WITH NUX VOMICA, GENTIAN, CAPSICUM AND CHLOROFORM
(R.B. II)

Tincture of Nux Vomica	40 cc.
Compound Tincture of Gentian	40 cc.
Tincture of Capsicum.	20 cc.
Spirit of Chloroform	30 cc.
Fluidextract of Cascara Sagrada	150 cc.
Compound Mixture of Rhubarb, a sufficient quantity,	
To make	1000 cc.

Mix the fluidextract of cascara sagrada with 500 cc. of the compound mixture of rhubarb. When effervescence has ceased, add the tinctures and spirit of chloroform, and finally sufficient compound mixture of rhubarb to make the product measure 1000 cc.

AVERAGE DOSE—Metric, 8 cc.—Apothecaries, 2 fluidrachms.

RHUBARB AND SODIUM SALICYLATE MIXTURE
(N.Y.H.F.)

Sodium Salicylate . . . . 160 Gm.
Compound Mixture of Rhubarb, a sufficient quantity,

To make . . . . 1000 cc.

Dissolve.

AVERAGE DOSE—Metric, 4 cc.—Apothecaries, 1 fluidrachm.

NOTE—This mixture should be freshly prepared.

COMPOUND RHUBARB AND SODIUM SALICYLATE MIXTURE WITH NUX VOMICA, CASCARA AND CAPSICUM
(B.N.Y.)

Fluidextract of Cascara Sagrada . . . . 120 cc.
Sodium Salicylate . . . . 62.5 Gm.
Tincture of Nux Vomica . . . . 15 cc.
Tincture of Capsicum. . . . . 15 cc.
Compound Mixture of Rhubarb, a sufficient quantity,

To make . . . . 1000 cc.

Dissolve the sodium salicylate in 500 cc. of the compound mixture of rhubarb. Add the other ingredients and sufficient compound mixture of rhubarb to make the product measure 1000 cc.

AVERAGE DOSE—Metric, 4 cc.—Apothecaries, 1 fluidrachm.

SEDATIVE MIXTURE
(N.Y.P.G.H.)

Sodium Bromide. . . . . 175 Gm.
Tincture of Valerian . . . . 175 cc.
Distilled Water, a sufficient quantity,

To make . . . . 1000 cc.

Dissolve the sodium bromide in 500 cc. of distilled water, add the tincture of valerian, and sufficient distilled water to make the product measure 1000 cc.

AVERAGE DOSE—Metric, 4 cc.—Apothecaries, 1 fluidrachm.

SEDATIVE MIXTURE, BROWN-SEQUARD
(V.C.N.Y.)

Potassium Iodide . . . . 40.5 Gm.
Potassium Bromide . . . . 81 Gm.
Ammonium Bromide . . . . 81 Gm.
Sodium Bicarbonate . . . . 32.5 Gm.
Tincture of Nux Vomica . . . . 46 cc.
Compound Tincture of Gentian . . . . 62 cc.
Distilled Water, a sufficient quantity,

To make . . . . 1000 cc.

Dissolve the salts in 500 cc. of distilled water, add the tinctures and sufficient distilled water to make the product measure 1000 cc.

AVERAGE DOSE—Metric, 8 cc.—Apothecaries, 2 fluidrachms.

AMMONIATED MIXTURE OF SENEGA, IPECAC AND PAREGORIC
(L.H.F.)

Aromatic Spirit of Ammonia.	25 cc.
Syrup of Senega	60 cc.
Syrup of Ipecac	60 cc.
Syrup of Tolu Balsam	60 cc.
Camphorated Tincture of Opium.	15 cc.
Compound Tincture of Cardamom	350 cc.
Anise Water, a sufficient quantity,	
To make	1000 cc.

Mix.

AVERAGE DOSE—Metric, 4 cc.—Apothecaries, 1 fluidrachm.

NOTE—This preparation is intended for administration to children.

SODA, NUX VOMICA AND CAPSICUM MIXTURE
(R.B. I)

Sodium Bicarbonate	95 Gm.
Tincture of Nux Vomica	25 cc.
Spirit of Chloroform	50 cc.
Tincture of Capsicum.	25 cc.
Compound Tincture of Gentian, a sufficient quantity,	
To make	1000 cc.

Add the finely powdered sodium bicarbonate to the mixed liquids and allow the effervescence to cease before placing in a stoppered container.

Dispense with a "shake well" label.

AVERAGE DOSE—Metric, 4 cc.—Apothecaries, 1 fluidrachm.

SODIUM BENZOATE AND BELLADONNA MIXTURE
(N.Y.H.F.)

Sodium Benzoate	250 Gm.
Tincture of Belladonna	130 cc.
Peppermint Water, a sufficient quantity,	
To make	1000 cc.

Dissolve the sodium benzoate in 600 cc. of peppermint water, add the tincture of belladonna and sufficient peppermint water to make the product measure 1000 cc.

AVERAGE DOSE—Metric, 4 cc.—Apothecaries, 1 fluidrachm.

AROMATIC SODIUM BENZOATE MIXTURE

White Cough Mixture

(R.B. I)

Sodium Benzoate . . . .   125 Gm.
Aromatic Elixir . . . .   250 cc.
Distilled Water, a sufficient quantity,

To make . . . .   1000 cc.

Dissolve the sodium benzoate in 600 cc. of distilled water, add the aromatic elixir and sufficient distilled water to make the product measure 1000 cc.

AVERAGE DOSE—Metric, 4 cc.—Apothecaries, 1 fluidrachm.

SODIUM BENZOATE, SALICYLATE AND BELLADONNA MIXTURE

(P.H.N.Y.)

Sodium Benzoate   15   Gm.
Sodium Salicylate   15   Gm.
Tincture of Belladonna . . . .   7.5 cc.
Distilled Water, a sufficient quantity,

To make   1000   cc.

Dissolve the sodium benzoate and sodium salicylate in 500 cc. of distilled water, add the tincture of belladonna and sufficient distilled water to make the product measure 1000 cc.

AVERAGE DOSE—Metric, 4 cc.—Apothecaries, 1 fluidrachm.

MIXTURE OF SODIUM BICARBONATE AND PEPPERMINT

(B.N.Y.)

Sodium Bicarbonate . . . .   40 Gm.
Spirit of Peppermint . . . .   20 cc.
Tincture of Caramel, a sufficient quantity,
Distilled Water, a sufficient quantity,

To make . . . .   1000 cc.

Dissolve the sodium bicarbonate in 500 cc. of distilled water, add the spirit of peppermint and the tincture of caramel, and sufficient water to make 1000 cc.

AVERAGE DOSE—Metric, 15 cc.—Apothecaries, ½ fluidounce.

SODIUM BROMIDE AND CHLORAL MIXTURE

(B.N.Y.)

Chloral Hydrate   30   Gm.
Sodium Bromide . . . .   100 Gm.
Spirit of Anise . . . .   1.5 cc.
Chloroform Water, a sufficient quantity,

To make   1000   cc.

Dissolve the sodium bromide and chloral hydrate in 500 cc. of chloroform water and add the spirit of anise.   Finally add sufficient chloroform water to make the product measure 1000 cc.

Average dose—Metric, 4 cc.—Apothecaries, 1 fluidrachm.

SODIUM BROMIDE, IRON AND QUININE MIXTURE
(b.n.y.)

Sodium Bromide	50 Gm.
Iron and Quinine Citrate	50 Gm.
Syrup of Senega	225 cc.
Syrup of Wild Cherry	325 cc.
Syrup of Acacia	125 cc.
Distilled Water, a sufficient quantity,	
To make	1000 cc.

Dissolve the iron and quinine citrate and sodium bromide in 200 cc. of distilled water.   Add the syrups and sufficient distilled water to make the product measure 1000 cc.

Average dose—Metric, 4 cc.—Apothecaries, 1 fluidrachm.

Note—This mixture must be freshly prepared.

SODIUM SALICYLATE MIXTURE
I
(n.y.p.g.h.)

Salicylic Acid	37.5	Gm.
Sodium Bicarbonate	75	Gm.
Glycerin	250	cc.
Distilled Water, a sufficient quantity,		
To make	1000	cc.

Mix the salicylic acid and sodium bicarbonate in a capacious mortar, add gradually 500 cc. of distilled water, triturating until the reaction is complete.   Add the glycerin and sufficient distilled water to make the product measure 1000 cc.

Average dose—Metric, 4 cc.—Apothecaries, 1 fluidrachm.

II
(n.y.h.f.)

Sodium Salicylate	150 Gm.
Sodium Bicarbonate	150 Gm.
Red Aromatic Elixir, a sufficient quantity,	
To make	1000 cc.

Dissolve the salts in the red aromatic elixir.

Average dose—Metric, 4 cc.—Apothecaries, 1 fluidrachm.

SODIUM SALICYLATE AND GLYCYRRHIZA MIXTURE
(v.c.n.y).

Sodium Salicylate	162 Gm.
Extract of Glycyrrhiza	25 Gm.
Distilled Water, a sufficient quantity,	
To make	1000 cc.

Dissolve the extract of glycyrrhiza in 500 cc. of warm distilled water, add the sodium salicylate dissolved in 200 cc. of distilled water, and then sufficient distilled water to make the product measure 1000 cc.

AVERAGE DOSE—Metric, 8 cc.—Apothecaries, 2 fluidrachms.

STOMACHIC MIXTURE
(v.c.n.y.)

Tincture of Nux Vomica	75 cc.
Compound Tincture of Gentian	250 cc.
Chloroform Water, a sufficient quantity,	
To make	1000 cc.

Mix the tinctures and add sufficient chloroform water to make the product measure 1000 cc.

AVERAGE DOSE—Metric, 8 cc.—Apothecaries, 2 fluidrachms.

COMPOUND THYME MIXTURE
(g.h.n.y.)

Fluidextract of Thyme	120 cc.
Fluidextract of Grindelia	120 cc.
Fluidextract of Castanea	240 cc.
Fluidextract of Senega	20 cc.
Honey, a sufficient quantity,	
To make	1000 cc.

Mix.

AVERAGE DOSE—Metric, 4 cc.—Apothecaries, 1 fluidrachm.

TRITICUM MIXTURE
Mistura Tritici
(Taylor)
(v.c.n.y.)

Fluidextract of Triticum	300	cc.
Fluidextract of Uva Ursi	300	cc.
Potassium Hydroxide	0.4	Gm
Distilled Water, a sufficient quantity,		
To make	1000	cc.

Dissolve the potassium hydroxide in 300 cc. of distilled water, add the fluidextracts and sufficient distilled water to make the product measure 1000 cc.

AVERAGE DOSE—Metric, 4 cc.—Apothecaries, 1 fluidrachm.

MUCILAGES

MUCILAGE OF ALTHEA
Mucilago Althææ
(R.B. I)

Althea, in small pieces	50 Gm.
Benzoic Acid	2 Gm.
Distilled Water	1000 cc.

Wash the althea with a small quantity of cold water and drain. Then add 1000 cc. of distilled water containing the benzoic acid and macerate for 3 hours. Strain without pressure.

AVERAGE DOSE—Metric, 8 cc.—Apothecaries, 2 fluidrachms.

NOTE—This mucilage should be freshly prepared.

MUCILAGE OF QUINCE SEED
Mucilago Cydonii
Mucilage of Cydonium
(U.S.P. VI)

Quince Seed	20 Gm.
Methyl Parahydroxybenzoic Acid	1 Gm.
Distilled Water	1000 cc.

Macerate the quince seed for half an hour, in a covered vessel containing the methyl parahydroxybenzoic acid and the distilled water, agitating frequently. Then strain the liquid through muslin, without pressure.

NOTE—This mucilage should be freshly prepared.

MUCILAGE OF SALEP
Mucilago Salep
(D.A.B. VI)

Salep, in moderately fine powder	10 Gm.
Methyl Parahydroxybenzoic Acid	1 Gm.
Alcohol	10 cc.
Distilled Water, boiling, a sufficient quantity,	
To make	1000 cc.

Place the salep and the methyl parahydroxybenzoic acid in a dry flask, add the alcohol and shake. Add 100 cc. of boiling distilled water, shake well, add the remainder of the boiling distilled water and shake occasionally until cold.

AVERAGE DOSE—Metric, 15 cc.—Apothecaries, 4 fluidrachms.

NOTE—This mucilage should be freshly prepared.

MUCILAGE OF STARCH
Mucilago Amyli
(B.P.C.)

Starch	25 Gm.
Distilled Water, a sufficient quantity,	
To make	1000 cc.

Rub the starch to a smooth paste with the distilled water and heat the mixture to boiling.

NOTE—This mucilage should be freshly prepared.

MEDICATED OILS

BAUNSCHEIDT OIL
(R.B. I)

Euphorbia Pilulifera, in coarse powder	50 Gm.
Cantharides, in coarse powder	30 Gm.
Olive Oil or Peanut Oil, a sufficient quantity,	
To make	1000 cc.

Digest the powders with the oil on a water bath for 4 hours and filter.

This oil is used as a counterirritant after the skin has been punctured by a special instrument.

BRITISH OIL
Oil of Petre, Oil of Stone
(P.F.)

Crude Petroleum	35 cc.
Coal Tar	105 cc.
Crude Oil of Amber	140 cc.
Oil of Juniper	140 cc.
Linseed Oil	280 cc.
Oil of Turpentine, a sufficient quantity,	
To make	1000 cc.

Mix.

CALOT'S CREOSOTED OIL

Calot's Solution
(Ext. Ph.)

Guaiacol . . . .   1 cc.
Creosote . . . .   5 cc.
Ethyl Oxide . . . .   30 cc.
Iodoform . . . .   10 Gm.
Olive Oil or Peanut Oil, a sufficient quantity,
                        To make . . . .   100 cc.

Add the ingredients to the olive oil in the following order: the creosote, guaiacol, iodoform and ethyl oxide.

CHLOROFORM OIL

Oleum Chloroformi
(D.A.B. V)

Chloroform . . . .   500 cc.
Peanut Oil, a sufficient quantity,
                        To make . . . .   1000 cc.

Mix.

AROMATIC COD LIVER OIL

Saccharin . . . .   0.5 Gm.
Compound Spirit of Orange   20   cc.
Cod Liver Oil, a sufficient quantity,
                        To make   1000   cc.

Dissolve the saccharin in the compound spirit of orange and mix with sufficient cod liver oil to make the product measure 1000 cc. Chill in an ice-box and filter through paper, returning the first portions of the filtrate until it filters clear.

Keep in completely filled, well-stoppered bottles in a cool place.

AVERAGE DOSE—Metric, 10 cc.—Apothecaries, 2½ fluidrachms.

DUTCH DROPS

Oleum Empyreumaticum

Haarlem Drops, Haarlem Oil, Tilly Drops

I
(P.F.)

Linseed Oil . . . .   200 Gm.
Sulfur . . . .   50 Gm.
Oil of Turpentine, a sufficient quantity,
                        To make . . . .   1000 Gm.

Mix the linseed oil and sulfur in an iron vessel large enough to allow some frothing. Heat to a temperature of 165° C., stirring well all the time, until the mixture drops from the stirrer with a glassy appearance.   Remove from the fire, and add the oil of turpentine and agitate until solution is effected or nearly so.   Filter.   The liquid should be limpid and of a brownish red color.

II

Linseed Oil . . . .   300 cc.
Oil of Turpentine, a sufficient quantity,
            To make . . . .   1000 cc.
Mix.

GRAY OIL
Oleum Hydrargyri Cinereum
Oleum Cinereum
(R.B. I)

Mercury . . . .   390 Gm.
Strong Mercurial Ointment . . . .   20 Gm.
White Petrolatum, sterile . . . .   190 Gm.
Heavy Liquid Petrolatum, heavy, sterile . . . .   400 Gm.
            To make . . . .   1000 Gm.

Triturate the mercury, strong mercurial ointment and 2.5 Gm. of white petrolatum in a sterile mortar under aseptic conditions until the mercury is extinguished, then incorporate the remainder of the white petrolatum and the liquid petrolatum.

INFANT ANOINTING OIL
Compound Liquid Petrolatum
(N.Y.H.F.)

Sesame Oil . . . .   100 cc.
Olive Oil . . . .   100 cc.
Heavy Liquid Petrolatum, a sufficient quantity,
            To make . . . .   1000 cc.
Mix.

INFUSED OILS
Olea Infusa
(N.F. V)

The Air Dried Drug, in moderately coarse powder . . . .   100 Gm.
Alcohol . . . .   100 cc.
Diluted Solution of Ammonia . . . .   2 cc.
Sesame Oil . . . .   1000 cc.
          To make about . . . .   1000 cc.

Moisten the drug with the alcohol and diluted solution of ammonia, previously mixed; macerate for 6 hours in a covered vessel and add the sesame oil. Warm this mixture on a water bath in an open vessel at a temperature between 60° and 70° C., stirring frequently, until the alcohol and diluted solution of ammonia are dissipated. Then transfer the mixture to a strainer, express the residue and filter the strained oil.

Keep in small, amber-colored bottles in a cool place.

NOTE—Other bland oils may be used.

ZINC OXIDE IN OIL
(E.B. IV)

Zinc Oxide . . . .   850 Gm.
Olive Oil or Peanut Oil, a sufficient quantity,
            To make . . . .   1000 cc.

Sift the zinc oxide through bolting cloth and incorporate sufficient olive oil, by thorough trituration in a mortar, to make the product measure 1000 cc.

OINTMENTS

ALOE VERA OINTMENT

Aloe Vera Pulp . . . .   500 Gm.
Soluble Ointment Base, R.B. . . . .   500 Gm.
Methyl Parahydroxybenzoate . . . .   1 Gm.

Strain the aloe pulp through gauze, thoroughly mix the strained material with the soluble ointment base, and incorporate the methyl parahydroxybenzoate.

ANALGESIC OINTMENT
(P.H.N.Y.)

Menthol . . . .   0.75 Gm.
Chloral Hydrate   100   Gm.
Camphor   100   Gm.
Wool Fat   800   Gm.
          To make about   1000   Gm.

Triturate together the menthol, chloral hydrate and camphor until liquefied, then incorporate with the wool fat.

ASTRINGENT OINTMENT
Unguentum Adstringens
(G.H.N.Y.)

Zinc Oxide . . . .   20 Gm.
Bismuth Subnitrate . . . .   20 Gm.
Peruvian Balsam. . . . .   190 Gm.
Petrolatum . . . .   770 Gm.
          To make . . . .   1000 Gm.

Incorporate the powders in the peruvian balsam and petrolatum, previously mixed.

PERUVIAN BALSAM OINTMENT
(B.N.Y.)

Peruvian Balsam	100 Gm.
Solid Petroxolin	900 Gm.
To make	1000 Gm.

Incorporate the peruvian balsam in divided portions with the solid petroxolin.

COMPOUND OINTMENT OF PERUVIAN BALSAM
(P.H.C.)

Peruvian Balsam	100 Gm.
Zinc Oxide	400 Gm.
Castor Oil	500 Gm.
To make	1000 Gm.

Mix the peruvian balsam intimately with the castor oil and gradually incorporate the zinc oxide.

BETANAPHTHOL OINTMENT
I
(G.H.N.Y.)

Betanaphthol	85 Gm.
Precipitated Calcium Carbonate	75 Gm.
Medicinal Soft Soap	300 Gm.
Petrolatum	540 Gm.
To make	1000 Gm.

Incorporate the betanaphthol and precipitated calcium carbonate with the soft soap and petrolatum, previously mixed.

II
(B.N.Y.)

Betanaphthol	100 Gm.
Petrolatum	900 Gm.
To make	1000 Gm.

Melt the petrolatum with the aid of gentle heat, add the betanaphthol and stir until the mixture congeals.

COMPOUND BETANAPHTHOL OINTMENT
(N.Y.P.G.H.)

Betanaphthol . . . . 62.5 Gm.
Precipitated Sulfur. . . . . 187.5 Gm.
Hydrous Wool Fat 375   Gm.
Petrolatum 375   Gm.

To make 1000   Gm.

Melt the petrolatum and add the betanaphthol, stir until the mixture congeals, and then incorporate the precipitated sulfur, triturating until smooth. Finally add the hydrous wool fat and mix thoroughly.

BISMUTH OLEATE OINTMENT
Anderson's Ointment
(Ext. Ph.)

Bismuth Oxide . . . . 48 Gm.
Oleic Acid . . . . 430 cc. 9
White Wax . . . . 144 Gm.
White Petrolatum, a sufficient quantity,

To make . . . . 1000 Gm.

Warm the bismuth oxide and oleic acid on a water bath for 1 hour before adding the other ingredients. Triturate thoroughly until cold.

BISMUTH SUBCARBONATE OINTMENT
Unguentum Bismuthi
Bismuth Ointment
(B.P.C. 1934)

Bismuth Subcarbonate . . . . 125 Gm.
White Petrolatum . . . . 875 Gm.

To make . . . . 1000 Gm.

Incorporate the bismuth subcarbonate with the petrolatum in divided portions, triturating after each addition until a smooth ointment is obtained.

BISMUTH SUBNITRATE OINTMENT
(B.N.Y.)

Bismuth Subnitrate . . . . 100 Gm.
White Petrolatum . . . . 900 Gm.

To make . . . . 1000 Gm.

Incorporate the bismuth subnitrate with the petrolatum in divided portions, triturating after each addition until a smooth ointment is obtained.

COMPOUND BISMUTH OINTMENT
(N.Y.P.G.H.)

Salicylic Acid, in very fine powder	25 Gm.
Bismuth Subnitrate	100 Gm.
Zinc Oxide	100 Gm.
Hydrous Wool Fat	100 Gm.
Petrolatum	675 Gm.
To make	1000 Gm.

Incorporate the salicylic acid with 200 Gm. of petrolatum, and rub the zinc oxide and bismuth subnitrate with the remainder of the petrolatum until smooth. Then mix the two ointments and incorporate with the hydrous wool fat.

NOTE—This ointment must not be allowed to come in contact with iron utensils.

BISMUTH, RESORCINOL, ZINC OXIDE AND CAMPHOR OINTMENT
(R.B. II)

Bismuth Subnitrate	65 Gm.
Resorcinol	25 Gm.
Starch	65 Gm.
Zinc Oxide	65 Gm.
Camphor, in fine powder	65 Gm.
Rose Water Ointment	715 Gm.
To make	1000 Gm.

Mix the dry ingredients and incorporate them with the rose water ointment.

BISMUTH TRIBROMOPHENATE OINTMENT
Xeroform Ointment
(U.C.H.)

Bismuth Tribromophenate	30 Gm.
Paraffin	10 Gm.
Yellow Wax	10 Gm.
Petrolatum	950 Gm.
To make	1000 Gm.

Melt together the paraffin, yellow wax and 750 Gm. of the petrolatum. Mix the bismuth tribromophenate to a smooth ointment with the remainder of the petrolatum, add it to the melted mixture, and stir until cold.

BISMUTH AND ZINC OINTMENT
(P.H.N.Y.)

Zinc Oxide	56 Gm.
Bismuth Subcarbonate	28 Gm.
Starch	106 Gm.
Rose Water Ointment	810 Gm.
To make	1000 Gm.

Mix the dry ingredients by trituration and pass through a No. 60 sieve, then incorporate the mixed powders with the ointment.

OINTMENT FOR BURNS
Burn Ointment

Chlorobutanol	20 Gm.
Oil of Eucalyptus	14 cc.
Zinc Oxide	73 Gm.
Bismuth Subnitrate	37 Gm.
White Petrolatum	290 Gm.
Wool Fat	293 Gm.
Distilled Water	273 cc.
To make about	1000 Gm.

Melt the wool fat and white petrolatum and stir until well blended, then add the distilled water, previously warmed, and pass the mixture through a homogenizer or mix in an electric mixer. Incorporate the zinc oxide and bismuth subnitrate into the warm creamy mixture and again homogenize.

NOTE—Useful in first degree burns or when skin is reddened but not blistered.

CALENDULA OINTMENT
Unguentum Calendulæ
(R.B. II)

Fluidextract of Calendula	100 cc.
White Ointment, a sufficient quantity,	
To make	1000 Gm.

Evaporate the fluidextract on a water bath to form a semi-fluid extract and incorporate it with the ointment.

COMPOUND OINTMENT OF CALOMEL AND PHENOL
(B.N.Y.)

Phenol	25 Gm.
Mild Mercurous Chloride	35 Gm.
Zinc Oxide Ointment	470 Gm.
Petrolatum	470 Gm.
To make	1000 Gm.

Melt 200 Gm. of petrolatum, add the phenol and when dissolved mix with the remainder of the petrolatum. Add the mild mercurous chloride, rubbing until a smooth ointment is obtained, and incorporate with the zinc oxide ointment.

CAMPHOR OINTMENT
Unguentum Camphoræ
(B.P.C. 1934)

Camphor, in fine powder	100 Gm.
White Petrolatum	900 Gm.
To make	1000 Gm.

Dissolve the camphor in the white petrolatum, previously melted at as low a temperature as possible, and stir until cold.

COMPOUND OINTMENT OF CAMPHOR, PHENOL AND ZINC OXIDE
(R.B. I)

Camphor	30 Gm.
Phenol	30 Gm.
Zinc Oxide	470 Gm.
Petrolatum	470 Gm.
To make	1000 Gm.

Triturate the camphor and phenol until liquefied and add gradually the previously mixed petrolatum and zinc oxide.

CEVADILLA OINTMENT
Unguentum Sabadillæ
(Ph. Aust.)

Cevadilla Seed, in fine powder	200 Gm.
Oil of Lemon	12 cc.
Petrolatum	790 Gm.
To make about	1000 Gm.

Incorporate the cevadilla seed and oil of lemon in the petrolatum.

COMPOUND CHRYSAROBIN OINTMENT
(G.H.N.Y., with Chloroform)

Chrysarobin	50 Gm.
Salicylic Acid, in fine powder	20 Gm.
Chloroform	22 cc.
Ichthammol	50 Gm.
Petrolatum, a sufficient quantity,	
To make	1000 Gm.

Triturate the powders with the chloroform and ichthammol, and add gradually the petrolatum until thoroughly mixed.

GUY'S COAL TAR OINTMENT

Solution of Aluminum Acetate . . . .   100 cc.
Coal Tar . . . .   40 Gm.
Wool Fat . . . .   200 Gm.
Ointment of Zinc Oxide, a sufficient quantity,
                              To make . . . .   1000 Gm.

Triturate the crude coal tar with the wool fat and incorporate the solution of aluminum acetate; add the ointment of zinc oxide and triturate until the ointment is uniformly mixed.

COMPOUND OINTMENT OF COAL TAR

White's Ointment
(N.Y.H.F.)

Coal Tar . . . .   50 Gm.
Zinc Oxide . . . .   50 Gm.
Starch . . . .   450 Gm.
Petrolatum, a sufficient quantity,
                              To make . . . .   1000 Gm.

Triturate the zinc oxide and starch together until a uniform powder results and incorporate it in a portion of the petrolatum.   Mix the coal tar with the remainder of the petrolatum and triturate the powder mixture with the coal tar mixture.

NOTE—This ointment is not to be confused with White Ointment of the U.S.P. XII, page 533, which is Unguentum Album.

OINTMENT OF COD LIVER OIL (Anhydrous)
I

Sodium Lauryl Sulfate* . . . .   28 Gm.
Cetyl Alcohol . . . .   172 Gm.
Stearyl Alcohol† . . . .   86 Gm.
White Ceresin . . . .   74 Gm.
Cod Liver Oil . . . .   640 cc.
Chlorobutanol . . . .   5 Gm.
                              To make about . . . .   1000 Gm.

Heat the ceresin, cetyl alcohol, stearyl alcohol and sodium lauryl sulfate on a water bath and stir until dissolved.   Dissolve the chlorobutanol in the cod liver oil and add to the warm liquid.   Stir until a uniform mixture results.

NOTE—This preparation is readily removed with water.

* DUPANOL—du Pont.
† STENOL—du Pont.

II

Cod Liver Oil	500 cc.
Petrolatum, a sufficient quantity,	
To make	1000 Gm.

Incorporate the oil in the petrolatum and mix until a uniform ointment results.

COMPOUND OINTMENT OF COD LIVER OIL
(U.C.H.)

Allantoin, in fine powder	10 Gm.
Cod Liver Oil	500 cc.
White Wax	50 Gm.
Hydrous Wool Fat	250 Gm.
Essential Oil, a sufficient quantity,	
Petrolatum, a sufficient quantity,	
To make	1000 Gm.

Melt the white wax, hydrous wool fat and petrolatum on a water bath, allow to cool, and incorporate the cod liver oil and then the allantoin. When the ointment is cold add the essential oil for improving the odor and triturate until a uniform ointment results.

COPPER OLEATE OINTMENT WITH PROCAINE
(S.H.F.)

Copper Oleate.	133 Gm.
Procaine Hydrochloride.	13 Gm.
Distilled Water	10 cc.
Lard	422 Gm.
Petrolatum	422 Gm.
To make	1000 Gm.

Fuse the copper oleate and 300 Gm. of lard with the aid of gentle heat. Powder the procaine hydrochloride, dissolve it in the distilled water and incorporate with the remainder of the lard. Mix thoroughly with the oleate and lard mixture and incorporate the petrolatum.

DEEK'S OINTMENT
(S.H.F.)

Salicylic Acid, in fine powder	40 Gm.
Bismuth Subnitrate.	100 Gm.
Mercuric Salicylate.	40 Gm.
Oil of Eucalyptus.	35 Gm.
Petrolatum	400 Gm.
Wool Fat	385 Gm.
To make	1000 Gm.

Incorporate the finely triturated powders with the petrolatum, mixing in the oil of eucalyptus and wool fat.

In a variation of this formula, the mercuric salicylate may be replaced by an equal weight of ammoniated mercury.

HEBRA'S DIACHYLON OINTMENT
(P.H.C.)

Olive Oil	450 Gm.
Lead Monoxide, in fine powder	114 Gm.
Distilled Water	436 cc.
To make	1000 Gm.

Mix the olive oil with the distilled water and heat on a steam bath until the water is boiling. Sift in the lead oxide and stir continually. Boil until all particles have disappeared, adding boiling distilled water to replace that lost by evaporation, and stir until cool.

NOTE—This ointment should be freshly prepared.

DIACHYLON AND TAR OINTMENT
(G.H.N.Y.)

Ointment of Lead Oleate,
Pine Tar Ointment, of each, an equal weight.

Mix intimately.

ERGOT OINTMENT
Unguentum Ergotae Compositum
(Levin)

Phenol	10 Gm.
Fluidextract of Ergot	90 cc.
Starch	90 Gm.
Zinc Oxide	90 Gm.
Rose Water Ointment	180 Gm.
Hydrous Wool Fat	540 Gm.
To make about	1000 Gm.

Incorporate the fluidextract of ergot with the hydrous wool fat. Add the starch and zinc oxide, followed by the rose water ointment. Finally add the phenol and mix thoroughly by trituration.

OINTMENT OF ETHYL AMINOBENZOATE (20 per cent)
(U.C.H.)

Ethyl Aminobenzoate	200 Gm.
White Petrolatum, a sufficient quantity,	
To make	1000 Gm.

Triturate the ethyl aminobenzoate with the petrolatum until a uniform ointment results.

COMPOUND OINTMENT OF ETHYL AMINOBENZOATE
(U.C.H.)

Ethyl Aminobenzoate . . . . 10 Gm.
Phenol . . . . 1 Gm.
Benzyl Alcohol . . . . 50 cc.
Zinc Oxide . . . . 50 Gm.
Methyl Salicylate . . . . 10 cc.
Paraffin . . . . 20 Gm.
Petrolatum, a sufficient quantity,

To make . . . . 1000 Gm.

Melt the paraffin on a water bath and add the petrolatum. Dissolve the ethyl aminobenzoate, phenol and methyl salicylate in the benzyl alcohol and incorporate this solution in the mixture of zinc oxide, paraffin and petrolatum. Triturate until a uniform ointment results. The amount of paraffin may be increased or decreased to produce an ointment of any desired consistency.

FUCHSIN OINTMENT
Unguentum Rosanilini
(S. and C.H.N.Y.)

Basic Fuchsin, in fine powder . . . . 20 Gm.
Phenol . . . . 20 Gm.
Petrolatum . . . . 960 Gm.

To make . . . . 1000 Gm.

Incorporate the basic fuchsin with the melted phenol and mix with the petrolatum.

OINTMENT OF GALL AND OPIUM
Unguentum Gallæ et Opii
(B.P.C. 1934)

Opium, in fine powder . . . . 75 Gm.
Nutgall Ointment . . . . 925 Gm.

To make . . . . 1000 Gm.

Triturate the opium with a portion of the nutgall ointment until smooth, then gradually add the remainder, mixing thoroughly by trituration.

NOTE—To be dispensed on prescription only.

CAUTION—*Do not permit to come in contact with iron utensils.*

COMPOUND OINTMENT OF GALL AND OPIUM
(R.B. I)

Acetanilid . . . . 50 Gm.
Ointment of Gall and Opium, R.B. . . . . 950 Gm.

To make . . . . 1000 Gm.

Mix intimately.

NOTE—To be dispensed on prescription only.

CAUTION—*Do not permit to come in contact with iron utensils.*

OINTMENT OF GALLIC ACID
Unguentum Acidi Gallici
(U.S.P. VI)

Gallic Acid	100 Gm.
Benzoinated Lard	900 Gm.
To make	1000 Gm.

Rub the gallic acid with the benzoinated lard, added gradually, until they are thoroughly mixed, avoiding the use of an iron spatula.

HOLOCAINE OINTMENT
(R.B. II)

Holocaine Hydrochloride	10 Gm.
Distilled Water	50 cc.
Solution of Epinephrine Hydrochloride	40 cc.
Wool Fat	100 Gm.
White Petrolatum	800 Gm.
To make about	1000 Gm.

Dissolve the holocaine hydrochloride in warm distilled water and add the solution of epinephrine hydrochloride. Incorporate the liquid with the wool fat, add the white petrolatum and mix.

HUFELAND'S OINTMENT
(Ph. Dan.)

Camphor, in fine powder	15 Gm.
Ammonium Carbonate, in fine powder	15 Gm.
Extract of Ox Bile, in fine powder	180 Gm.
Petrolatum	90 Gm.
Lard	700 Gm.
To make	1000 Gm.

Mix the powdered drugs and incorporate the mixture with the petrolatum and lard.

STRONGER ICHTHAMMOL OINTMENT
(R.B. II)

Ichthammol	200 Gm.
Hydrous Wool Fat	800 Gm.
To make	1000 Gm.

Mix intimately.

UNNA'S ICHTHAMMOL OINTMENT
(R.B. II)

Ichthammol	40 Gm.
Hydrous Wool Fat	250 Gm.
Petrolatum	710 Gm.
To make	1000 Gm.

Mix the ichthammol with the hydrous wool fat and incorporate the petrolatum.

ICHTHAMMOL AND EUCALYPTOL OINTMENT
Nasal Ointment
(N.Y.P.G.H.)

Ichthammol	85 Gm.
Eucalyptol	15 cc.
Hydrous Wool Fat	450 Gm.
Petrolatum	450 Gm.
To make about	1000 Gm.

Mix the ichthammol with the hydrous wool fat and then incorporate the petrolatum with which the eucalyptol has been previously mixed.

ICHTHAMMOL AND METHYL SALICYLATE OINTMENT
(R.B. II)

Methyl Salicylate	200 Gm.
Ointment of Ichthammol	800 Gm.
To make	1000 Gm.

Incorporate the methyl salicylate with the ointment of ichthammol.

ICHTHAMMOL AND SALICYLIC ACID OINTMENT WITH PHENOL
(N.Y.P.G.H.)

Phenol	40 Gm.
Ichthammol	75 Gm.
Salicylic Acid, in fine powder	75 Gm.
Hydrous Wool Fat	410 Gm.
Petrolatum	400 Gm.
To make	1000 Gm.

Dissolve the phenol in the melted petrolatum, add the salicylic acid and cool. Add the hydrous wool fat with which the ichthammol has been mixed.

JUNIPER TAR OINTMENT
(B.N.Y.)

Juniper Tar	100 Gm.
Ointment of Zinc Oxide	900 Gm.
To make	1000 Gm.

Incorporate the juniper tar in the zinc oxide ointment.

COMPOUND OINTMENT OF JUNIPER TAR
(P.H.C.)

Salicylic Acid, in fine powder	6 Gm.
Menthol, in fine powder	6 Gm.
Precipitated Sulfur.	67 Gm.
Zinc Oxide	133 Gm.
Juniper Tar	119 Gm.
Starch	233 Gm.
Petrolatum	436 Gm.
To make	1000 Gm.

Triturate the powders together and add the petrolatum, triturating until a smooth uniform product is obtained. Lastly, add the juniper tar and continue the trituration until uniform.

JUNIPER TAR AND TANNIC ACID OINTMENT
(G.H.N.Y.)

	5 per cent	10 per cent
Juniper Tar	50 Gm.	100 Gm.
Tannic Acid	50 Gm.	50 Gm.
Zinc Oxide, free from gritty particles	180 Gm.	170 Gm.
Benzoinated Lard	720 Gm.	680 Gm.
To make	1000 Gm.	1000 Gm.

Melt the benzoinated lard and triturate about 180 Gm. of it in a warmed mortar with the zinc oxide. Add the remainder of the benzoinated lard, incorporate the tannic acid and juniper tar and stir until the ointment congeals.

LEAD IODIDE OINTMENT
(B.N.Y.)

Lead Iodide, in fine powder	100 Gm.
Petrolatum	100 Gm.
Hydrous Wool Fat	800 Gm.
To make	1000 Gm.

Rub the lead iodide with the petrolatum until a smooth ointment is obtained, then incorporate the hydrous wool fat.

MENTHOL OINTMENT
Unguentum Mentholis
(G.H.N.Y.)

Menthol, in fine powder.	10 Gm.
Salicylic Acid, in fine powder	10 Gm.
Petrolatum	980 Gm.
To make	1000 Gm.

Triturate the menthol with the salicylic acid and incorporate the mixture with the petrolatum.

MENTHOL AND BORIC ACID OINTMENT
(P.H.N.Y.)

Menthol . . . . 6 Gm.
Boric Acid, in fine powder. . . . . 156 Gm.
Heavy Liquid Petrolatum . . . . 395 Gm.
Oil of Myristica . . . . 3 cc.
White Petrolatum . . . . 440 Gm.

To make about . . . . 1000 Gm.

Dissolve the menthol in a small quantity of the liquid petrolatum. Add the oil of myristica and the remainder of the liquid petrolatum and incorporate with the previously melted white petrolatum. Add this mixture gradually to the boric acid contained in a mortar, triturating thoroughly until the ointment congeals.

MENTHOL, CAMPHOR AND EUCALYPTOL OINTMENT
(N.Y.P.G.H.)

Menthol . . . . 8 Gm.
Camphor . . . . 8 Gm.
Eucalyptol . . . . 28 cc.
Petrolatum . . . . 956 Gm.

To make about . . . . 1000 Gm.

Triturate the menthol and camphor until liquefied. Add the eucalyptol and then incorporate the mixture with the petrolatum.

MENTHOL AND EUCALYPTOL OINTMENT
(G.H.N.Y.)

Menthol . . . . 10 Gm.
Eucalyptol . . . . 30 cc.
White Petrolatum . . . . 960 Gm.

To make about . . . . 1000 Gm.

Dissolve the menthol in the eucalyptol and incorporate the solution with the white petrolatum.

MENTHOL AND PHENOL OINTMENT
(R.B. I)

Phenol . . . . 20 Gm.
Menthol . . . . 60 Gm.
Wool Fat . . . . 320 Gm.
Petrolatum . . . . 600 Gm.

To make . . . . 1000 Gm.

Rub the phenol and menthol together until liquefied, then incorporate with the petrolatum and wool fat.

MERCURIC OLEATE OINTMENT
Unguentum Hydrargyri Oleati
(B.P. 1932)

Oleate of Mercury	200 Gm.
Wool Fat	40 Gm.
Paraffin.	80 Gm.
Petrolatum	680 Gm.
To make	1000 Gm.

Melt together the wool fat, paraffin and petrolatum and stir until cold.   Mix with the oleate of mercury by trituration.

COMPOUND MERCURY OLEATE OINTMENT
Brooke's Ointment
(Ext. Ph.)

Mercury Oleate Ointment	100 Gm.
Salicylic Acid	60 Gm.
Ichthammol	120 Gm.
White Petrolatum	300 Gm.
Paste of Zinc Oxide, a sufficient quantity,	
To make	1000 Gm.

Incorporate the salicylic acid and ichthammol in the mixture of mercury oleate ointment, zinc oxide paste, and white petrolatum.

MERCURIC SALICYLATE OINTMENT
Unguentum Hydrargyri Salicylatis
(R.B. I)

Mercuric Salicylate	100 Gm.
Petrolatum	450 Gm.
Hydrous Wool Fat	450 Gm.
To make	1000 Gm.

Triturate the mercury salt with the base until a smooth, uniform product is obtained.

MERCURY SUBSULFATE OINTMENT
Unguentum Hydrargyri Sulfatis Flavæ
Bazin's Ointment
(P.F.)

Mercury Subsulfate	35 Gm.
Benzoinated Lard	965 Gm.
To make	1000 Gm.

Triturate the mercury salt with the base until a smooth, uniform product is obtained.

NUTGALL OINTMENT
Unguentum Gallæ
(U.S.P. XI)

Nutgall, in very fine powder.	200 Gm.
Wool Fat	50 Gm.
Yellow Wax	50 Gm.
Petrolatum	700 Gm.
To make	1000 Gm.

Melt the yellow wax in a suitable dish on a water bath, then add the wool fat and petrolatum, and continue the heating until the mixture is liquefied. Stir until congealed and incorporate the nutgall.

CAUTION—*During its manufacture and storage this ointment must not come in contact with iron utensils or containers.*

OXYQUINOLINE OINTMENT
(R.B. II)

Oxyquinoline Sulfate	10 Gm.
Oil of Thyme	5 cc.
Oil of Eucalyptus	5 cc.
Hydrous Wool Fat	490 Gm.
Petrolatum	490 Gm.
To make about	1000 Gm.

Mix the oxyquinoline sulfate with the petrolatum and incorporate the hydrous wool fat with which the oils have been previously mixed.

PARAFFIN OINTMENT
Unguentum Paraffini
(B.P.)

White Wax	30 Gm.
Paraffin	270 Gm.
Petrolatum	700 Gm.
To make	1000 Gm.

Melt together and stir until cold.

For white ointments use white petrolatum and for colored ointments use the yellow variety.

HARD PARAFFIN OINTMENT
Unguentum Paraffini
Paraffin Salbe, Unguentum Durum
(D.A.B. V)

Ceresin.	400 Gm.
Heavy Liquid Petrolatum.	500 Gm.
Wool Fat.	100 Gm.
To make	1000 Gm.

Fuse the ceresin on a water bath. Add the wool fat and continue to heat until liquefied. Then add the liquid petrolatum and stir until the ointment congeals.

PHENOL AND CAMPHOR OINTMENT
(R.B. II)

Phenol.	50 Gm.
Camphor.	100 Gm.
Hydrous Wool Fat.	200 Gm.
White Wax.	130 Gm.
Petrolatum.	520 Gm.
To make	1000 Gm.

Melt together the white wax, hydrous wool fat and petrolatum. Stir until congealed, then add the phenol and camphor, previously triturated together until liquefied.

PHENOL, MENTHOL AND EUCALYPTUS OINTMENT
(B.N.Y.)

Phenol.	22 Gm.
Menthol.	22 Gm.
Oil of Eucalyptus.	65 cc.
Yellow Wax.	55 Gm.
Petrolatum.	418 Gm.
Wool Fat.	418 Gm.
To make about	1000 Gm.

Fuse the yellow wax with the aid of gentle heat, add the petrolatum and wool fat and continue warming until all are melted. Then add the oil of eucalyptus in which the phenol and menthol have been previously dissolved. Stir until the ointment congeals.

PROCAINE OINTMENT
(R.B. II)

Procaine Hydrochloride.	40 Gm.
Distilled Water	50 cc.
Hydrous Wool Fat.	150 Gm.
Petrolatum.	760 Gm.
To make	1000 Gm.

Dissolve the procaine hydrochloride in the distilled water and incorporate the solution with the hydrous wool fat.   Lastly add the petrolatum and mix thoroughly.

STRONG PROTEIN SILVER OINTMENT
(R.B. I)

Strong Protein Silver.	250 Gm.
Hydrous Wool Fat.	150 Gm.
Distilled Water, a sufficient quantity,	
Petrolatum, a sufficient quantity,	
To make	1000 Gm.

Moisten the strong protein silver with sufficient distilled water to produce a paste. Incorporate the wool fat and finally add sufficient petrolatum to make the product weigh 1000 Gm. and mix thoroughly.

RESORCINOL, SALICYLIC ACID AND ICHTHAMMOL OINTMENT
(G.H.N.Y.)

Resorcinol, in fine powder.	50 Gm.
Salicylic Acid, in fine powder	20 Gm.
Ichthammol.	50 Gm.
Petrolatum	880 Gm.
To make	1000 Gm.

Triturate the salicylic acid and resorcinol with the petrolatum, then incorporate the ichthammol.

RESORCINOL AND SULFUR OINTMENT
(N.Y.P.G.H.)

Resorcinol, in fine powder.	135 Gm.
Precipitated Sulfur.	270 Gm.
Rose Water Ointment	595 Gm.
Alcohol.	60 cc.
To make about	1000 Gm.

Triturate the resorcinol with the alcohol and incorporate with 300 Gm. of rose water ointment.   Rub the sulfur with the remainder of the ointment until smooth and finally mix the two portions.

CAUTION—*This ointment must not be allowed to come in contact with metallic utensils.*

RESORCINOL AND ZINC OINTMENT
(B.N.Y.)

Resorcinol, in fine powder.	100 Gm.
Hydrous Wool Fat	20 Gm.
Water, a sufficient quantity,	
Zinc Oxide Ointment, a sufficient quantity,	
To make	1000 Gm.

Moisten the resorcinol with sufficient distilled water to produce a paste. Incorporate the wool fat, and finally add sufficient zinc oxide ointment to make the product weigh 1000 Gm. and mix thoroughly.

RESORCINOL, ZINC OXIDE AND STARCH OINTMENT
(B.N.Y.)

Resorcinol, in fine powder	45 Gm.
Zinc Oxide	250 Gm.
Starch	250 Gm.
Petrolatum	455 Gm.
To make	1000 Gm.

Triturate the resorcinol with the petrolatum previously melted, then incorporate the zinc oxide and starch, rubbing until a smooth ointment is obtained.

SALICYLIC ACID OINTMENT
Unguentum Acidi Salicylici
(B.P.)

Salicylic Acid, in very fine powder	20 Gm.
White Paraffin Ointment, R.B.	980 Gm.
To make	1000 Gm.

Melt the paraffin ointment, add the salicylic acid and stir until cold.

SALICYLIC AND BENZOIC ACID OINTMENT WITH THYMOL
Whitfield's Ointment with Thymol
Modified Whitfield's Ointment
(R.B. II)

Salicylic Acid	60 Gm.
Benzoic Acid	120 Gm.
Thymol	12 Gm.
Yellow Wax	50 Gm.
Wool Fat	350 Gm.
Petrolatum	408 Gm.
To make	1000 Gm.

Melt together the yellow wax, wool fat and petrolatum. Powder the salicylic acid, benzoic acid and thymol very finely and triturate with the base until it congeals.

OINTMENT OF SALICYLIC ACID AND CHRYSAROBIN WITH OIL OF BIRCH TAR

Modified Dreuw's Ointment

Salicylic Acid, in fine powder	100 Gm.
Rectified Oil of Birch Tar	100 Gm.
Liniment of Soft Soap	200 Gm.
Chrysarobin	200 Gm.
Wool Fat	400 Gm.
Chloroform	80 cc.
To make about	1000 Gm.

Make the chrysarobin into a paste with 80 cc. of chloroform and mix into 200 Gm. of the wool fat. Warm to volatilize the chloroform. Add the salicylic acid and rectified oil of birch tar to the liniment of soft soap and incorporate with the remainder of the wool fat, and mix with the chrysarobin and wool fat.

CAUTION—*This preparation must not be allowed to come in contact with iron utensils.*

OINTMENT OF SALICYLATED SULFUR

Unguentum Sulfuris Salicylicum
(PH. DAN.)

Salicylic Acid	20 Gm.
Precipiated Sulfur	100 Gm.
Zinc Oxide	88 Gm.
Petrolatum	352 Gm.
Wool Fat, a sufficient quantity,	
To make	1000 Gm.

Triturate the salicylic acid, sulfur and zinc oxide with the petrolatum, and then add the wool fat and triturate the ointment until uniformly mixed.

OINTMENT OF SALICYLIC ACID AND SULFUR
(B.N.Y.)

Salicylic Acid	20 Gm.
Precipitated Sulfur	30 Gm.
Petrolatum	950 Gm.
To make	1000 Gm.

Triturate the powders together and incorporate with the petrolatum, triturating until a uniform ointment results.

COMPOUND OINTMENT OF SALICYLIC ACID AND ZINC OXIDE
(R.B. I)

Salicylic Acid, in very fine powder	20 Gm.
Zinc Oxide Ointment	125 Gm.
Wool Fat	125 Gm.
Solution of Calcium Hydroxide	150 cc.
White Petrolatum	580 Gm.
To make about	1000 Gm

Incorporate the salicylic acid with the zinc oxide ointment and the solution of calcium hydroxide with the wool fat, mix the two, and incorporate the mixture thoroughly with the petrolatum.

SCARLET RED AND ZINC OXIDE OINTMENT
(L.H.F.)

Scarlet Red	80 Gm.
Castor Oil	100 Gm.
Zinc Oxide Ointment	820 Gm.
To make	1000 Gm.

Triturate the scarlet red with the castor oil and incorporate with the zinc oxide ointment.

SOFT OINTMENT
Unguentum Molle

Weiche Salbe
(D.A.B. V)

Petrolatum,
Hydrous Wool Fat, of each, an equal weight.
Mix.

STARCH AND ZINC OXIDE OINTMENT
(N.Y.H.F.)

Zinc Oxide	150 Gm.
Starch	150 Gm.
White Petrolatum	700 Gm.
To make	1000 Gm.

Triturate the zinc oxide and starch with the white petrolatum until a smooth ointment is obtained.

MILD OINTMENT OF SULFUR AND PERUVIAN BALSAM
(N.Y.P.G.H.)

Peruvian Balsam.	125 Gm.
Precipitated Sulfur.	125 Gm.
Hydrous Wool Fat	375 Gm.
Petrolatum	375 Gm.
To make	1000 Gm.

Rub the sulfur with 200 Gm. of the petrolatum until smooth. Incorporate the peruvian balsam with the remainder of the petrolatum and add the hydrous wool fat. Finally mix the two portions of ointment.

STRONG OINTMENT OF SULFUR AND PERUVIAN BALSAM
Brown Ointment
(G.H.N.Y.)

Peruvian Balsam.	250 Gm.
Sulfur Ointment	750 Gm.
To make	1000 Gm.

Mix.

SULFUR OINTMENT WITH BETANAPHTHOL
(G.H.N.Y.)

Betanaphthol	50 Gm.
Sulfur Ointment	950 Gm.
To make	1000 Gm.

Mix.

OINTMENT OF SULFUR AND KAOLIN
Sulfur-Kaolin Ointment
(U.C.H.)

Precipitated Sulfur	100 Gm.
Kaolin	100 Gm.
Ointment of Zinc Oxide, a sufficient quantity,	
To make	1000 Gm.

Mix the two powders together intimately and incorporate the mixed powders in the ointment of zinc oxide.

OINTMENT OF SULFUR AND PINE TAR
(N.Y.P.G.H.)

Storax	130 Gm.
Sulfur Ointment	260 Gm.
Pine Tar Ointment.	130 Gm.
Medicinal Soft Soap	130 Gm.
Petrolatum	350 Gm.
To make	1000 Gm.

Warm the storax and incorporate it with the petrolatum, then add the sulfur ointment, pine tar ointment, and medicinal soft soap and mix thoroughly.

OINTMENT OF THYMOL IODIDE
(R.B. II)

Thymol Iodide.	200 Gm.
Heavy Liquid Petrolatum	135 Gm.
Hydrous Wool Fat	100 Gm.
Petrolatum	565 Gm.
To make	1000 Gm.

Triturate the thymol iodide with the liquid petrolatum to a smooth paste and incorporate with the petrolatum.   Lastly add the hydrous wool fat and mix.

ZINC OXIDE OINTMENT WITH CALOMEL AND LEAD ACETATE
Walker's Ointment
(R.B. I)

Zinc Oxide Ointment.	400 Gm.
Mild Mercurous Chloride.	45 Gm.
Lead Acetate, in fine powder	45 Gm.
Hydrous Wool Fat	510 Gm.
To make	1000 Gm.

Rub the mild mercurous chloride and lead acetate into a smooth ointment with the zinc oxide ointment, then incorporate the wool fat.

WAX OINTMENT
Unguentum Cereum
Wachssalbe
(D.A.B. V)

Peanut Oil	700 Gm.
Yellow Wax.	300 Gm.
To make	1000 Gm.

Melt the wax and incorporate with the peanut oil.   Stir while cooling.

WITCH HAZEL OINTMENT
Unguentum Hamamelidis
(B.P.C.)

Fluidextract of Hamamelis Leaf	100 cc.
Wool Fat	600 Gm.
Petrolatum, a sufficient quantity,	
To make about	1000 Gm.

Mix by trituration in a warm mortar.

COMPOUND ZINC OXIDE OINTMENT

Wilson's Ointment

(R.B. I)

Benzoin, in fine powder.	32 Gm.
Zinc Oxide	200 Gm.
Lard	768 Gm.
To make	1000 Gm.

Incorporate the zinc oxide and benzoin with the lard.

COMPOUND OINTMENT OF ZINC, BORIC ACID AND AMMONIATED MERCURY

(R.B. I)

Boric Acid Ointment	235 Gm.
Zinc Oxide Ointment.	475 Gm.
Ammoniated Mercury Ointment	235 Gm.
Solution of Coal Tar	20 cc.
Liquefied Phenol	35 cc.
To make about	1000 Gm.

Incorporate the liquids thoroughly in the mixed ointments.

OINTMENT OF ZINC OLEATE
Unguentum Zinci Oleatis

(B.P.)

Zinc Oleate,
White Paraffin Ointment, R.B., of each, an equal weight.

Mix with the aid of gentle heat.

OINTMENT OF SULFURATED ZINC
Unguentum Zinci Sulfurati

Ointment of Lotio Alba

(R.B. II)

Sulfurated Potash	130 Gm.
Zinc Sulfate.	130 Gm.
Distilled Water	200 cc.
Wool Fat	130 Gm.
White Petrolatum	410 Gm.
To make about	1000 Gm.

Dissolve the sulfurated potash and zinc sulfate, each separately, in 100 cc. of distilled water and filter each solution. Add the first solution to the second in a mortar and triturate thoroughly for several minutes until the mixture becomes uniform in consistence and nearly white in color. Incorporate the wool fat, add the white petrolatum and mix thoroughly.

PARENOL

Parenol Spissum

Solid Parenol

(B.P.C. 1934)

Petrolatum, white or yellow	650 Gm.
Wool Fat	150 Gm.
Distilled Water	200 cc.
To make	1000 Gm.

Melt the petrolatum and wool fat, pour the mixture into a warm mortar and incorporate gradually the warmed distilled water.

NOTE—Parenol is a stable emulsion of petrolatum. It does not become rancid on keeping and forms a useful vehicle for the application of various medicaments for which rapid absorption is desired. Parenol can be made to take up more than its own weight of water and mixes readily with all fats.

PETROLANUM

(B.P.C.)

Wool Fat	650 Gm.
Distilled Water	220 cc.
Light Liquid Petrolatum	130 Gm.
To make about	1000 Gm.

Melt the wool fat by means of gentle heat and add to it the liquid petrolatum and finally the warmed, distilled water; stir vigorously in order to obtain a homogeneous product.

NOTE—This formula gives an ointment base which is not so sticky as Hydrous Wool Fat.

SPECIAL OINTMENT BASE

(R.B. II)

White Wax	165 Gm.
Heavy Liquid Petrolatum	580 Gm.
Rose Water	247 cc.
Sodium Borate	8 Gm.
To make about	1000 Gm.

Melt the white wax, add the liquid petrolatum and continue the heat until the mixture is uniform and cool to 70° C. Dissolve the sodium borate in the rose water and bring this solution to the same temperature as that of the oily solution. Add the aqueous solution all at once to the oily solution and stir until congealed.

SOLUBLE OINTMENT BASE
(A.PH.A. 1940)

Glyceryl Monostearate . . . .   100 Gm.
Glycerin . . . .   250 Gm.
Bentonite . . . .   20 Gm.
Distilled Water, a sufficient quantity,
                        To make . . . .   1000 Gm.

Sprinkle the bentonite on 500 cc. of distilled water and after it is thoroughly wetted stir until a uniform magma results. Heat the glyceryl monostearate, the glycerin and the remainder of the distilled water on a water bath to 85° C. Add the bentonite magma, previously heated to the same temperature and stir vigorously until cooled.

OLEATES

OLEATE OF ATROPINE
Oleatum Atropinæ
(N.F. IV)

Atropine . . . .   20 Gm.
Alcohol . . . .   20 cc.
Oleic Acid . . . .   500 Gm.
Olive Oil or Peanut Oil . . . .   480 Gm.
                        To make . . . .   1000 Gm.

Triturate the atropine in a mortar with the alcohol, then add about an equal volume of the oleic acid, and, after warming the mortar, stir until the alcohol has evaporated. Now add the remainder of the oleic acid, and continue stirring until the atropine is dissolved. Finally add the olive oil.

MEDICATED PAINTS

BOHLMAN'S VIOLET
(R.B. I)

Methylrosaniline . . . .   2 Gm.
Monohydrated Sodium Carbonate . . . .   0.1 Gm.
Distilled Water . . . .   35 cc.
Acetone . . . .   10 cc.
Alcohol . . . .   55 cc.
                        To make about . . . .   100 cc.

Dissolve the methylrosaniline in the alcohol and the sodium carbonate in the distilled water. Mix these solutions and add the acetone.

CASTELLANI'S STAIN

Castellani's Lotion, Fuchsin Paint
(R.B. I)

Boric Acid	1 Gm.
Acetone	5 cc.
Resorcinol	10 Gm.

Solution of Carbol-Fuchsin (Ziehl-Neelsen), a sufficient quantity,

To make . . . .   100 cc.

Dissolve the boric acid in 80 cc. of the solution of carbol-fuchsin, add the acetone, the resorcinol, and sufficient solution of carbol-fuchsin to make the product measure 100 cc.

COMPOUND IODINE PAINT

Pigmentum Iodi Compositum

Mandl's Paint
(B.P.C. 1934)

Iodine	12.5 Gm.
Potassium Iodide	25 Gm.
Distilled Water	25 cc.
Oil of Peppermint	7.5 cc.

Glycerin, a sufficient quantity,

To make   1000   cc.

Dissolve the iodine and potassium iodide in the distilled water, add 500 cc. of glycerin, the oil of peppermint, and then sufficient glycerin to make the product measure 1000 cc.

Dispense with a "shake well" label.

COMPOUND IODOFORM PAINT

Pigmentum Iodoformi Compositum

Whitehead's Varnish
(B.P.C. 1934)

Siam Benzoin, coarsely powdered	100 Gm.
Storax	75 Gm.
Tolu Balsam	50 Gm.
Iodoform	100 Gm.

Ethyl Oxide, a sufficient quantity,

To make . . . .   1000 cc.

Macerate the benzoin, storax and tolu balsam with 800 cc. of ethyl oxide for 7 days, agitating frequently, filter, dissolve the iodoform in the filtrate and pass sufficient ethyl oxide through the filter to make the product measure 1000 cc.

MENTHOL AND TOLUENE PAINT
Loeffler's Paint
(B.P.C.)

Menthol	100 Gm.
Dehydrated Alcohol	600 cc.
Solution of Ferric Chloride	60 cc.
Toluene, a sufficient quantity,	
To make	1000 cc.

Dissolve the menthol in the dehydrated alcohol, add the solution of ferric chloride and sufficient toluene to make the product measure 1000 cc.

MEDICATED PASTES

PASTE BASE
(R.B. I)

Tragacanth, powdered	40 Gm.
Methyl Parahydroxybenzoic Acid	1 Gm.
Glycerin	150 Gm.
Distilled Water	810 cc.
To make	1000 Gm.

Dissolve the acid in 600 cc. of distilled water, add the glycerin, and heat with the tragacanth until a mucilage is formed, cool and add the remainder of the distilled water.

This preparation is used as a base for the incorporation of medicaments.

BETANAPHTHOL PASTE
Pasta Betanaphtholis

Pasta Naphtholis, Lassar; Lassar's Naphthol Paste
(N.F. V)

Betanaphthol, in very fine powder	100 Gm.
Precipitated Sulfur	500 Gm.
Petrolatum	200 Gm.
Medicinal Soft Soap	200 Gm.
To make	1000 Gm.

Triturate the betanaphthol and sulfur with the petrolatum and incorporate the medicinal soft soap with the mixture.

LASSAR'S BETANAPHTHOL AND PERUVIAN BALSAM PASTE
Lassar's Betanaphthol Paste
(R.B. I)

Betanaphthol, in fine powder	400 Gm.
Peruvian Balsam	200 Gm.
Liniment of Soft Soap	400 Gm.
To make	1000 Gm.

Triturate the betanaphthol with the peruvian balsam and add the liniment of soft soap.

B. I. P. PASTE
(S.H.F.)

Bismuth Subnitrate.	262 Gm.
Iodoform	262 Gm.
Heavy Liquid Petrolatum	476 Gm.
To make	1000 Gm.

Incorporate the powders with the liquid petrolatum.

Dispense in a wide-mouthed bottle.

CARBAMIDE (UREA) PASTE
(Fantus)

Benzoic Acid	2 Gm.
Citric Acid	10 Gm.
Carbamide (Urea)	20 Gm.
Tragacanth, in fine powder	100 Gm.
Glycerin	100 cc.
Ringer's Solution (Bodanksy formula), R.B., a sufficient quantity,	
To make	1000 Gm.

Dissolve the carbamide, citric acid and benzoic acid in the Ringer's solution and add the glycerin. To this solution add the tragacanth, allow to swell and homogenize by straining through cheesecloth or, if possible, by means of an homogenizer.

ETHYL AMINOBENZOATE PASTE
(Fantus)

Benzoic Acid	2 Gm.
Ethyl Aminobenzoate	10 Gm.
Chloroform	20 cc.
Glycerin	100 cc.
Tragacanth, powder	100 Gm.
Ringer's Solution (Bodansky formula), R.B., a sufficient quantity,	
To make	1000 Gm.

Dissolve the benzoic acid in the Ringer's solution and add the glycerin. To this solution add the tragacanth, allow to swell and homogenize by straining through cheesecloth or by means of an homogenizer. Dissolve the ethyl aminobenzoate in the chloroform and add this solution slowly and with constant stirring to the tragacanth mixture and triturate until the chloroform is completely evaporated.

ICHTHAMMOL PASTE
Pasta Ichthammolis
Gelatinum Ichthammol, Ammonium Ichthosulfonate Paste
(B.P.C. 1934)

Ichthammol	95 Gm.
Gelatin	95 Gm.
Glycerin	570 Gm.
Distilled Water	240 cc.
To make	1000 Gm.

Soak the gelatin in the distilled water until softened; then heat it on a water bath until dissolved, replace the water lost by evaporation, add the glycerin and finally the ichthammol, and mix.

COMPOUND ICHTHAMMOL PASTE
Pasta Ichthammolis Composita
(B.P.C. 1923)

Ichthammol	250 Gm.
Phenol	25 Gm.
Starch	500 Gm.
Distilled Water	225 cc.
To make	1000 Gm.

Dissolve the ichthammol and phenol in the warmed distilled water, and mix with the starch.

MAGNESIUM SULFATE PASTE
Pasta Magnesii Sulfatis
Morison's Paste
(B.P.C. 1934)

Magnesium Sulfate, dried at 100° C.	450 Gm.
Glycerin	550 Gm.
Phenol	5 Gm.

Dissolve the phenol in the glycerin and mix with the dried magnesium sulfate in a warm mortar.

NOTE—This paste should be stored in well-closed containers.

POTASSA AND LIME PASTE
Pasta Potassæ cum Calce
Pasta Viennensis, Vienna Paste
(B.P.C. 1923)

Potassa with Lime, R.B.,
Alcohol, of each, a sufficient quantity.

Mix the potassa with lime together with sufficient alcohol to make a paste. Glycerin may be used to replace the alcohol.

NOTE—This paste should be freshly prepared.

SODA AND LIME PASTE
Pasta Sodæ cum Calce
Pasta Londonensis, London Paste
(P.F.)

Soda Lime
Distilled Water, of each, a sufficient quantity.

Mix the soda lime with sufficient distilled water to make a paste.

NOTE—This paste should be freshly prepared.

STARCH AND ALUM PASTE
(R.B. I)

Starch	100 Gm.
Alum.	5 Gm.
Phenol	10 Gm.
Distilled Water, a sufficient quantity,	
To make	1000 Gm.

Mix the starch with 100 cc. of distilled water, and stir into 800 cc. of boiling distilled water in which the alum is dissolved. Continue heating until the mixture is homogeneous, add the phenol and sufficient distilled water to make the product weigh 1000 Gm.

TRAGACANTH PASTE
(Fantus)

Benzoic Acid	2 Gm.
Glycerin	100 cc.
Tragacanth, in fine powder	100 Gm.
Ringer's Solution (Bodansky formula), R.B., a sufficient quantity,	
To make	1000 Gm.

Dissolve the benzoic acid in the Ringer's solution, add the glycerin and tragacanth, allow to swell and homogenize by straining through cheesecloth or, if possible, by means of an homogenizer.

MODIFIED LASSAR'S ZINC PASTE
(R.B. I)

Zinc Oxide	125 Gm.
Starch	125 Gm.
Rose Water Ointment	750 Gm.
To make	1000 Gm.

Mix thoroughly.

UNNA'S ZINC GELATIN PASTE
(Hager)

Zinc Oxide	150 Gm.
Gelatin	150 Gm.
Glycerin	250 Gm.
Water, a sufficient quantity,	
To make	1000 Gm.

Rub the zinc oxide and glycerin to a smooth paste and add the hot solution of gelatin and water and triturate the paste until cool.

PASTE OF ZINC OXIDE AND STARCH
Simple Paste
(E.H.P.)

Zinc Oxide	266 Gm.
Starch	266 Gm.
Petrolatum	468 Gm.
To make	1000 Gm.

Triturate the zinc oxide with the starch and incorporate the mixed powders in the petrolatum.

SULFURATED ZINC PASTE
Pasta Zinci Sulfurata

Pasta Zinci Sulfurata, Unna, Unna's Sulfurated Zinc Paste
(N. F. V)

Zinc Oxide, in very fine powder	150 Gm.
Precipitated Sulfur	100 Gm.
Purified Siliceous Earth	50 Gm.
Benzoinated Lard	700 Gm.
To make	1000 Gm.

Mix the powders and triturate them with about an equal weight of benzoinated lard until a smooth mixture is obtained. Then incorporate the remainder of the benzoinated lard.

MODIFIED SULFURATED ZINC PASTE
(N.Y.P.G.H.)

Precipitated Sulfur	100 Gm.
Kaolin	100 Gm.
Zinc Oxide Ointment	800 Gm.
To make	1000 Gm.

Mix intimately.

ZINC PEROXIDE PASTE
(Meleney and Johnson)

Zinc Peroxide . . . .   10 Gm.
Distilled Water, a sufficient quantity to make a paste.
NOTE—This paste should be freshly prepared.

PETROXOLINS

IODOFORM PETROXOLIN
Petroxolinum Iodoformi

Iodoform Petrox
(N.F. IV)

Iodoform . . . .   30 Gm.
Acetone . . . .   200 cc.
Oleic Acid . . . .   100 cc.
Eucalyptol . . . .   30 cc.
Liquid Petroxolin, a sufficient quantity,

To make . . . .   1000 cc.

Dissolve the iodoform in the acetone, add the eucalyptol, oleic acid and sufficient liquid petroxolin, to make the product measure 1000 cc.; mix the ingredients thoroughly.

NOTE—This petroxolin should be freshly prepared.

TAR PETROXOLIN
Petroxolinum Picis

Tar Petrox
(N.F. IV)

Rectified Oil of Tar . . . .   250 cc.
Liquid Petroxolin . . . .   750 cc.

To make . . . .   1000 cc.

Mix.

PILLS

COMPOUND PILLS OF ALOE, MERCURY AND SCAMMONY
Pilulæ Aloes, Hydrargyri et Scammonii Compositæ

Francis' "Triplex" Pills
(N.F. IV)

Aloe, in fine powder	5	Gm.
Resin of Ipomea	5	Gm.
Mass of Mercury	5	Gm.
Croton Oil	0.32	cc.
Oil of Caraway	1	cc.
Tincture of Aloe and Myrrh, a sufficient quantity,		
To make	100	Pills

Incorporate the oils with the other ingredients, add sufficient tincture to form a mass and divide it into 100 pills.

AVERAGE DOSE—1 pill.

COMPOUND PILLS OF ALOIN
Pilulæ Aloini Compositæ
(N.F. V)

Aloin	3	Gm.
Resin of Podophyllum	0.8	Gm.
Pilular Extract of Belladonna	1	Gm.
To make	100	Pills

Mix intimately, form a mass and divide it into 100 pills.

AVERAGE DOSE—1 pill.

COMPOUND PILLS OF ANTIMONY
Pilulæ Antimonii Compositæ

Plummer's Pills
(N.F. IV)

Sulfurated Antimony	4 Gm.
Mild Mercurous Chloride	4 Gm.
Guaiac, in fine powder	8 Gm.
Castor Oil, a sufficient quantity,	
To make	100 Pills

Mix the solid ingredients intimately, form a mass with sufficient castor oil and divide it into 100 pills.

AVERAGE DOSE—1 pill.

ANTIPERIODIC PILLS
Pilulæ Antiperiodicæ
Warburg's Pills
(N.F. V)

Aloe, in fine powder	13 Gm.
Rhubarb, in fine powder	3.2 Gm.
Angelica Fruit, in fine powder	3.2 Gm.
Inula, in fine powder	1.6 Gm.
Crocus, in fine powder	1.6 Gm.
Fennel, in fine powder	1.6 Gm.
Zedoary, in fine powder	0.8 Gm.
Cubeb, in fine powder	0.8 Gm.
Myrrh, in fine powder	0.8 Gm.
Agaric, in fine powder	0.8 Gm.
Camphor, in fine powder	0.8 Gm.
Quinine Sulfate	9.0 Gm.
Extract of Gentian, a sufficient quantity,	
To make	100 Pills

Mix the powders and quinine sulfate intimately, make into a mass with the extract of gentian and divide it into 100 pills.

AVERAGE DOSE—1 pill.

ARSENICAL PILLS

Tanjore Pills, Asiatic Pills, Oriental Pills
(R.B. I)

	No. 1	No. 2	Stronger
Arsenic Trioxide	0.4 Gm.	0.2 Gm.	0.72 Gm.
Pepper, in fine powder	3.2 Gm.	1.6 Gm.	6.4 Gm.
Acacia, in fine powder	1.2 Gm.	1.2 Gm.	1.2 Gm.
Distilled Water, a sufficient quantity,			
To make	100 Pills	100 Pills	100 Pills

Mix the powders intimately, incorporate a sufficient quantity of distilled water to form a mass and divide it into 100 pills.

AVERAGE DOSE—1 pill.

Each No. 1 pill contains about 0.004 Gm. ($\frac{1}{15}$ grain) of arsenic trioxide.
Each No. 2 pill contains about 0.002 Gm. ($\frac{1}{30}$ grain) of arsenic trioxide.
Each stronger pill contains about 0.0072 Gm. ($\frac{3}{25}$ grain) of arsenic trioxide.

BARKER'S PILLS
Pilulæ Laxitivæ Post Partum
(N.F. IV)

Compound Extract of Colocynth	11 Gm.
Aloe, in fine powder	5.5 Gm.
Extract of Nux Vomica	2.5 Gm.
Resin of Podophyllum	0.5 Gm.
Ipecac, in fine powder	0.5 Gm.
Pilular Extract of Hyoscyamus	4 Gm.
Diluted Alcohol, a sufficient quantity,	
To make	100 Pills

Mix the solid ingredients intimately, form a mass with the diluted alcohol and divide it into 100 pills.

AVERAGE DOSE—1 pill.

CAMPHOR PILLS
(R.B. I)

Camphor, in fine powder	30 Gm.
Purified Talc	10 Gm.
Hard Soap, in fine powder,	
Water, of each, a sufficient quantity,	
To make	100 Pills

Mix the camphor and purified talc intimately, form a mass with the hard soap and water and divide it into 100 pills.

AVERAGE DOSE—1 pill.

COMPOUND PILLS OF COLOCYNTH
Pilulæ Colocynthidis Compositæ
Pilulæ Cocciæ; Cochia Pills
(N.F. IV)

Extract of Colocynth	1 Gm.
Aloe, in fine powder	13 Gm.
Resin of Ipomea	13 Gm.
Oil of Clove	2 cc.
Diluted Alcohol, a sufficient quantity,	
To make	100 Pills

Mix the solid ingredients intimately, incorporate the oil, form a mass with the diluted alcohol and divide it into 100 pills.

AVERAGE DOSE—1 pill.

COLOCYNTH AND HYOSCYAMUS PILLS
Pilulæ Colocynthidis et Hyoscyami
(N.F. IV)

Extract of Colocynth	0.6	Gm.
Aloe, in fine powder	10	Gm.
Resin of Ipomea	10	Gm.
Pilular Extract of Hyoscyamus	10	Gm.
Oil of Clove	1	cc.
Diluted Alcohol, a sufficient quantity,		
To make	100	Pills

Mix the solid ingredients intimately, incorporate the oil, form a mass with the diluted alcohol and divide it into 100 pills.

AVERAGE DOSE—1 pill.

COLOCYNTH AND PODOPHYLLIN PILLS
Pilulæ Colocynthidis et Podophyllini
(N.F. IV)

Compound Extract of Colocynth	16.2 Gm.
Resin of Podophyllum	1.6 Gm.
Syrup, a sufficient quantity,	
To make	100 Pills

Mix the solid ingredients intimately, form a mass with the syrup and divide it into 100 pills.

AVERAGE DOSE—1 pill.

WOLFF'S CREOSOTE PILLS
Pilulæ Creosoti
(R.B. I)

Creosote	2.7	cc.
Althea, in fine powder	2	Gm.
Gentian, in fine powder	2.7	Gm.
Extract of Glycyrrhiza, in fine powder	4	Gm.
Glycerin	1.5	cc.
Glycyrrhiza, in fine powder, a sufficient quantity,		
To make	100	Pills

Mix the althea, gentian and extract of glycyrrhiza intimately, and incorporate the creosote and glycerin. Add sufficient glycyrrhiza to make a mass and divide it into 100 pills.

AVERAGE DOSE—1 pill.

DIGITALIS, SQUILL AND MERCURY PILLS
Pilulæ Digitalis, Scillæ et Hydrargyri
Niemeyer's Pills; Guy's Pills
(N.F. V)

Digitalis, in fine powder	6.5 Gm.
Squill, in fine powder.	6.5 Gm.
Mass of Mercury	6.5 Gm.
Honey, a sufficient quantity,	
To make	100 Pills

Mix the solid ingredients intimately, form a mass with the honey and divide it into 100 pills.

AVERAGE DOSE—1 pill.

FOTHERGILL'S PILLS
(P.F.)

Ipecac, in fine powder	6.5 Gm.
Strychnine	0.3 Gm.
Oil of Black Pepper	12.5 cc.
Pill Mass of Aloes and Mastic, N. F.	16 Gm.
To make	100 Pills

Mix intimately, form a mass with the pill mass of aloes and mastic and divide into 100 pills.

AVERAGE DOSE—1 pill.

NOTE—Each pill contains 0.003 Gm. or $\frac{1}{20}$ grain of strychnine.

CAUTION—*Oil of black pepper is not to be confused with oleoresin of black pepper.*

PILLS OF GUAIACOL
(P.F.)

Guaiacol	6 cc.
Hard Soap, in fine powder	6 Gm.
Glycyrrhiza, in powder,	
Extract of Glycyrrhiza,	
Water, of each, a sufficient quantity,	
To make	100 Pills

Triturate the guaiacol with the hard soap until thoroughly mixed. Add sufficient glycyrrhiza, extract of glycyrrhiza and water to form a mass and divide it into 100 pills.

AVERAGE DOSE—1 pill.

HUFELAND'S PILLS
(R.B. I)

Extract of Ox Bile . . . . 3.3 Gm.
Hard Soap, in fine powder. . . . . 3.3 Gm.
Extract of Taraxacum. . . . . 3.3 Gm.
Rhubarb, in fine powder . . . . 3.3 Gm.
Syrup, a sufficient quantity,

To make . . . . 100 Pills

Mix the powders intimately, incorporate sufficient syrup to form a mass and divide it into 100 pills.

AVERAGE DOSE—1 pill.

IRON, QUININE AND STRYCHNINE PILLS
(N.Y.P.G.H.)

Soluble Iron Pyrophosphate . . . . 6 Gm.
Quinine Sulfate . . . . 3 Gm.
Strychnine Sulfate . . . . 0.1 Gm.
Acacia, in fine powder,
Syrup, of each, a sufficient quantity,

To make . . . . 100 Pills

Mix the first three ingredients intimately, form a mass with acacia and syrup and divide it into 100 pills.

AVERAGE DOSE—1 pill.

Each pill contains about 0.001 Gm. ($\frac{1}{60}$ grain) of strychnine sulfate.

LAXATIVE PILLS, CHAPMAN
(N.F. IV)

Aloe, in fine powder . . . . 10 Gm.
Mastic, in fine powder . . . . 10 Gm.
Ipecac, in fine powder. . . . . 6.5 Gm.
Oil of Fennel . . . . 1.5 cc.
Diluted Alcohol, a sufficient quantity,

To make . . . . 100 Pills

Mix the ingredients intimately, form a mass with the diluted alcohol and divide it into 100 pills.

AVERAGE DOSE—1 pill.

LAXATIVE PILLS, COLE
(N.F. IV)

Aloe, in fine powder . . . . 7.80 Gm.
Mass of Mercury. . . . . 7.80 Gm.
Jalap, in fine powder . . . . 7.80 Gm.
Antimony and Potassium Tartrate . . . . 0.13 Gm.
Syrup, a sufficient quantity,

To make . . . . 100 Pills

Mix the powdered ingredients intimately with the mass of mercury, form a mass with the syrup and divide it into 100 pills.

AVERAGE DOSE—1 pill.

MERCURIC SALICYLATE PILLS
Pilulæ Hydrargyri Salicylatis
(P.F.)

Mercuric Salicylate.	2 Gm.
Extract of Gentian	7 Gm.
Syrup, a sufficient quantity,	
To make	100 Pills

Mix the solid ingredients intimately, form a mass with the syrup and divide it into 100 pills.

AVERAGE DOSE—1 pill.

PILLS OF NITROGLYCERIN
Pilulæ Glycerylis Nitratis
Pilulæ Glonoini, Pills of Glonoin
(N.F. IV)

Spirit of Glyceryl Trinitrate	6.5 cc.
Althea, in fine powder	6.5 Gm.
Confection of Rose, R.B., a sufficient quantity,	
To make	100 Pills

Mix the spirit of glyceryl trinitrate intimately with the althea, expose the mixture for a short time to the air, avoiding heat, in order that the alcohol may evaporate, then make a mass with the confection of rose and divide it into 100 pills.

NOTE—Protect the hands with rubber gloves.

AVERAGE DOSE—1 pill.

PHOSPHORUS PILLS
Pilulæ Phosphori
(U.S.P. X)

Phosphorus	0.06	Gm.
Althea, in very fine powder	6	Gm.
Acacia, in very fine powder	3	Gm.
Chloroform,		
Glycerin,		
Water,		
Tolu Balsam,		
Ethyl Oxide, of each, a sufficient quantity,		
To make	100	Pills

Dissolve the phosphorus in a test tube in 5 cc. of chloroform, with the aid of very gentle heat, replacing from time to time any of the chloroform which may be lost by evaporation.   Mix the althea and acacia in a mortar, add the solution of phosphorus, then immediately afterwards a sufficient quantity (about 4 cc.) of a mixture of 2 volumes of glycerin and 1 volume of water and quickly form a mass.   Divide it into 100 pills.

Dissolve 10 Gm. of tolu balsam in 15 cc. of ethyl oxide, shake the pills with a sufficient quantity of this solution until they are uniformly coated and put them on a plate to dry, occasionally rolling them about until the drying is completed.

Keep in a well-stoppered bottle.

AVERAGE DOSE—1 pill.

Each pill contains about 0.0006 Gm. ($\frac{1}{100}$ grain) of phosphorus.

STRONG PROTEIN SILVER PILLS
(R.B. I)

Strong Protein Silver.	10 Gm.
Kaolin	10 Gm.
Petrolatum, a sufficient quantity,	
To make	100 Pills

Triturate the strong protein silver with the kaolin and work into a mass with sufficient petrolatum.   Divide it into 100 pills.

AVERAGE DOSE—1 pill.

ZINC PHOSPHIDE PILLS
(R.B. I)

Zinc Phosphide	0.8 Gm.
Glycyrrhiza, in fine powder	6 Gm.
Althea, in fine powder	1 Gm.
Glycerin	1.5 cc.
Syrup of Acacia, a sufficient quantity,	
To make	100 Pills

Mix the powders, incorporate the glycerin and sufficient syrup of acacia to form a mass and divide it into 100 pills.

AVERAGE DOSE—1 pill.

PLASTERS

SALICYLIC ACID PLASTER
(B.N.Y.)

Salicylic Acid	50 Gm.
Plaster of Lead Oleate	600 Gm.
Soap Plaster, R.B.	250 Gm.
Yellow Wax	20 Gm.
Petrolatum	80 Gm.
To make	1000 Gm.

Fuse the plaster of lead oleate on a water bath, add the soap plaster and wax. Continue warming until all are fused, then add the petrolatum and the salicylic acid, previously mixed with the aid of heat. Mix intimately and allow to congeal.

SOAP PLASTER
Emplastrum Saponis
(N.F. V)

Hard Soap, dried, and in coarse powder . . . .   100 Gm.
Plaster of Lead Oleate . . . .   900 Gm.
Water, a sufficient quantity,
                 To make about . . . .   1000 Gm.

Rub the hard soap with enough water to reduce it to a semi-liquid, mix it with the plaster of lead oleate, previously melted, incorporate thoroughly by stirring and evaporate the mixture to the consistence of a plaster.

POULTICES

BORIC ACID POULTICE
(S.H.F.)

Boric Acid . . . .   8 Gm.
Starch . . . .   30 Gm.
Water, a sufficient quantity,
                 To make about . . . .   1000 Gm.

Mix the boric acid and starch with 50 cc. of cold water. Pour the mixture into 1000 cc. of boiling water and stir until a semi-transparent jelly is formed. Allow to stand until cold.

BREAD POULTICE
Cataplasma Panis
(S.H.F.)

Bread Crumbs. . . . .   550 Gm.
Water, boiling. . . . .   450 cc.
                 To make . . . .   1000 Gm.

Mix the bread crumbs, gradually, with the boiling water in a basin and let the mixture stand in a warm place for 15 minutes. Drain off the water and spread.

LINSEED POULTICE
Flaxseed Poultice
(S.H.F.) *

Linseed Meal . . . .   225 Gm.
Water, boiling . . . .   775 cc.
                 To make . . . .   1000 Gm.

Add the linseed meal gradually, with constant stirring, to the boiling water.

MUSTARD POULTICE
(S.H.F.)

Black Mustard, in coarse powder . . . .   90 Gm.
Linseed Poultice, R.B..   910 Gm.
To make . . . .   1000 Gm.

Incorporate the mustard with the recently prepared linseed poultice while it is yet lukewarm, but not hot.

PHENOL AND LINSEED POULTICE
(S.H.F.)

Linseed Meal . . . .   230 Gm.
Liquefied Phenol. . . . .   12 cc.
Water, boiling . . . .   758 cc.
To make about . . . .   1000 Gm.

Dissolve the liquefied phenol in the boiling water and add the linseed meal gradually, with constant stirring.

SLIPPERY ELM POULTICE
(B.P.C.)

Elm, in coarse powder . . . .   240 Gm.
Boric Acid . . . .   40 Gm.
Activated Charcoal . . . .   40 Gm.
Water, boiling. . . . .   680 cc.
To make . . . .   1000 Gm.

Mix the powders and add the boiling water gradually.

MEDICATED POWDERS

POWDER OF ALOE AND CANELLA
Pulvis Aloes et Canellæ

Hiera Picra
(N.F. V)

Aloe, in fine powder . . . .   800 Gm.
Canella, in fine powder . . . .   200 Gm.
To make . . . .   1000 Gm.

Mix intimately.

AVERAGE DOSE—Metric, 0.3 Gm.—Apothecaries, 5 grains.

ANTACID TRIBASIC POWDER
(U.C.H.)

Magnesium Trisilicate	330 Gm.
Tribasic Magnesium Phosphate	330 Gm.
Tribasic Calcium Phosphate	340 Gm.
To make	1000 Gm.

Mix the powders intimately.

AVERAGE DOSE—1 teaspoonful.

ASCORBIC ACID POWDERS (Chocolate Flavor)

Ascorbic Acid	0.25 Gm.
Cacao, powdered	1.2 Gm.
Tincture of Vanilla	0.30 cc.
Sucrose	3 Gm.

Mix well and divide into 10 powders.

AVERAGE DOSE—1 powder.

ASCORBIC ACID POWDERS (Lemon Flavor)

Ascorbic Acid	0.25 Gm.
Citric Acid	0.30 Gm.
Tincture of Lemon	0.30 cc.
Sucrose	3 Gm.

Mix well and divide into 10 powders.

AVERAGE DOSE—1 powder.

BISMUTH-KAOLIN POWDER
(U.C.H.)

Bismuth Subcarbonate	250 Gm.
Vanillin	1 Gm.
Kaolin	749 Gm.
To make	1000 Gm.

Mix intimately the bismuth subcarbonate and the kaolin in a mortar and add the vanillin dissolved in 5 cc. of alcohol; continue the trituration until the alcohol is evaporated and the vanillin is uniformly dispersed in the mixed powders.

AVERAGE DOSE—1 teaspoonful.

CERIUM AND BISMUTH POWDER
(B.N.Y.)

Cerium Oxalate	150 Gm.
Bismuth Subcarbonate	275 Gm.
Magnesium Carbonate	575 Gm.
To make	1000 Gm.

Mix by trituration and pass through a No. 60 sieve.

AVERAGE DOSE—Metric, 1 Gm.—Apothecaries, 15 grains.

CERIUM AND SODA POWDER
(V.C.N.Y.)

Cerium Oxalate	330 Gm.
Sodium Bicarbonate	670 Gm.
To make	1000 Gm.

Mix by trituration and pass through a No. 60 sieve.

AVERAGE DOSE—Metric, 2 Gm.—Apothecaries, 30 grains.

COMPOUND POWDER OF GAMBIR
Pulvis Gambir Compositus
Pulvis Catechu Compositus
(N.F. IV)

Gambir, in fine powder	400 Gm.
Kino, in fine powder	200 Gm.
Krameria, in fine powder	200 Gm.
Cinnamon, in fine powder	100 Gm.
Myristica, in fine powder	100 Gm.
To make	1000 Gm.

Mix the powders intimately, pass through a No. 60 sieve and afterwards rub lightly in a mortar.

Keep in a stoppered bottle.

AVERAGE DOSE—Metric, 1.25 Gm.—Apothecaries, 20 grains.

COMPOUND IODINE POWDER
(N.Y.H.F.)

Iodine, crystals	10 Gm.
Boric Acid, finely powdered	990 Gm.
To make	1000 Gm.

An alcoholic solution of the iodine is mixed with the boric acid powder and the alcohol allowed to evaporate completely.

NOTE—Especially prepared for Otolaryngology. A 2% powder is also used.

LENITIVE POWDER
Pulvis Lenitivus
(P.F.)

Potassium Bitartrate	350 Gm.
Senna, in fine powder	350 Gm.
Cinnamon, in fine powder	100 Gm.
Fennel, in fine powder	100 Gm.
Anise, in fine powder	100 Gm.
To make	1000 Gm.

Mix intimately.

AVERAGE DOSE—Metric, 2 Gm.—Apothecaries, 30 grains.

COMPOUND MAGNESIA POWDER
Pulvis Magnesiæ Compositus
(N.Y.P.G.H.)

Heavy Magnesium Oxide,
Monohydrated Sodium Carbonate,
Sodium Bicarbonate,
Lactose, of each, an equal weight.

Mix thoroughly by trituration and pass through a No. 40 sieve.

AVERAGE DOSE—Metric, 2 Gm.—Apothecaries, 30 grains.

MAGNESIA AND BISMUTH POWDER
(G.H.N.Y.)

Heavy Magnesium Oxide	250 Gm.
Sodium Bicarbonate	375 Gm.
Bismuth Subnitrate	375 Gm.
To make	1000 Gm.

Mix thoroughly by trituration and pass through a No. 40 sieve.

AVERAGE DOSE—Metric, 1 to 2 Gm.—Apothecaries, 15 to 30 grains.

COMPOUND POWDER OF MAGNESIUM CARBONATE
(V.C.N.Y.)

Prepared Chalk,
Sodium Bicarbonate, in fine powder,
Magnesium Carbonate, of each, an equal weight.

Mix by trituration and pass through a No. 40 sieve.

AVERAGE DOSE—Metric, 6 Gm.—Apothecaries, 1½ drachms.

COMPOUND POWDER OF MORPHINE
Tully's Powder
(U.S.P. VIII)

Morphine Sulfate	1.5 Gm.
Camphor	32 Gm.
Precipitated Calcium Carbonate	33.5 Gm.
Glycyrrhiza, powdered	33 Gm.
Alcohol, a sufficient quantity,	
To make	100 Gm.

Triturate the camphor with the alcohol and gradually add the other ingredients.
Triturate until the alcohol is evaporated and the powder is uniformly mixed.

AVERAGE DOSE—Metric, 0.5 Gm.—Apothecaries, 8 grains.

NOTE—This powder must be dispensed on prescription only.

SIPPY POWDERS
(B.N.Y.)
Powder A or No. 1

Precipitated Calcium Carbonate . . . .   0.6 Gm.
Sodium Bicarbonate   2   Gm.
To make . . . .   1 Powder
Mix.
AVERAGE DOSE—1 powder.

Powder B or No. 2

Heavy Magnesium Oxide . . . .   0.6 Gm.
Sodium Bicarbonate . . . .   0.6 Gm.
To make . . . .   1 Powder
Mix.
AVERAGE DOSE—1 powder.
These powders are taken alternately.

STARR'S POWDER
(R.B. I)

Exsiccated Sodium Phosphate . . . .   250 Gm.
Exsiccated Sodium Sulfate . . . .   625 Gm.
Sodium Salicylate, in fine powder . . . .   125 Gm.
To make . . . .   1000 Gm.
Mix thoroughly by trituration and pass through a No. 40 sieve.
AVERAGE DOSE—Metric, 4 to 8 Gm.—Apothecaries, 1 to 2 drachms.

SULFUR, MAGNESIUM CARBONATE, AND MAGNESIUM SULFATE POWDER
(N.Y.H.F.)

Oil of Anise . . . .   2.5 cc.
Precipitated Sulfur . . . .   47.5 Gm.
Magnesium Carbonate   475   Gm.
Exsiccated Magnesium Sulfate   475   Gm.
To make about   1000   Gm.
Mix the powders thoroughly, incorporate the oil by trituration and pass through a No. 40 sieve.
AVERAGE DOSE—Metric, 4 Gm.—Apothecaries, 1 drachm.

COMPOUND TRI-PHOSPHATE POWDER
Pulvis Phosphatum Trium Compositus
(R.B. II)

Tribasic Magnesium Phosphate	20 Gm.
Precipitated Calcium Phosphate	80 Gm.
Calcium Glycerophosphate	80 Gm.
Potassium Bicarbonate	320 Gm.
Sodium Bicarbonate	500 Gm.
To make	1000 Gm.

Mix thoroughly by trituration.

AVERAGE DOSE—Metric, 2 Gm.—Apothecaries, 30 grains.

MEDICATED DUSTING POWDERS

COMPOUND ALUM DUSTING POWDER
Pulvis Aluminis Compositus
(R.B. I)

Phenol, in fine powder	10 Gm.
Camphor, in fine powder	30 Gm.
Exsiccated Alum	960 Gm.
To make	1000 Gm.

Mix the phenol with part of the alum and separately mix the camphor with the remainder of the alum. Pass both powders through a No. 60 sieve and mix lightly, but well.

Keep in well-closed containers.

COMPOUND AMMONIATED MERCURY DUSTING POWDER WITH ZINC OXIDE, BORIC ACID AND ZINC CARBONATE
(U.C.H.)

Ammoniated Mercury	20 Gm.
Zinc Oxide	235 Gm.
Boric Acid, powder	235 Gm.
Precipitated Zinc Carbonate	235 Gm.
Purified Talc	275 Gm.
To make	1000 Gm.

Mix intimately in a mortar and pass through a No. 60 sieve. To be used as a dusting powder.

ANDERSON'S DUSTING POWDER
Pulvis Inspersorius, Andersonii
(P.F.)

Camphor, in fine powder	120 Gm.
Starch	580 Gm.
Zinc Oxide	300 Gm.
To make	1000 Gm.

Mix intimately and pass through a No. 60 sieve.

ASTRINGENT DUSTING POWDER
Tannic Acid, Alum and Boric Acid Dusting Powder
(G.H.N.Y.)

Tannic Acid	100 Gm.
Alum	100 Gm.
Boric Acid	800 Gm.
To make	1000 Gm.

Mix thoroughly and pass through a No. 60 sieve.

BISMUTH SUBGALLATE DUSTING POWDER
(E.B. IV)

Bismuth Subgallate	200 Gm.
Starch	100 Gm.
Purified Talc	700 Gm.
To make	1000 Gm.

Mix intimately and pass through a No. 60 sieve.

BORATED DUSTING POWDER
(F.M.G.)

Boric Acid, in fine powder	100 Gm.
Purified Talc	200 Gm.
Rice Starch	700 Gm.
To make	1000 Gm.

Mix intimately and pass through a No. 60 sieve.

BORIC ACID, BISMUTH AND CALOMEL DUSTING POWDER
A.B.C. Powder
(P.F.)

Boric Acid, in fine powder,
Bismuth Subnitrate,
Mild Mercurous Chloride, of each, an equal weight.

Mix intimately and pass through a No. 60 sieve.

BORIC ACID AND IODOFORM DUSTING POWDER
Pulvis Iodoformi et Acidi Borici
(B.P.C. 1934)

Iodoform, in fine powder	250 Gm.
Boric Acid, in fine powder.	750 Gm.
To make	1000 Gm.

Mix intimately and pass through a No. 60 sieve.

COMPOUND BORIC ACID AND LYCOPODIUM DUSTING POWDER WITH BISMUTH SUBNITRATE AND ZINC OXIDE
Pulvis Acidi Borici et Lycopodii Compositus
(P.F.)

Boric Acid, in fine powder,
Bismuth Subnitrate,
Zinc Oxide,
Lycopodium, of each, an equal weight.

Mix intimately and pass through a No. 60 sieve.

BORIC ACID AND MENTHOL DUSTING POWDER
(R.B. I)

Menthol, in fine powder.	6 Gm.
Boric Acid, in fine powder	400 Gm.
Purified Talc	594 Gm.
To make	1000 Gm.

Mix intimately and pass through a No. 60 sieve.

BORIC ACID AND STARCH DUSTING POWDER
Pulvis Acidi Borici et Amyli
(B.P.C. 1934)

Boric Acid, in fine powder.
Starch, of each, an equal weight.

Mix intimately and pass through a No. 60 sieve.

BORIC ACID AND TALC DUSTING POWDER WITH MENTHOL AND THYMOL
(R.B. I)

Menthol, in fine powder.	5 Gm.
Thymol, in fine powder	5 Gm.
Boric Acid, in fine powder.	200 Gm.
Purified Talc	790 Gm.
Oil of Rose Geranium	2 cc.
To make about	1000 Gm.

Mix the menthol, thymol and oil with 500 Gm. of purified talc, add the boric acid and the remainder of the purified talc and pass through a No. 60 sieve.

COMPOUND BORIC ACID AND ZINC DUSTING POWDER
Pulvis Acidi Borici et Zinci Oxidi Compositus
(P.F.)

Boric Acid, in fine powder.	100 Gm.
Zinc Oxide	300 Gm.
Starch	600 Gm.
To make	1000 Gm.

Mix intimately and pass through a No. 60 sieve.

The starch may be replaced by purified talc if desired.

COMPOUND CALOMEL AND BISMUTH SUBNITRATE DUSTING POWDER
(B.N.Y.)

Mild Mercurous Chloride,
Bismuth Subnitrate,
Starch, of each, an equal weight.

Mix intimately and pass through a No. 60 sieve.

CALOMEL, ZINC AND STARCH DUSTING POWDER
(N.Y.H.F.)

Mild Mercurous Chloride,
Zinc Oxide,
Starch, of each, an equal weight.

Mix thoroughly and pass through a No. 60 sieve.

COMPOUND SALICYLIC ACID DUSTING POWDER WITH BORIC ACID, THYMOL, AND ZINC OXIDE
Pulvis Acidi Salicylici Compositus
(R.B. I)

Thymol, in fine powder	10 Gm.
Salicylic Acid, in fine powder	30 Gm.
Boric Acid	150 Gm.
Zinc Oxide	120 Gm.
Purified Talc	690 Gm.
To make	1000 Gm.

Triturate the thymol with the purified talc, add the salicylic acid and then the boric acid and zinc oxide. Mix and pass through a No. 60 sieve.

SALICYLIC AND BENZOIC ACID DUSTING POWDER
(U.C.H.)

Salicylic Acid	25	Gm.
Benzoic Acid	25	Gm.
Chlorothymol	0.4	Gm.
Purified Talc	949.6	Gm.
To make about	1000	Gm.

Mix the powders intimately and pass through a No. 60 sieve.

S.B.Z. DUSTING POWDER
(P.H.N.Y.)

Salicylic Acid, in fine powder	250 Gm.
Bismuth Subnitrate	250 Gm.
Zinc Oxide	500 Gm.
To make	1000 Gm.

Mix thoroughly and pass through a No. 60 sieve.

BORO-SALICYLATED TALC DUSTING POWDER
Pulvis Talci Compositus

Pulvis Talci Salicylicus, Boro-Salicylated Powder of Talc
(N.F. V)

Salicylic Acid, in very fine powder	30 Gm.
Boric Acid, in very fine powder	100 Gm.
Purified Talc, in very fine powder	870 Gm.
To make	1000 Gm.

Mix intimately and pass through a No. 60 sieve.

COMPOUND TALC DUSTING POWDER
(R.B. I)

Boric Acid, in fine powder	100 Gm.
Zinc Stearate	100 Gm.
Magnesium Carbonate	100 Gm.
Zinc Oxide	200 Gm.
Purified Talc	500 Gm.
To make	1000 Gm.

Mix intimately and pass through a No. 60 sieve.

THIERSCH'S POWDER
Pulvis Boro-Salicylatus
Boro-Salicylated Powder

Salicylic Acid, in fine powder	110 Gm.
Boric Acid, in fine powder.	890 Gm.
To make	1000 Gm.

Mix intimately and pass through a No. 60 sieve.

THYMOL IODIDE DUSTING POWDER WITH BORIC ACID AND TALC
(U.C.H.)

Thymol Iodide	250 Gm.
Boric Acid, in fine powder.	250 Gm.
Purified Talc, a sufficient quantity,	
To make	1000 Gm.

Mix the powders intimately and pass through a No. 60 sieve.

THYMOL IODIDE DUSTING POWDER WITH BISMUTH SUBGALLATE AND BORIC ACID
(N.Y.H.F.)

Thymol Iodide	100 Gm.
Bismuth Subgallate	200 Gm.
Boric Acid, in fine powder.	700 Gm.
To make	1000 Gm.

Mix intimately and pass through a No. 60 sieve.

ZINC AND BORIC ACID DUSTING POWDER
Pulvis Zinci et Acidi Borici
(B.P.C. 1934)

Zinc Oxide,
Boric Acid, in fine powder, of each, an equal weight.

Mix intimately and pass through a No. 60 sieve.

ZINC AND STARCH DUSTING POWDER
Pulvis Zinci et Amyli
(B.P.C. 1934)

Zinc Oxide,
Starch, of each, an equal weight.

Mix intimately and pass through a No. 60 sieve.

BENZOINATED ZINC AND STARCH DUSTING POWDER WITH BORIC ACID
(Lux. F.)

Zinc Oxide	300 Gm.
Starch	300 Gm.
Purified Talc	300 Gm.
Tincture of Benzoin	100 cc.
Theobroma Oil, grated	60 Gm.
Boric Acid	30 Gm.
To make about	1000 Gm.

Triturate the first four ingredients together and allow to dry. Add the other ingredients, mix thoroughly and pass through a No. 60 sieve.

COMPOUND ZINC AND STARCH DUSTING POWDER
Pulvis Zinci et Amyli Compositus
(B.P.C. 1934)

Zinc Oxide	250 Gm.
Starch	250 Gm.
Boric Acid, in fine powder	250 Gm.
Purified Talc	250 Gm.
Oil of Rose Geranium	2 cc.
To make about	1000 Gm.

Triturate the oil of rose geranium with the powders until mixed intimately, then pass through a No. 60 sieve.

SALICYLATED ZINC, STARCH AND TALC DUSTING POWDER
(Ph. Aust.)

Salicylic Acid, in fine powder	20 Gm.
Orris, in fine powder	100 Gm.
Zinc Oxide	200 Gm.
Starch	280 Gm.
Purified Talc	400 Gm.
To make	1000 Gm.

Mix intimately and pass through a No. 60 sieve.

COMPOUND ZINC OLEOSTEARATE DUSTING POWDER
(B.P.C. 1934)

Zinc Oleostearate, in fine powder	250 Gm.
Boric Acid, in fine powder	250 Gm.
Starch	500 Gm.
Oil of Rose Geranium	1 cc.
To make about	1000 Gm.

Triturate the oil of rose geranium with the powders, then pass through a No. 60 sieve.

COMPOUND ZINC STEARATE DUSTING POWDER
Pulvis Zinci Stearatis Compositus
(Austral. Ph. F.)

Zinc Stearate	247 Gm.
Starch	247 Gm.
Boric Acid, in fine powder.	247 Gm.
Lycopodium.	247 Gm.
Camphor, in fine powder	12 Gm.
To make	1000 Gm.

Mix intimately and pass through a No. 60 sieve.

POWDERS, MISCELLANEOUS

ALKALINE POWDER
N. B. B. C. Powder
(G.H.N.Y.)

Sodium Bicarbonate,
Sodium Borate,
Sodium Chloride, of each, an equal weight.

Mix intimately and pass through a No. 60 sieve.

For use as a nose wash or gargle, 1 teaspoonful is dissolved in a tumblerful of warm water.

COMPOUND LOBELIA POWDER
(Sir M. Mackenzie)

Lobelia, in coarse powder	230 Gm.
Stramonium, in coarse powder.	230 Gm.
Tea Leaves, in coarse powder	230 Gm.
Potassium Nitrate, in coarse powder	230 Gm.
Anise, in coarse powder.	40 Gm.
Fennel, in coarse powder	40 Gm.
To make	1000 Gm.

Mix intimately.

For use, ½ to 1 teaspoonful is burned and the fumes are inhaled.

LOBELIA AND STRAMONIUM POWDER
I
(Ext. Ph.)

Lobelia, in coarse powder,
Stramonium, in coarse powder,
Black Tea Leaves, in coarse powder,
Potassium Nitrate, in coarse powder, of each, an equal weight.

Mix intimately.

For use, ½ to 1 teaspoonful is burned and the fumes are inhaled.

II
(Ext. Ph.)

Lobelia, in coarse powder	250 Gm.
Stramonium, in coarse powder	250 Gm.
Tea Leaves, in coarse powder	250 Gm.
Potassium Nitrate, in coarse powder	250 Gm.
Oil of Anise	4 cc.
Oil of Fennel	4 cc.
To make about	1000 Gm.

Mix the powdered drugs intimately and incorporate the oils of anise and fennel.

For use, ½ to 1 teaspoonful is burned and the fumes are inhaled.

COMPOUND STRAMONIUM POWDER
Pulvis Stramonii Compositus
I
(B.P.C. 1934)

Stramonium, in coarse powder	500 Gm.
Anise, in coarse powder	120 Gm.
Lobelia, in coarse powder	60 Gm.
Tea Leaves, in coarse powder	60 Gm.
Oil of Eucalyptus	10 cc.
Potassium Nitrate, in coarse powder	260 Gm.
To make about	1000 Gm.

Mix the oil with the vegetable powders, add the potassium nitrate and pass through a coarse sieve.

For use, ½ teaspoonful is burned and the fumes are inhaled.

II
(P.F.)

Stramonium, in coarse powder	500 Gm.
Potassium Nitrate, in coarse powder	250 Gm.
Anise, in coarse powder	250 Gm.
To make	1000 Gm.

Mix intimately.

For use, ½ to 1 teaspoonful is burned and the fumes are inhaled.

COMPOUND STRAMONIUM AND CASCARILLA POWDER
(P.H.N.Y.)

Stramonium, in coarse powder.	440 Gm.
Cascarilla, in coarse powder	120 Gm.
Potassium Nitrate, in coarse powder	220 Gm.
Ipecac, in coarse powder	220 Gm.
To make	1000 Gm.

Mix on a flat surface or pass repeatedly through a sieve.

For use, ½ to 1 teaspoonful is burned and the fumes are inhaled.

SOAPS

LIQUID SOAP
Sapo Liquidus
(R.B. I)

Sodium Hydroxide.	16 Gm.
Potassium Hydroxide	16 Gm.
Coconut Oil	40 Gm.
Cottonseed Oil	175 cc.
Alcohol	100 cc.
Water, a sufficient quantity,	
To make	1000 cc.

Dissolve the potassium hydroxide and sodium hydroxide in 100 cc. of water, add the alcohol and then the mixed oils in three or four portions, agitating frequently until saponification has been completed. Then add sufficient water to make the product measure 1000 cc. and mix.

ETHEREAL LIQUID SOAP
(R.B. I)

Soft Soap	320 Gm.
Alcohol	200 cc.
Ethyl Oxide, a sufficient quantity,	
To make	1000 cc.

Digest the soap in the alcohol, using gentle heat. When solution is effected and the liquid has cooled, add sufficient ethyl oxide to make the product measure 1000 cc. and mix thoroughly.

COMPOUND ETHEREAL LIQUID SOAP
(R.B. I)

Oleic Acid.	220 cc.
Alcohol	95 cc.
Oil of Lavender	2 cc.
Potassium Hydroxide, the required quantity,	
Ethyl Oxide, a sufficient quantity,	
To make	1000 cc.

Mix the oleic acid and alcohol and neutralize the mixture with a saturated solution of potassium hydroxide (of which about 47 cc., equivalent to 47 Gm. KOH, is required), using phenolphthalein as indicator. Allow the neutralized product to cool and add the oil and sufficient ethyl oxide to make the product measure 1000 cc.

SURGICAL LIQUID SOAP
(R.B. I)

Cottonseed Oil . . . .   210 cc.
Coconut Oil . . . .   95 Gm.
Alcohol . . . .   190 cc.
Sodium Hydroxide . . . .   43 Gm.
Potassium Carbonate . . . .   10 Gm.
Ethyl Oxide . . . .   15 cc.
Liquefied Phenol . . . .   25 cc.
Water, a sufficient quantity,

To make . . . .   1000 cc.

Mix the oils thoroughly with the alcohol and 100 cc. of water. Dissolve the potassium carbonate and sodium hydroxide in 300 cc. of water. Mix the two solutions and warm until saponification is complete. Cool, add the ethyl oxide, phenol and sufficient water to make the product measure 1000 cc.

COTTONSEED OIL SOFT SOAP
(R.B. II)

Cottonseed Oil . . . .   430 Gm.
Potassium Hydroxide . . . .   86 Gm.
Alcohol . . . .   50 cc.
Water, a sufficient quantity,

To make . . . .   1000 Gm.

Dissolve the potassium hydroxide in 100 cc. of water in a tared, capacious dish with the aid of heat. Add the cottonseed oil immediately to the hot solution and stir the mixture actively for a few moments. Reapply the heat and, at the first evidence of froth from boiling, pour in the alcohol, stir it actively until the froth suddenly rises, then withdraw the heat and again stir until the soap assumes the consistency of a paste. Determine* whether the product will contain the required excess of potassium hydroxide when distilled water is added to make 1000 Gm. If the product does not meet the requirements, add more potassium hydroxide or cottonseed oil as may be needed and again heat until saponification is complete. Finally add sufficient water to make the product weigh 1000 Gm. and warm gently, stirring carefully, until the water is all absorbed and a clear soap results.

*Dissolve about 5 Gm. of the soap, accurately weighed, in 100 cc. of hot alcohol, collect the residue, if any, on a filter, wash thoroughly with hot alcohol and dry to constant weight at 100° C. The dried residue is not more than 3 per cent of the weight of soap taken. The combined filtrate and washings, on the addition of 0.5 cc. of phenolphthalein T.S. and titration with tenth-normal sulfuric acid, show not less than 0.1 per cent and not more than 0.25 per cent of KOH. One cc. of tenth-normal sulfuric acid is equivalent to 0.0056 Gm. of KOH.

UNNA'S SALVE SOAP
Mollinum
(R.B. I)

Lard	382 Gm.
Potassium Hydroxide.	54 Gm.
Alcohol	38 Gm.
Water	382 cc.
Glycerin	144 Gm.
To make	1000 Gm.

Dissolve the potassium hydroxide in the water at about 70° C. and add the alcohol. Add to this the melted lard, little by little, shaking frequently until saponification is complete. Set aside for 12 hours at 50° to 60° C. and add the glycerin.

NOTE—This white soap, containing about 12 per cent excess of fat, is used as a basis for ointments for rapid absorption. It is readily washed off with water with which it forms a lather, leaving the skin fresh and supple. It leaves no grease spots on linens.

SOLUTIONS

ADLER'S SOLUTION
(P.F.)

Sodium Chloride.	5.90 Gm.
Sodium Bicarbonate	3.51 Gm.
Potassium Chloride.	0.40 Gm.
Calcium Chloride.	0.40 Gm.
Magnesium Chloride	0.25 Gm.
Sodium Biphosphate	0.12 Gm.
Dextrose	1.50 Gm.
Ampul Water, a sufficient quantity,	
To make	1000 cc.

Dissolve the salts in 750 cc. of distilled water with as little agitation as possible. Add the dextrose and sufficient ampul water to make the product measure 1000 cc. Strain through gauze and sterilize by Process D (see N.F. VII, page 35).

SOLUTION OF ALUMINUM ACETICO-TARTRATE
Liquor Aluminis Acetico-Tartratis
(N.F. IV)

Ammonium Alum	750 Gm.
Monohydrated Sodium Carbonate	300 Gm.
Glacial Acetic Acid.	150 Gm.
Tartaric Acid	135 Gm.
Water, a sufficient quantity,	
To make	1000 Gm.

Dissolve the alum and monohydrated sodium carbonate each in 10,000 cc. of water, mix the solutions and wash the precipitate with water, first by decantation, and afterwards on a strainer, until the washings are free from sulfate. Allow the precipitate to drain and to shrink in volume by exposure on the strainer, then transfer it to a tared dish, add the glacial acetic acid and the tartaric acid and apply heat until solution is effected. Finally, evaporate the liquid until it weighs 1000 Gm.

SOLUTION OF AMMONIUM CHLORIDE

Ammonium Chloride	50 Gm.
Glycerin	500 cc.
Anise Water	250 cc.
Peppermint Water, a sufficient quantity,	
To make	1000 cc.

Dissolve the ammonium chloride in the anise water, add the glycerin and sufficient peppermint water to make 1000 cc.

AVERAGE DOSE—Metric, 4 cc.—Apothecaries, 1 fluidrachm.

NOTE—A sugar-free solution of ammonium chloride intended for diabetics.

SOLUTION OF AMMONIUM CITRATE
Liquor Ammonii Citratis
(N.F. IV)

Citric Acid	125 Gm.
Diluted Solution of Ammonia, the required quantity,	
Distilled Water, a sufficient quantity,	
To make	1000 cc.

Dissolve the citric acid in 600 cc. of distilled water and cautiously add sufficient diluted solution of ammonia to produce a solution neutral to litmus paper. Cool the solution, add sufficient distilled water to make the product measure 1000 cc. and filter.

Keep in bottles free from lead.

AVERAGE DOSE—Metric, 4 cc.—Apothecaries, 1 fluidrachm.

CLEMENS' SOLUTION OF ARSENIC
Liquor Arsenicalis, Clemens
Liquor Potassii Arsenatis et Bromidi

Solution of Potassium Arsenate and Bromide
(N.F. IV)

Arsenic Trioxide	10 Gm.
Potassium Bicarbonate	40.5 Gm.
Bromine	5 cc.
Distilled Water, a sufficient quantity,	
To make	1000 cc.

Boil the arsenic trioxide with the potassium bicarbonate and 200 cc. of distilled water, until solution is effected. Allow this to cool, add 500 cc. of distilled water, then the bromine and afterwards sufficient distilled water to make the product measure 1000 cc. Allow the mixture to stand during 12 hours, agitating occasionally, then filter.

AVERAGE DOSE—Metric, 0.2 cc.—Apothecaries, 3 minims.

COMPOUND SOLUTION OF ATROPINE SULFATE
(R.B. I)

Atropine Sulfate	2	Gm.
Salicylic Acid	0.25	Gm.
Distilled Water, a sufficient quantity,		
To make	100	cc.

Dissolve and filter.

SOLUTION OF BISMUTH AND AMMONIUM CITRATE
Liquor Bismuthi et Ammonii Citratis
(B.P.C. 1934)

Bismuth Subnitrate.	70 Gm.
Citric Acid, in powder.	52 Gm.
Diluted Solution of Ammonia, the required quantity,	
Distilled Water, a sufficient quantity,	
To make	1000 cc.

Mix the citric acid with the bismuth subnitrate and 2 cc. of distilled water. Heat on a water bath until a small portion is completely soluble in diluted solution of ammonia. Transfer to a filter and wash with distilled water until the washings give no reaction for nitrate. Add to the washed residue just sufficient diluted solution of ammonia to dissolve it and then add sufficient distilled water to make the product measure 1000 cc.

AVERAGE DOSE—Metric, 2 to 4 cc.—Apothecaries, ½ to 1 fluidrachm.

NOTE—It is necessary that the citric acid contain its exact requirement for water of crystallization.

BONAIN'S SOLUTION
Bonain's Mixture
(Cod. Fr.)

Phenol,
Cocaine,
Menthol, of each, an equal weight.

Mix until liquefied.

BORO-SALICYLATED SOLUTION
Liquor Boro-Salicylatus
(Thiersch)

Salicylic Acid	2 Gm.
Boric Acid, crystals	12 Gm.
Distilled Water, a sufficient quantity,	
To make	1000 cc.

Dissolve and filter if necessary.

SOLUTION OF THREE BROMIDES
(N.Y.H.F.)

Sodium Bromide.	80 Gm.
Potassium Bromide.	80 Gm.
Ammonium Bromide	80 Gm.
Distilled Water, a sufficient quantity,	
To make	1000 cc.

Dissolve, and filter if necessary.

AVERAGE DOSE—Metric, 4 cc.—Apothecaries, 1 fluidrachm.

NOTE—This preparation is not to be confused with Elixir of Three Bromides, N.F. VII.

COMPOUND SOLUTION OF BROMIDES WITH POTASSIUM ARSENITE
(V.C.N.Y.)

Sodium Bromide.	162 Gm.
Potassium Bromide.	162 Gm.
Ammonium Bromide	81 Gm.
Sodium Bicarbonate	32 Gm.
Solution of Potassium Arsenite	15 cc.
Distilled Water, a sufficient quantity,	
To make	1000 cc.

Dissolve the bromides and the sodium bicarbonate in 750 cc. of distilled water. Add the solution of potassium arsenite and sufficient distilled water to make the product measure 1000 cc. Filter if necessary.

AVERAGE DOSE—Metric, 4 cc.—Apothecaries, 1 fluidrachm.

SOLUTION OF BROMINE
Liquor Bromi

Smith's Solution of Bromine
(N.F. IV)

Bromine . . . .   83 cc.
Potassium Bromide.   125 Gm.
Distilled Water, a sufficient quantity,

　　　　　　　To make . . . .   1000 cc.

Dissolve the potassium bromide in 800 cc. of distilled water contained in a bottle, add the bromine and shake the mixture until solution is effected.   Finally add sufficient distilled water to make the product measure 1000 cc.

Keep in glass-stoppered bottles in a dark place.

SOLUTION OF CALCIUM CHLORIDE
(N.Y.H.F.)

Calcium Chloride . . . .   150 Gm.
Distilled Water, a sufficient quantity,

　　　　　　　To make . . . .   1000 cc.

Dissolve and filter if necessary.

AVERAGE DOSE—Metric, 4 cc.—Apothecaries, 1 fluidrachm.

SOLUTION OF CALCIUM HYDROCHLOROPHOSPHATE
Liquor Calcii Hydrochlorophosphatis

Soluté Calcii Chlorhydrophosphatis

Solution de chlorhydrophosphate calcique, Pautauberge
(Lux. F.)

Precipitated Calcium Phosphate . . . .   20 Gm.
Hydrochloric Acid . . . .   15 cc.
Distilled Water, a sufficient quantity,

　　　　　　　To make . . . .   1000 cc.

Dissolve the calcium phosphate in the mixed liquids without the application of heat.

AVERAGE DOSE—Metric, 4 cc.—Apothecaries, 1 fluidrachm.

SOLUTION OF CAMPHOR AND PHENOL
(Chlumsky)
(P.H.N.Y.)

Camphor . . . .   600 Gm.
Phenol . . . .   300 Gm.
Alcohol . . . .   125 cc.

　　　　　　　To make about . . . .   1000 Gm.

Triturate the camphor and phenol together and then add the alcohol.

CASEIN SOLUTION
(R.B. I)

Casein	1 Gm.
Monohydrated Sodium Carbonate	1 Gm.
Chloroform	1 cc.
Distilled Water, a sufficient quantity,	
To make	1000 cc.

Dissolve the casein with the aid of the monohydrated sodium carbonate in 900 cc. of distilled water. Add the chloroform and sufficient distilled water to make the product measure 1000 cc. Filter if necessary.

SOLUTION OF CHLORINATED LIME AND BORIC ACID

Eusol
(B.P.C. 1934)

Chlorinated Lime	12.5 Gm.
Boric Acid	12.5 Gm.
Distilled Water, a sufficient quantity,	
To make	1000 cc.

Mix. Allow to stand 12 hours and filter.

SOLUTION OF CHLORAL AND SODIUM BROMIDE
(B.N.Y.)

Chloral Hydrate	60 Gm.
Sodium Bromide	120 Gm.
Distilled Water, a sufficient quantity,	
To make	1000 cc.

Dissolve the chloral hydrate and sodium bromide in the distilled water.

AVERAGE DOSE—Metric, 4 cc.—Apothecaries, 1 fluidrachm.

DEODORIZING CLEANSING SOLUTION
(R.B. I)

Thymol.	2 Gm.
Oil of Dwarf Pine Needles	2 cc.
Oil of Peppermint	2 cc.
Alcohol	60 cc.
Liniment of Soft Soap	30 cc.
Water, a sufficient quantity,	
To make	1000 cc.

Dissolve the thymol and oils in the alcohol. Add the liniment and finally sufficient water to make the product measure 1000 cc.

COMPOUND SOLUTION OF CREOSOTE
(R.B. I)

Calcium Hydrochlorophosphate	30	Gm.
Hydrochloric Acid	6	cc.
Creosote	7.5	cc.
Glycerin	100	cc
Alcohol	100	cc.
Crocated Tincture of Opium, R.B.	5	cc.
Distilled Water, a sufficient quantity,		
To make	1000	cc.

Dissolve the creosote in the alcohol and glycerin and the calcium hydrochlorophosphate in 500 cc. of distilled water, adding the hydrochloric acid and crocated tincture of opium. Mix the two liquids and add sufficient distilled water to make the product measure 1000 cc.

AVERAGE DOSE—Metric, 8 cc.—Apothecaries, 2 fluidrachms.

DAKIN'S SOLUTION
(Original)
(R.B. I)

Boric Acid	4 Gm.
Chlorinated Lime	20 Gm.
Exsiccated Sodium Carbonate	14 Gm.
Distilled Water	1000 cc.
To make about	1000 cc.

Dissolve the exsiccated sodium carbonate in the distilled water and add the chlorinated lime. Set aside for about 1 hour, siphon off the clear liquid and in this dissolve the boric acid.

NOTE—This preparation is not to be confused with Diluted Solution of Sodium Hypochlorite (Modified Dakin's Solution), N.F. VII, which is to be dispensed when Dakin's Solution is ordered.

DORANTI'S SOLUTION
(R.B. II)

Iodine	9 Gm.
Guaiacol	18 cc.
Creosote	44 cc.
Alcohol	50 cc.
Glycerin, a sufficient quantity,	
To make	1000 cc.

Triturate the iodine well with the guaiacol and creosote in a glass mortar and pour into a bottle. Mix the alcohol with any undissolved iodine remaining in the mortar and add to the first solution. Add sufficient glycerin to make the product measure 1000 cc. and mix thoroughly by shaking.

SAPONACEOUS SOLUTION OF EUCALYPTUS
Liquor Eucalypti Saponatus
(Austral. Ph. F.)

Oil of Eucalyptus.	765 cc.
Medicinal Soft Soap	31 Gm.
Distilled Water	204 cc.
To make about	1000 cc.

Triturate the medicinal soft soap thoroughly in a mortar with a small quantity of the oil until a thin transparent paste is produced. Add to this a small quantity of the distilled water so as to form an emulsion. Add more oil gradually with constant stirring till the emulsion is at the breaking point. Thin this with a few drops of distilled water and continue to add the oil and water alternately, until all the oil has been added; finally incorporate the remainder of the distilled water.

SOLUTION OF FERRIC ACETATE
Liquor Ferri Acetatis
(N.F. IV)

Solution of Ferric Sulfate	800 Gm.
Glacial Acetic Acid.	260 Gm.
Diluted Solution of Ammonia	850 cc.
Water, the required quantity,	
Distilled Water, a sufficient quantity,	
To make	1000 Gm.

Mix the diluted solution of ammonia with 3000 cc. of cold water and the solution of ferric sulfate with 10,000 cc. of cold water. Add the latter solution slowly to the diluted ammonia solution, stirring constantly. Allow the mixture to stand until the precipitate has subsided as far as practicable and decant the supernatant liquid. Add to the precipitate 6000 cc. of boiling water, mix well, again set the mixture aside and decant as before. Repeat the washing with successive portions of boiling water, in the same manner, until the washings are no longer effected by barium chloride T.S. Transfer the mixture to a wet muslin strainer, allow the precipitate to drain completely and press it, folded in the strainer, until its weight is reduced to 700 Gm. or less. Now add the precipitate gradually to the glacial acetic acid, contained in a tared jar provided with a glass stopper, stirring the mixture after each addition until the magma added is nearly dissolved before adding another portion. Finally, add sufficient distilled water to make the product weigh 1000 Gm., allow it to become clear by subsidence and decant the clear solution.

Keep in well-stoppered bottles, in a cool place, protected from light.

AVERAGE DOSE—Metric, 0.3 cc.—Apothecaries, 5 minims.

SOLUTION OF FERRIC CITRATE
Liquor Ferri Citratis
(N.F. V)

Solution of Ferric Sulfate	730 cc.
Citric Acid	375 Gm.
Diluted Solution of Ammonia	1100 cc.
Water, a sufficient quantity,	
Distilled Water, a sufficient quantity,	
To make	1000 cc.

Mix the diluted solution of ammonia with 3000 cc. of cold water, and the solution of ferric sulfate with 10,000 cc. of cold water. Add the latter solution slowly to the dilute ammonia solution, stirring constantly. Pour the mixture upon a wet muslin strainer, and allow the liquid to run off and the precipitate to drain. Remove the moist mass from the strainer, mix it well with 6000 cc. of cold water, again pour it on the strainer and let it drain. Repeat this washing with several successive portions of cold distilled water, in the same manner, until the washings cease to produce more than a faint cloudiness with barium chloride T.S. Allow the precipitate to drain completely, transfer it to a porcelain dish, add the citric acid and heat the mixture on a water bath to 60° C., stirring constantly until the magma is dissolved. Lastly, filter the liquid and evaporate it, at the above-mentioned temperature, until it measures 1000 cc.

AVERAGE DOSE—Metric, 0.6 cc.—Apothecaries, 10 minims.

SOLUTION OF FERRIC OXYCHLORIDE
Liquor Ferri Oxychloridi
(N.F. IV)

Solution of Ferric Chloride	300 cc.
Diluted Solution of Ammonia	600 cc.
Glycerin	125 cc.
Hydrochloric Acid	30 cc.
Water, a sufficient quantity,	
Distilled Water, a sufficient quantity,	
To make	1000 cc.

Add the solution of ferric chloride, previously diluted with 1500 cc. of distilled water, to the diluted solution of ammonia, previously diluted with 3000 cc. of distilled water, with constant stirring. Allow the mixture to stand until the precipitate has subsided, then decant the supernatant liquid and repeat the washing by decantation with water 3 times. Now collect the precipitate on a strainer and wash it with distilled water until the washings give only a faint opalescence with silver nitrate T.S. Drain the precipitate, express and discard the excess of liquid, transfer it to an evaporating dish, add the hydrochloric acid, and stir the mixture occasionally during 3 days. If necessary, warm the mixture to 40° C. to effect solution. Allow it to cool, add the glycerin and then sufficient distilled water to make the product measure 1000 cc. and filter.

Keep in small, well-stoppered bottles in a cool place, protected from sunlight.

AVERAGE DOSE—Metric, 2 cc.—Apothecaries, 30 minims.

SOLUTION OF FERRIC OXYSULFATE
Liquor Ferri Oxysulfatis
(N.F. IV)

Ferrous Sulfate	165 Gm.
Nitric Acid	118 cc.
Distilled Water, a sufficient quantity,	
To make	1000 cc.

Dissolve the ferrous sulfate in 850 cc. of boiling distilled water in a flask, add gradually the nitric acid and heat until the escaping vapors cease to have a nitrous odor. When the reaction is complete, allow the liquid to cool and add sufficient distilled water to make the product measure 1000 cc.

SOLUTION OF FERROUS CHLORIDE
Liquor Ferri Protochloridi
Solution of Protochloride of Iron
(N.F. IV)

Iron, in the form of bright, fine wire	160 Gm.
Hydrochloric Acid	540 cc.
Glycerin	250 cc.
Hypophosphorous Acid	3 cc.
Distilled Water, a sufficient quantity,	
To make	1000 cc.

To the iron contained in a flask add 350 cc. of distilled water and the hydrochloric acid, and apply gentle heat until effervescence ceases. Then heat the liquid to boiling, keep it at this temperature for a short time so that the iron may be brought into solution as far as possible and filter the solution through purified cotton, washing the flask and cotton with a little distilled water. Evaporate the filtrate on a steam bath until crystals begin to form and the escaping vapors cease to redden, or only slightly affect moistened blue litmus paper. Add the glycerin and hypophosphorous acid and continue the heat, if necessary, until the crystals are redissolved. When the liquid is cool, add sufficient distilled water to make the product measure 1000 cc.

AVERAGE DOSE—Metric, 0.6 cc.—Apothecaries, 10 minims.

NOTE—This solution should be freshly prepared.

FISCHER'S SOLUTION
(R.B. I)

Monohydrated Sodium Carbonate	5 Gm.
Sodium Chloride	14 Gm.
Ampul Water, a sufficient quantity,	
To make	1000 cc.

Dissolve the salts in the ampul water, strain through fine gauze and sterilize by Process D (see N.F. VII, page 35).

SOLUTION OF GELATIN FOR INJECTION
Soluté de Gélatine Injectable
Soluté Salin de Gélatine
(Cod. Fr.)

Gelatin	10 Gm.
Sodium Chloride.	8 Gm.
Distilled Water, a sufficient quantity,	
To make	1000 Gm.

Introduce successively into a tared flat-bottomed flask of 1500 cc. capacity the gelatin, sodium chloride and 500 cc. of distilled water, and heat on a water bath. Test the reaction with litmus paper; if it be acid, neutralize accurately by the addition, drop by drop, of tenth-normal sodium hydroxide, then add sufficient distilled water to make the product weigh 1000 Gm.   Maintain the flask for 15 minutes at 115° C. in an autoclave, calculating the time from the moment when this temperature is reached.   Filter the liquid while hot through a germ-proof filter and fill it into previously sterilized 100 cc. containers, seal and place them in an autoclave for 15 minutes at 115° C., counting the time from the moment when this temperature is reached.

GLYCERINATED SOLUTION OF GUAIACOL
(P.H.N.Y.)

Guaiacol	430 cc.
Glycerin	430 cc.
Tincture of Myrrh	130 cc.
Oil of Cinnamon.	10 cc.
To make about	1000 cc.

Mix.

For use, 1 teaspoonful is diluted with a tumblerful of water.

SOLUTION OF GUTTA PERCHA
Liquor Guttæ Perchæ
Traumaticin
(N.F. IV)

Gutta Percha, in thin slices	150 Gm.
Chloroform	1000 cc.
Lead Carbonate, in fine powder	170 Gm.
To make about	1000 cc.

Add the gutta percha to 750 cc. of the chloroform contained in a bottle, stopper tightly and shake occasionally until the gutta percha is dissolved.   Then add the lead carbonate, previously mixed with the remainder of the chloroform, and, having shaken the whole together several times, at intervals of half an hour, set the mixture aside until the insoluble matter has subsided and the solution has become clear.   Decant the clear liquid.

Keep in small, cork-stoppered bottles.

COMPOUND GUTTA PERCHA SOLUTION WITH CHRYSAROBIN
Liquor Guttæ Perchæ Compositus
Chrysarobin Traumaticin
(R.B. I)

Chrysarobin.	50 Gm.
Solution of Gutta Percha, R.B., a sufficient quantity,	
To make	1000 cc.

Dissolve.

HARRINGTON'S SOLUTION
(R.B. I)

Mercury Bichloride	0.8	Gm.
Hydrochloric Acid	60	cc.
Distilled Water	300	cc.
Alcohol, a sufficient quantity,		
To make	1000	cc.

Mix the hydrochloric acid with the distilled water and dissolve the mercury bichloride in the mixture. Add sufficient alcohol to make the product measure 1000 cc.

SOLUTION OF HYPOPHOSPHITES
Liquor Hypophosphitum
(N.F. IV)

Calcium Hypophosphite.	35	Gm.
Sodium Hypophosphite	20	Gm.
Potassium Hypophosphite.	17.5	Gm.
Hypophosphorous Acid	6	cc.
Distilled Water, a sufficient quantity,		
To make	1000	cc.

Dissolve the hypophosphites in the mixed liquids and filter.
AVERAGE DOSE—Metric, 4 cc.—Apothecaries, 1 fluidrachm.

IODINE AND GUAIACOL SOLUTION
(N.Y.H.F.)

Iodine	10 Gm.
Potassium Iodide	20 Gm.
Guaiacol	50 cc.
Glycerin, a sufficient quantity,	
To make	1000 cc.

Triturate the iodine and potassium iodide together, adding gradually 200 cc. of the glycerin. Add the guaiacol which has been previously mixed with 500 cc. of glycerin and then sufficient glycerin to make the product measure 1000 cc.

IODO-SALICYLATE SOLUTION
(N.Y.P.G.H.)

Sodium Salicylate . . . .   62.5 Gm.
Potassium Iodide   30   Gm.
Distilled Water, a sufficient quantity,
                        To make   1000   cc.

Dissolve.

AVERAGE DOSE—Metric, 4 cc.—Apothecaries, 1 fluidrachm.

SOLUTION OF ALBUMINIZED IRON
Liquor Ferri Albuminati

Solution of Iron Albuminate
(N.F. V)

Albuminized Iron . . . .   50 Gm.
Cinnamon Water . . . .   200 cc.
Aromatic Elixir . . . .   400 cc.
Alcohol . . . .   120 cc.
Distilled Water, a sufficient quantity,
                        To make . . . .   1000 cc.

Dissolve the albuminized iron in the cinnamon water and 150 cc. of distilled water, add the aromatic elixir, the alcohol and sufficient distilled water to make the product measure 1000 cc. Allow it to stand 12 hours, and filter.

AVERAGE DOSE—Metric, 8 cc.—Apothecaries, 2 fluidrachms.

AQUEOUS SOLUTION OF KRAMERIA

Krameria   1000   Gm.
Glycerin   300   cc.
Salicylic Acid . . . .   0.65 Gm.
Distilled Water, a sufficient quantity,
                        To make   1000   cc.

Macerate the krameria with a mixture of 300 cc. of glycerin and 700 cc. of distilled water for a period of 24 hours. Pack the macerated drug in a percolator and allow the liquid to drain. Reserve this first percolate. Continue the percolation of the drug with distilled water until the drug is exhausted. Evaporate this second fraction at a low temperature until when mixed with the first percolate the product measures 1000 cc. Add the salicylic acid to the solution.

AVERAGE DOSE—Metric, 1 cc.—Apothecaries, 15 minims.

LACTIC ACID BUFFER SOLUTION
(Hartmann)
(R.B. II)

Sodium Hydroxide	2 Gm.
Lactic Acid	15 cc.
Distilled water, a sufficient quantity,	
To make	1000 cc.

Dissolve the sodium hydroxide in 100 cc. of distilled water, add the lactic acid and sufficient distilled water to make the product measure 1000 cc.

NOTE—This solution is for oral use only and is not to be confused with Hartmann's Physiological Buffer Solution.

LAVAGE SOLUTION
(P.H.N.Y.)

Sodium Chloride.	267 Gm.
Monohydrated Sodium Carbonate	40 Gm.
Distilled Water, a sufficient quantity,	
To make	1000 cc.

Dissolve.

For use, 30 cc. is added to 1000 cc. of warm water.

LOCKWOOD'S SOLUTION
Lockwood's Gastric Solution

Strontium Bromide	100 Gm.
Chloral Hydrate	16.5 Gm.
Spirit of Anise.	2.5 cc.
Chloroform Water, a sufficient quantity,	
To make	1000 cc.

Mix and dissolve.

AVERAGE DOSE—Metric, 4 cc.—Apothecaries, 1 fluidrachm.

SOLUTION OF MAGNESIUM SULFATE
(N.Y.H.F.)

Magnesium Sulfate	500 Gm.
Distilled Water, a sufficient quantity,	
To make	1000 cc.

Dissolve.

AVERAGE DOSE—Metric, 30 cc. diluted to 100 cc. with water—Apothecaries, 1 fluidounce diluted to 3 or 4 fluidounces with water.

EFFERVESCENT SOLUTION OF MAGNESIUM SULFATE
Liquor Magnesii Sulfatis Effervescens
(N.F. IV)

Magnesium Sulfate.	25	Gm.
Citric Acid	4	Gm.
Syrup of Citric Acid	60	cc.
Potassium Bicarbonate	2.5	Gm.
Distilled Water, a sufficient quantity,		
To make about	350	cc.

Dissolve the magnesium sulfate and the citric acid in 250 cc. of distilled water, add the syrup of citric acid and filter the solution into a strong bottle of about 360 cc. capacity. Then add sufficient distilled water to make 350 cc., drop in the potassium bicarbonate and immediately stopper the bottle securely. Lastly, shake the bottle occasionally until the crystals are dissolved.

AVERAGE DOSE—Metric, 350 cc.—Apothecaries, 12 fluidounces.

SOLUTION OF MAGNESIUM, POTASSIUM AND SODIUM SULFATES
(G.H.N.Y.)

Magnesium Sulfate.	100 Gm.
Potassium Sulfate	20 Gm.
Sodium Sulfate	400 Gm.
Distilled Water, a sufficient quantity,	
To make	1000 cc.

Dissolve, and filter if necessary.

AVERAGE DOSE—Metric, 4 to 8 cc.—Apothecaries, 1 to 2 fluidrachms.

MEHU SOLUTION (Test for Albumin)
(Merck Index)

Phenol	250 Gm.
Glacial Acetic Acid.	250 cc.
Alcohol, 90%, a sufficient quantity,	
To make	1000 cc.

Mix and dissolve the phenol.

NOTE—This solution will precipitate albumin in the presence of nitric or sulfuric acid. The test is carried out as follows: Add 10 cc. of the reagent and 2 cc. of nitric acid to 100 cc. of the liquid to be tested. If albumin is present a flocculent precipitate will form.

MENCIERE'S SOLUTION
(R.B. I)

Guaiacol . . . . 45 cc.
Iodoform . . . . • . . . 50 Gm.
Eucalyptol . . . . 55 cc.
Alcohol . . . . 60 cc.
Peruvian Balsam. . . . . 150 Gm.
Ethyl Oxide, a sufficient quantity,

To make . . . . 1000 cc.

Mix.

SOLUTION OF MERCURIC NITRATE
Liquor Hydrargyri Nitratis
(R.B. II)

Red Mercuric Oxide . . . . 830 Gm.
Nitric Acid . . . . 660 cc.
Distilled Water . . . . 310 cc.

To make about . . . . 1000 cc.

Mix the nitric acid with the distilled water and dissolve the red mercuric oxide in the mixture.

Keep in glass-stoppered bottles.

SOLUTION OF MERCURIC AND POTASSIUM IODIDES
Liquor Hydrargyri et Potassii Iodidorum

Solution of Potassium Iodohydrargyrate, Channing's Solution
(N.F. IV)

Red Mercuric Iodide . . . . 10 Gm.
Potassium Iodide . . . . 8 Gm.
Distilled Water, a sufficient quantity,

To make . . . . 1000 cc.

Triturate the red mercuric iodide and potassium iodide with about 20 cc. of distilled water until solution has been effected, then add sufficient distilled water to make the product measure 1000 cc.

AVERAGE DOSE—Metric, 0.2 cc.—Apothecaries, 3 minims.

COMPOUND SOLUTION OF MERCURY BICHLORIDE
(N.Y.H.F.)

Mercuric Bichloride . . . . 0.5 Gm.
Boric Acid, crystals . . . . 40 Gm.
Distilled Water . . . . 500 cc.
Alcohol, 80%, a sufficient quantity;

To make . . . . 1000 cc.

Dissolve the boric acid and mercuric bichloride in a mixture of the water and 40 cc. of alcohol and adding sufficient 80% alcohol to make the product measure 1000 cc.

AVERAGE DOSE—2 drops into the external auditory canal.

SOLUTION OF MERCURIC OXYCYANIDE
(N.Y.P.G.H.)

Mercuric Oxycyanide.	0.25 Gm.
Distilled Water, a sufficient quantity,	
To make	1000 cc.

Dissolve.

OESCHNER'S SOLUTION
(R.B. II)

Liquefied Phenol.	4 cc.
Boric Acid.	19 Gm.
Alcohol	125 cc.
Distilled Water, a sufficient quantity,	
To make	1000 cc.

Dissolve the boric acid in 800 cc. of distilled water, add the liquefied phenol and the alcohol and then sufficient distilled water to make the product measure 1000 cc.

BUFFERED OPHTHALMIC SOLUTIONS

(Dr. Gifford)

STOCK SOLUTION OF SODIUM CARBONATE

Sodium Carbonate, anhydrous.	21.2 Gm.
Distilled Water, previously boiled, a sufficient quantity,	
To make	1000 cc.

Dissolve.

STANDARD ACID BUFFER SOLUTION NO. 1 (pH 5.0)

Boric Acid, crystals	12.4 Gm.
Potassium Chloride, anhydrous	7.4 Gm.
Distilled Water, previously boiled, a sufficient quantity,	
To make	1000 cc.

Dissolve the salts in the boiled distilled water.

NOTE—This solution is a suitable solvent for Butyn and Phenacaine.

ACID BUFFER SOLUTION NO. 2 (pH 6.0)

Stock Solution of Sodium Carbonate	0.05 cc.
Acid Buffer Solution No. 1	30 cc.

Mix well.

NOTE—This solution is a suitable solvent for Zinc salts, Cocaine and Epinephrine.

STANDARD ALKALINE BUFFER SOLUTION NO. 1 (pH 7.6)

Stock Solution of Sodium Carbonate . . . .   1.5 cc.
Acid Buffer Solution No. 1 . . . .   30 cc.
    Mix well.

NOTE—This solution is a suitable solvent for Atropine, Homatropine and Pilocarpine. Physostigmine solutions turn dark red almost immediately and such solutions have probably lost significant potency.

ALKALINE BUFFER SOLUTION NO. 2 (pH 8.4)

Stock Solution of Sodium Carbonate . . . .   4 cc.
Standard Acid Buffer Solution No. 1 . . . .   30 cc.
    Mix well.

NOTE—This solution is used as an eye wash in vernal conjunctivitis and certain cases of chronic conjunctivitis with tenacious and somewhat dry secretion.

ALKALINE BUFFER SOLUTION NO. 3 (pH 9.0)

Stock Solution of Sodium Carbonate . . . .   8 cc.
Standard Acid Buffer Solution No. 1 . . . .   30 cc.
    Mix well.

NOTE—This solution is a suitable solvent for Sodium Fluorescein.

BUFFER SOLUTION FOR EUPHTHALMIN

Boric Acid, crystals . . . .   12.4 Gm.
Anhydrous Sodium Borate . . . .   0.5 Gm.
Anhydrous Potassium Chloride . . . .   7.4 Gm.
Distilled Water, previously boiled, a sufficient quantity,
           To make . . . .   1000 cc.
Dissolve the salts in the distilled water.

OPHTHALMIC SOLUTIONS WITH SPECIAL REFERENCE TO pH AND ISOTONICITY

Colorimetric Determination of pH

Indicators used:			
Methyl Red T.S.	4.2–6.2	red–yellow
Bromthymol Blue T.S.	6.0–7.6	yellow–blue
Phenol Red T.S.	6.8–8.4	yellow–red
Thymol Blue T.S.	8.0–9.6	yellow–blue

BUFFER SOLUTIONS FOR OPHTHALMIC USE

1. Gifford Standard Acid Buffer Solution No. 1, R.B.
2. Gifford Standard Alkaline Buffer Solution No. 1, R.B.

NOTE—The special designated solutions (by Gifford) which are most often used are: Acid Buffer Solution No. 1, Acid Buffer Solution No. 2, Alkaline Buffer Solution No. 1 and Alkaline Buffer Solution No. 2. However, if a physician desires a solution with a pH other than those designated by Gifford, the pharmacist can prepare the desired solution by mixing the above standard buffered solutions in the proportions shown in the table which follows:

Desired pH		Gifford Standard No. 1 Acid Solution		Gifford Stock Sodium Carbonate Solution	Gifford Special Designation
5.0	Mix	30.0 cc.	+	0.00 cc.	Acid Buffer Solution No. 1
6.0	Mix	30.0 cc.	+	0.05 cc.	Acid Buffer Solution No. 2
6.2	Mix	30.0 cc.	+	0.10 cc.	
6.4	Mix	30.0 cc.	+	0.15 cc.	
6.6	Mix	30.0 cc.	+	0.20 cc.	
6.8	Mix	30.0 cc.	+	0.30 cc.	
7.0	Mix	30.0 cc.	+	0.60 cc.	
7.2	Mix	30.0 cc.	+	1.00 cc.	
7.4	Mix	30.0 cc.	+	1.25 cc.	Normal Lachrymal Fluid
7.6	Mix	30.0 cc.	+	1.50 cc.	Alkaline Buffer Solution No. 1
7.8	Mix	30.0 cc.	+	2.00 cc.	
8.0	Mix	30.0 cc.	+	2.50 cc.	
8.2	Mix	30.0 cc.	+	3.00 cc.	
8.4	Mix	30.0 cc.	+	4.00 cc.	Alkaline Buffer Solution No. 2
9.0	Mix	30.0 cc.	+	8.00 cc.	

Pharmaceutical applications of solutions above:

pH 5.0 Solvent for Butyn; Phenacaine.

pH 6.0 Solvent for Alum; Zinc salts; Epinephrine Hydrochloride; Procaine Hydrochloride; Ephedrine Hydrochloride; Cocaine and other Alkaloidal salts.

pH 7.6 Solvent for Atropine; Homatropine; Pilocarpine; Scopolamine and other alkaloids.

pH 9.0 Solvent for Soluble Fluorescein.

Therapeutic applications of solutions above:

pH 7.4 Eye Wash; Contact Lens Fluid.

pH 6.0 For Alkali Burns; Vernal Conjunctivitis; Pneumococcic Infections; Corneal Ulcers.

pH 8.0 For Streptococcic Infections.

LACHRYMAL-ISOTONIC SOLUTIONS

The lachrymal fluid is isotonic with a 1.4 per cent solution of sodium chloride. These fluids have the same osmotic pressure; also the same freezing point, $-0.80°$ C.

Table of Concentrations of Solutions Isotonic with Lachrymal Fluid
(Expressed in Grams per 100 cc. of aqueous solution)

Acid, Boric	3.1	Phenol	4.3
Alum, Ammonium	7.8	Pilocarpine Hydrochloride	7.0
Atropine Sulfate	15.0	Pontocaine Hydrochloride	8.2
Chlorobutanol	7.6	Potassium Chloride	1.8
Cocaine Hydrochloride	9.8	Potassium Nitrate	2.4
Copper Sulfate	11.0	Potassium Sulfate	3.3
Dextrose	7.5	Procaine Hydrochloride	7.5
Dionin	11.0	Silver Nitrate	4.0
Emetine Hydrochloride	12.0	Mild Silver Protein	45.0
Ephedrine Hydrochloride	5.8	Sodium Benzoate	2.8
Ephedrine Sulfate	9.2	Sodium Bicarbonate	2.0
Eserine Salicylate	17.8	Sodium Biphosphate	4.0
Eserine Sulfate	14.2	Sodium Borate	4.5
Homatropine Hydrobromide	10.2	Sodium Chloride	1.4
Hyoscine Hydrobromide	12.6	Sodium Nitrate	2.0
Lactose	14.0	Sodium Sulfate $\cdot$ 10H$_2$O	6.0
Metycaine Hydrochloride	8.2	Sucrose	15.0
Morphine Hydrochloride	10.8	Tannic Acid	13.9
Morphine Sulfate	16.3	Tutocaine Hydrochloride	8.6
Phenacaine	9.7	Zinc Sulfate	8.2

EXAMPLE (for use of above table for preparing a correct solution):

What quantity of potassium nitrate should be added to 100 cc. of a 1% solution of silver nitrate to make the finished solution isotonic with the lachrymal fluid?

1. Determine percentage of isotonicity of unadjusted solution. (Refer to silver nitrate in the table above.) } $\frac{1}{4} \times 100 = 25$ per cent isotonicity.

2. Determine percentage of isotonicity to be supplied by the isotonic agent. (Subtract first result from 100 per cent.) } 100 per cent $-$ 25 per cent $=$ 75 per cent isotonicity to be supplied.

3. Compute the weight of isotonic agent needed. (Refer to potassium nitrate in the table above.) } 2.4 Gm. $\times$ 0.75 $=$ 1.8 Gm.

4. Therefore 1.8 Gm. of potassium nitrate should be added to every 100 cc. of 1 per cent solution of silver nitrate to make the finished solution isotonic with lachrymal fluid.

OSLER'S SOLUTION

Alcohol	125 cc.
Liquefied Phenol	6 cc.
Saturated Solution of Boric Acid, a sufficient quantity,	
To make	1000 cc.

Mix the liquefied phenol with the alcohol and add this solution to the saturated solution of boric acid.

SOLUTION OF PEPSIN
Liquor Pepsini
(N.F. V)

Glycerite of Pepsin*	50 cc.
Diluted Hydrochloric Acid	5 cc.
Glycerin	315 cc.
Distilled Water, a sufficient quantity,	
To make	1000 cc.

Mix by very gentle agitation.

AVERAGE DOSE—Metric, 8 cc.—Apothecaries, 2 fluidrachms.

ACID SOLUTION OF PEPSIN
(P.H.N.Y.)

Pepsin*	30 Gm.
Diluted Hydrochloric Acid	150 cc.
Glycerin	75 cc.
Distilled Water, a sufficient quantity,	
To make	1000 cc.

Mix the pepsin with 500 cc. of distilled water and the acid, agitate gently until solution is complete, add the glycerin and sufficient distilled water to make the product measure 1000 cc.

AVERAGE DOSE—Metric, 4 cc.—Apothecaries, 1 fluidrachm.

---

* Pepsin solutions are reduced in proteolytic activity by agitation and storage, particularly when at or above normal room temperature. To insure the dispensing of this solution at standard strength it is strongly recommended that the quantity of pepsin in the formula be increased by 50 to 150 per cent to allow for such loss in activity, and that the solution be stored in a cool place.

ANTISEPTIC SOLUTION OF PEPSIN
Liquor Pepsini Antisepticus
(N.F. V)

Pepsin*	50	Gm.
Diluted Hydrochloric Acid	5	cc.
Glycerin	50	cc.
Alcohol	10	cc.
Menthol	0.5	Gm.
Eucalyptol	0.5	cc.
Methyl Salicylate	0.5	cc.
Distilled Water, a sufficient quantity,		
To make	1000	cc.

Mix the diluted hydrochloric acid with 800 cc. of cold distilled water and dissolve the pepsin in this liquid by gentle stirring; then add the glycerin. Dissolve the menthol, eucalyptol and methyl salicylate in the alcohol, add to the first solution, then add sufficient distilled water to make the product measure 1000 cc. Set aside for 24 hours, and filter.

NOTE—This preparation is used externally only, chiefly on sloughing wounds.

AROMATIC SOLUTION OF PEPSIN
Liquor Pepsini Aromaticus
(N.F. V)

Pepsin*	17.50	Gm.
Diluted Hydrochloric Acid	5	cc.
Glycerin	250	cc.
Alcohol	35	cc.
Oil of Cinnamon	0.25	cc.
Oil of Pimenta	0.25	cc.
Oil of Clove	0.50	cc.
Distilled Water, a sufficient quantity,		
To make	1000	cc.

Mix the diluted hydrochloric acid with 700 cc. of cold distilled water and dissolve the pepsin in this liquid by gentle stirring; then add the glycerin. Dissolve the oils in the alcohol and add to the aqueous solution, add sufficient distilled water to make the product measure 1000 cc. and mix thoroughly by gentle agitation. Set the mixture aside for 24 hours, then filter.

AVERAGE DOSE—Metric, 8 cc.—Apothecaries, 2 fluidrachms.

* Pepsin solutions are reduced in proteolytic activity by agitation and storage, particularly at or above normal room temperature. To insure the dispensing of this solution at standard strength it is strongly recommended that the quantity of pepsin directed in the formula be increased by 50 to 150 per cent to allow for such loss in activity, and that the solution be stored in a cool place.

COMPOUND PHENOL SOLUTION
(v.c.n.y.)

Liquefied Phenol.	3 cc.
Sodium Bicarbonate	5 Gm.
Sodium Borate	5 Gm.
Glycerin	125 cc.
Distilled Water, a sufficient quantity,	
To make	1000 cc.

Dissolve the liquefied phenol in the glycerin and add a solution of the sodium borate and sodium bicarbonate in 500 cc. of distilled water. When effervescence has subsided add sufficient distilled water to make the product measure 1000 cc.

PERFUSION SOLUTIONS

I

LOCKE'S SOLUTION

Reagent Sodium Chloride	9.20 Gm.
Reagent Potassium Chloride	0.42 Gm.
Reagent Calcium Chloride	0.12 Gm.
Reagent Sodium Bicarbonate	0.15 Gm.
Reagent Dextrose	1 Gm.
Distilled Water, a sufficient quantity,	
To make	1000 cc.

Dissolve, and filter if necessary. Sterilize by Process D (see N.F. VII, page 35).

Note—The constituents (except the dextrose) may be made up in more concentrated stock solutions and diluted as needed. This solution should be freshly prepared and dispensed only on prescription.

II

RINGER'S SOLUTION (Non-official)

Reagent Sodium Chloride.	6 Gm.
Reagent Potassium Chloride	0.075 Gm.
Reagent Calcium Chloride	0.10 Gm.
Sodium Bicarbonate	1 Gm.
Water, recently distilled from a hard glass flask, a sufficient quantity,	
To make	1000 cc.

Dissolve and filter if necessary. Sterilize the solution by placing in an autoclave and keeping at 15 pounds pressure for 15 minutes.

Note—This solution must be freshly prepared.

This solution should not be confused with the official "Ringer's Solution" the title of which is "Isotonic Solution of Three Chlorides," U.S.P. XII, page 261.

III
RINGER'S SOLUTION (Bodansky Formula)

Reagent Calcium Chloride	0.25 Gm.
Reagent Potassium Chloride	0.50 Gm.
Reagent Sodium Chloride	8 Gm.
Distilled Water, a sufficient quantity,	
To make	1000 cc.

Dissolve the salts in the distilled water.

IV
TYRODE SOLUTION

Reagent Sodium Chloride	8 Gm.
Reagent Potassium Chloride	0.20 Gm.
Reagent Calcium Chloride	0.10 Gm.
Monobasic Reagent Sodium Biphosphate	0.05 Gm.
Reagent Magnesium Chloride	0.10 Gm.
Sodium Bicarbonate	1 Gm.
Dextrose	1 Gm.
Water, recently distilled from a hard glass flask, a sufficient quantity,	
To make	1000 cc.

Dissolve and filter. Sterilize by Process D (see N.F. VII, page 35).

NOTE—This solution must be freshly prepared. The constituents (except the dextrose and sodium bicarbonate) may be made up in a more concentrated stock solution and diluted as needed.

SOLUTION OF PHOSPHORUS
Liquor Phosphori

Thompson's Solution of Phosphorus

(N.F. V)

Phosphorus	0.7 Gm.
Spirit of Peppermint	5 cc.
Glycerin	645 cc.
Dehydrated Alcohol, a sufficient quantity,	
To make	1000 cc.

Weigh the phosphorus in a dish containing water (which should be counter-balanced after each trial weighing), dry it carefully and quickly with blotting paper and introduce it into a flask containing 350 cc. of dehydrated alcohol. Into the neck of the flask insert a perforated cork stopper fitted with a glass tube about 50 cm. in length, to serve as a condenser. Place the flask on a water bath and heat it so that the alcohol shall be kept boiling gently, until the phosphorus is dissolved. Allow the solution to cool, add the spirit of peppermint and glycerin and then sufficient dehydrated alcohol to make the product measure 1000 cc.

AVERAGE DOSE—Metric, 0.6 cc.—Apothecaries, 10 minims

SOLUTION OF PHYSOSTIGMINE SALICYLATE
(R.B. II)

Physostigmine Salicylate	2.5 Gm
Boric Acid, crystals	55.5 Gm.
Distilled Water, a sufficient quantity,	
To make	1000 cc.

Dissolve and filter.

SOLUTION OF CHLORINATED POTASSA
Liquor Potassæ Chlorinatæ

Liquor Potassæ Chloratæ; Javelle Water
(N.F. IV)

Potassium Carbonate.	58 Gm.
Chlorinated Lime	80 Gm.
Distilled Water, a sufficient quantity,	
To make	1000 cc.

Mix the chlorinated lime intimately with 400 cc. of distilled water. Dissolve the potassium carbonate in 300 cc. of boiling distilled water, and pour the hot solution into the mixture first prepared. Shake the flask or bottle well, stopper it, set it aside to cool and then add sufficient distilled water to make the product measure 1000 cc. and filter.

Keep in well-stoppered bottles, in a cool place, protected from light.

SOLUTION OF POTASSIUM ACETATE, CITRATE AND POTASSIUM AND SODIUM TARTRATE
Alkaline Mixture
(N.Y.H.F.)

Potassium Acetate	120 Gm.
Potassium Citrate	120 Gm.
Potassium and Sodium Tartrate	120 Gm.
Distilled Water, a sufficient quantity,	
To make	1000 cc.

Dissolve and filter if necessary.

AVERAGE DOSE—Metric, 15 cc.—Apothecaries, 4 fluidrachms.

SOLUTION OF POTASSIUM CITRATE AND POTASSIUM AND SODIUM TARTRATE
(N.Y.H.F.)

Potassium Citrate	160 Gm.
Potassium and Sodium Tartrate	250 Gm.
Distilled Water, a sufficient quantity,	
To make	1000 cc.

Dissolve and filter if necessary.

AVERAGE DOSE—Metric, 4 cc.—Apothecaries, 1 fluidrachm.

SOLUTION OF POTASSIUM PERMANGANATE
Liquor Potassii Permanganatis
(B.P.C. 1934)

Potassium Permanganate	10 Gm.
Distilled Water, a sufficient quantity,	
To make	1000 cc.

Dissolve.

AVERAGE DOSE—Metric, 8 to 16 cc.—Apothecaries, 2 to 4 fluidrachms.

NOTE—This solution is comparable to that known as Condy's Fluid. Preserve in glass-stoppered bottles.

COMPOUND QUININE SOLUTION
Liquor Quininæ Compositus
(N.Y.P.G.H.)

Quinine Sulfate	22.5	Gm.
Diluted Sulfuric Acid	30	cc.
Tincture of Ferric Chloride	150	cc.
Spirit of Chloroform	125	cc.
Glycerin	150	cc.
Distilled Water, a sufficient quantity,		
To make	1000	cc.

Dissolve the quinine sulfate in the acid, add 500 cc. of distilled water, the glycerin, tincture of ferric chloride and spirit of chloroform. Finally add sufficient distilled water to make the product measure 1000 cc.

AVERAGE DOSE—Metric, 4 cc.—Apothecaries, 1 fluidrachm.

SOLUTION OF SALICYLIC ACID WITH THYMOL
(R.B. II)

Salicylic Acid	40 Gm.
Thymol	10 Gm.
Chlorobutanol	10 Gm.
Distilled Water	250 cc.
Alcohol, a sufficient quantity,	
To make	1000 cc.

Dissolve the salicylic acid, thymol and chlorobutanol in 650 cc. of alcohol. Add the distilled water little by little, shaking after each addition. Lastly, add sufficient alcohol to make the product measure 1000 cc.

SCHLESINGER'S SOLUTION
(R.B. I)

Scopolamine Hydrobromide.................	0.25 Gm.
Morphine Hydrochloride	20 Gm.
Ethylmorphine Hydrochloride	40 Gm.
Ampul Water, a sufficient quantity,	
To make	1000 cc.

Dissolve, filter and sterilize by Process F (see N.F. VII, page 36).

NOTE—This preparation must be dispensed on prescription only.

SEMMOLA'S SOLUTION
Semmola's Fluid
(R.B. I)

Sodium Iodide........................	2 Gm.
Sodium Phosphate.....................	4 Gm.
Sodium Chloride......................	8 Gm.
Distilled Water, a sufficient quantity,	
To make	1000 cc.

Dissolve, and filter.

AVERAGE DOSE—Metric, 60 cc.—Apothecaries, 2 fluidounces.

SENN'S SOLUTION
(R B. I)

Iodine	10 Gm.
Potassium Iodide	10 Gm.
Distilled Water, a sufficient quantity,	
To make	1000 cc.

Dissolve.

SOLUTION OF CHLORINATED SODA
Liquor Sodæ Chlorinatæ

Liq. Sod. Chlorinat.; Labarraque's Solution
(U.S.P. X)

Monohydrated Sodium Carbonate	70 Gm.
Chlorinated Lime.....................	100 Gm.
Water, a sufficient quantity,	
To make	1000 Gm.

Triturate the chlorinated lime with 500 cc. of water gradually added until a uniform mixture results. Dissolve the monohydrated sodium carbonate in 500 cc. of warm water, and add this solution to the chlorinated lime mixture contained in a suitable vessel. Stir or shake the mixture thoroughly, and if it becomes gelatinous warm the vessel very gently until its contents again liquefy. Then transfer the mixture to a wetted muslin strainer, and return the first portion until the liquid passes

through clear.   Add a few drops of sodium carbonate T.S. to 10 cc. of this clear filtrate.   If it remains clear on the addition of the reagent, continue the operation
without further treatment.   If the filtrate becomes cloudy, return the mixture to the
vessel, add sufficient monohydrated sodium carbonate to precipitate the excess of
lime and again filter, returning the first portions until the liquid passes through clear.
When no more liquid drains from the filter, wash the precipitate with sufficient water
to make the product weigh 1000 Gm.

DAUFRESNE SOLUTION OF CHLORINATED SODA
(B.P.C. 1934)

Chlorinated Lime	20 Gm.
Exsiccated Sodium Carbonate	10 Gm.
Sodium Bicarbonate	8 Gm.
Distilled Water	1000 cc.
To make about	1000 cc.

Mix the chlorinated lime with 500 cc. of distilled water in a 2-liter flask and set
aside overnight.   Dissolve the two sodium salts in 500 cc. of distilled water, add this
solution to the chlorinated lime mixture, agitate well and set aside.   When the calcium carbonate has completely precipitated, siphon off the clear liquid and filter.

Keep in well-stoppered bottles, protected from light.

NOTE—This preparation is not to be confused with Diluted Solution of Sodium
Hypochlorite (Modified Dakin's Solution), N.F. VII, which is to be dispensed when
Dakin's Solution is ordered.

COMPOUND SOLUTION OF SODIUM BIPHOSPHATE
Compound Solution of Sodium Acid Phosphate
(P.F.)

Boric Acid	25 Gm.
Sodium Biphosphate	500 Gm.
Distilled Water, a sufficient quantity,	
To make	1000 cc.

Dissolve.

This is used for rendering the urine acid in reaction prior to treatment with
methenamine.

AVERAGE DOSE—Metric, 2 cc.—Apothecaries, 30 minims.

SOLUTION OF STRYCHNINE AND QUININE
(N.Y.P.G.H.)

Strychnine Sulfate	0.325	Gm.
Quinine Sulfate	7	Gm.
Diluted Phosphoric Acid	125	cc.
Distilled Water, a sufficient quantity,		
To make	1000	cc.

Dissolve the strychnine sulfate and quinine sulfate in the diluted phosphoric acid, add sufficient distilled water to make the product measure 1000 cc., and filter.

AVERAGE DOSE—Metric, 4 cc.—Apothecaries, 1 fluidrachm.

COMPOUND SOLUTION OF TANNIC ACID
(Fantus)

Potassium Chloride	0.42 Gm.
Calcium Chloride	0.84 Gm.
Salicylic Acid	1 Gm.
Sodium Chloride	10.5 Gm.
Tannic Acid	100 Gm.
Distilled Water, a sufficient quantity,	
To make	1000 cc.

Mix the solids with the distilled water, shaking occasionally until solution is effected.   Filter.

SOLUBLE TAR
Solution of Tar
(Arny)

Oil of Tar	90 cc.
Alcohol	180 cc.
Magnesium Carbonate	75 Gm.
Glycerin	360 cc.
Distilled Water, a sufficient quantity,	
To make	1000 cc.

Dissolve the oil of tar in the alcohol and triturate this solution with the magnesium carbonate; add the other ingredients, macerate for several days and filter.

SOLUTION OF TAR
(R.B. I)

Pine Tar	10 Gm.
Monohydrated Sodium Carbonate	10 Gm.
Distilled Water, a sufficient quantity,	
To make	1000 cc.

Dissolve the sodium carbonate in 950 cc. of distilled water heated to about 50° C. Add the pine tar and shake vigorously until the mixture is homogeneous.   Set aside for 12 hours and filter, then add sufficient distilled water, through the filter, to make the product measure 1000 cc.

ALKALINE SOLUTION OF TAR
Liquor Picis Alkalinus
(N.F. IV)

Pine Tar	250 Gm.
Potassium Hydroxide	125 Gm.
Distilled Water, a sufficient quantity,	
To make	1000 cc.

Dissolve the potassium hydroxide in 625 cc. of distilled water, add the pine tar and agitate until solution is effected. Allow it to stand 24 hours, then strain the solution through purified cotton and pass sufficient distilled water through the strainer to make the product measure 1000 cc.

COMPOUND SOLUTION OF TRICHLOROACETIC ACID
(R.B. I)

Trichloroacetic Acid	330 Gm.
Magnesium Sulfate.	500 Gm.
Distilled Water, a sufficient quantity,	
To make	1000 cc.

Dissolve.

ULZMAN'S SOLUTION
(R.B. I)

Zinc Sulfate.	4.3 Gm.
Alum.	4.3 Gm.
Liquefied Phenol.	2.2 cc.
Distilled Water, a sufficient quantity,	
To make	1000 cc.

Dissolve.

WRIGHT'S ARSENICAL SOLUTION WITH GOLD BROMIDE
(R.B. I)

Arsenic Trioxide.	5.5 Gm.
Potassium Carbonate.	5.5 Gm.
Bromine	5 cc.
Gold, in leaf.	1.8 Gm.
Distilled Water, a sufficient quantity,	
To make	1000 cc.

Boil the arsenic trioxide and potassium carbonate with 250 cc. of distilled water in a flask until solution has been effected. Place the gold leaf in a bottle, add 600 cc. of distilled water, then add the bromine carefully and shake until solution is effected. Add the first solution, mix well, transfer to a flask or retort and boil until bromine fumes are no longer evolved. When cool, add sufficient distilled water to make the product measure 1000 cc. Filter if necessary.

AVERAGE DOSE—Metric, 0.3 cc.—Apothecaries, 5 minims.

NOTE—This preparation is not to be confused with Wright's Surgical Solution, R.B.

WRIGHT'S SURGICAL SOLUTION
(R.B. I)

Sodium Citrate	8.5 Gm.
Sodium Chloride	34 Gm.
Distilled Water, a sufficient quantity,	
To make	1000 cc.

Dissolve, filter and sterilize by Process C (see N.F. VII, page 35).

This solution is used as a wet dressing for wounds to prevent clotting and thereby promote free drainage.

NOTE—This preparation is not to be confused with Wright's Arsenical Solution, R.B.

COMPOUND SOLUTION OF ZINC AND ALUMINUM
Liquor Zinci et Alumini Compositus
(N.F. IV)

Zinc Sulfate	200 Gm.
Aluminum Sulfate	200 Gm.
Betanaphthol	0.6 Gm.
Oil of Thyme	2 cc.
Distilled Water, a sufficient quantity,	
To make	1000 cc.

Dissolve the zinc sulfate and the aluminum sulfate in 800 cc. of distilled water, by the aid of heat, add the betanaphthol and oil of thyme and shake the mixture occasionally, in a stoppered bottle, until it is cold. Add sufficient distilled water to make the product measure 1000 cc., mix well, set aside for 2 days and then filter through a wetted filter.

COMPOUND SOLUTION OF ZINC AND IRON
Liquor Zinci et Ferri Compositus
Deodorant Solution
(N.F. IV)

Zinc Sulfate	200 Gm.
Ferrous Sulfate	200 Gm.
Cupric Sulfate	65 Gm.
Betanaphthol	0.6 Gm.
Oil of Thyme	2 cc.
Hypophosphorous Acid	4 cc.
Distilled Water, a sufficient quantity,	
To make	1000 cc.

Dissolve the zinc sulfate, ferrous sulfate and cupric sulfate in 800 cc. of boiling distilled water, add the betanaphthol and oil of thyme and shake the mixture occasionally, in a stoppered bottle, until it is cold. Then add the hypophosphorous acid and sufficient distilled water to make the product measure 1000 cc. and filter.

SPECIES

TEAS

Teas, although one of the oldest forms of household remedies, are still largely in use.

Teas are mixtures of whole or comminuted plant drugs. They may be employed for the preparation of internal medicines, for external applications and for baths. When used for infusions or decoctions or for baths, the drugs are cut or bruised. When intended to be placed into flannel bags, to be heated and applied dry as a cataplasm, the drugs should be finely cut or coarsely ground. Teas which are to be mixed with hot water to form a poultice should be in the form of a coarse powder.

As a general rule, flowers, leaves, stems and rhizomes should be cut; some fruits, barks, roots and woods may be cut while others require to be bruised; seeds should be bruised and hard woods rasped.

SPECIES OF ABSINTHIUM, COLTSFOOT, SANTONICA AND MATRICARIA

Worm Species

(D.M.)

Absinthium,
Coltsfoot,
Santonica,
Matricaria, of each, an equal weight.

Cut or bruise and mix intimately.

AVERAGE DOSE—2 teaspoonfuls made into a decoction with 8 fluidounces of boiling water and strained.

COMPOUND SPECIES OF ALOE, MYRRH AND RHUBARB

Schwedische Kräuter, Bitter Ansatz

(E.B. III)

Aloe, granulated	400 Gm.
Myrrh, granulated	67 Gm.
Rhubarb	67 Gm.
Gentian	67 Gm.
Galangal	67 Gm.
Zedoary	67 Gm.
Crocus	67 Gm.
Honey	67 Gm.
Agaric	131 Gm.
To make	1000 Gm.

Triturate the coarsely ground agaric with the honey and mix with the aloe and myrrh; add the other drugs, previously cut.

AVERAGE DOSE—2 teaspoonfuls made into an infusion with 8 fluidounces of boiling water and strained.

SPECIES OF ALPINE HERBS
Species Herbarum Alpinarum
Species Alpinæ, Alpenkräutertee, Alpine Tea
(P.F.)

Frangula	400 Gm.
Senna	200 Gm.
Tilia Flowers (Linden Flowers)	100 Gm.
Sambucus	100 Gm.
Mullein Flowers	50 Gm.
Acacia Flowers*	50 Gm.
Rest Harrow Root	50 Gm.
Lovage Root	50 Gm.
To make	1000 Gm.

Cut or bruise and mix intimately.

AVERAGE DOSE—2 teaspoonfuls made into an infusion with 8 fluidounces of boiling water and strained.

SPECIES OF ALTHEA LEAVES, ALTHEA, GLYCYRRHIZA AND MALLOW FLOWERS
Species Althææ
Eibischtee, Marshmallow Tea, Althea Tea
(Ph. Aust.)

Althea Leaves	550 Gm.
Althea	250 Gm.
Glycyrrhiza	150 Gm.
Mallow Flowers	50 Gm.
To make	1000 Gm.

Cut or bruise and mix intimately.

AVERAGE DOSE—2 teaspoonfuls made into an infusion with 8 fluidounces of boiling water and strained.

COMPOUND SPECIES OF ALTHEA LEAVES AND LINSEED
Species Emollientes
(N.F. V)

Althea Leaves, in coarse powder,
Mallow Leaves, in coarse powder,
Melilot, in coarse powder,
Matricaria, in coarse powder,
Linseed, in coarse powder, of each, an equal weight.

Mix intimately.

This specie is used, mixed with a suitable quantity of hot water, as a poultice

* Flowers of *Prunus spinosa*.

SPECIES OF ALTHEA, COLTSFOOT AND GLYCYRRHIZA

Pectoral Species, Breast Tea
(N.F. V)

Althea	400 Gm.
Coltsfoot	200 Gm.
Glycyrrhiza, peeled	150 Gm.
Anise	100 Gm.
Mullein Flowers	100 Gm.
Orris	50 Gm.
To make	1000 Gm.

Cut or bruise and mix intimately.

AVERAGE DOSE—2 teaspoonfuls made into an infusion with 8 fluidounces of boiling water and strained.

SPECIES OF ALTHEA, COLTSFOOT AND GLYCYRRHIZA WITH FRUITS
(D.M.)

Species of Althea, Coltsfoot and Glycyrrhiza, R.B.	550 Gm.
Barley	140 Gm.
St. John's Bread*	210 Gm.
Fig	100 Gm.
To make	1000 Gm.

Cut the fig and St. John's bread coarsely and mix with the other ingredients.

AVERAGE DOSE—2 teaspoonfuls made into an infusion with 8 fluidounces of boiling water and strained.

SPECIES OF ALTHEA, GLYCYRRHIZA AND FENNEL

Hustentee
(D.M.)

Althea	450 Gm.
Glycyrrhiza	450 Gm.
Fennel	100 Gm.
To make	1000 Gm.

Cut or bruise and mix intimately.

AVERAGE DOSE—2 teaspoonfuls made into an infusion with 8 fluidounces of boiling water and strained.

* The fruit of *Ceratonia Siliqua*.

SPECIES OF ALTHEA, GLYCYRRHIZA AND TRITICUM WITH MATRICARIA AND FENNEL

Carminative Tea
(Ph. Aust.)

Althea	250 Gm.
Glycyrrhiza	250 Gm.
Triticum	250 Gm.
Matricaria	125 Gm.
Fennel	125 Gm.
To make	1000 Gm.

Cut or bruise and mix intimately.

AVERAGE DOSE—2 teaspoonfuls made into an infusion with 8 fluidounces of boiling water and strained.

SPECIES OF ALTHEA LEAVES, GLYCYRRHIZA AND TRITICUM WITH MATRICARIA, FENNEL AND PARSLEY FRUIT

(Ph. Aust.)

Matricaria	117.5 Gm.
Fennel	117.5 Gm.
Althea Leaves	235 Gm.
Glycyrrhiza	235 Gm.
Triticum	235 Gm.
Parsley Fruit	60 Gm.
To make	1000 Gm.

Cut or bruise and mix intimately.

AVERAGE DOSE—2 teaspoonfuls made into an infusion with 8 fluidounces of boiling water and strained.

NOTE—This preparation is intended for administration to children.

SPECIES OF ALTHEA, GLYCYRRHIZA AND TRITICUM WITH WATERMELON SEED AND MULLEIN FLOWERS

(Ph. Aust.)

Watermelon Seed	100 Gm.
Mullein Flowers	100 Gm.
Glycyrrhiza	200 Gm.
Triticum	200 Gm.
Althea Tea, R.B.	400 Gm.
To make	1000 Gm.

Cut or bruise and mix intimately.

AVERAGE DOSE—2 teaspoonfuls made into an infusion with 8 fluidounces of boiling water and strained.

SPECIES OF PEPPERMINT, LAVENDER FLOWERS, WILD THYME, THYME, CLOVE AND CUBEB

Species Aromaticæ

Aromatic Species

(D.A.B. VI)

Peppermint	200 Gm.
Lavender Flowers	200 Gm.
Wild Thyme	200 Gm.
Thyme	200 Gm.
Clove	100 Gm.
Cubeb, in coarse powder	100 Gm.
To make	1000 Gm.

Cut the first five ingredients in fine pieces and mix with the cubeb.

This specie is used in the form of a dry or wet poultice.

SPECIES OF STRAMONIUM, LOBELIA AND POTASSIUM NITRATE

Asthma Spasm Species

(E.B. III)

Stramonium	630	Gm.
Lobelia	120	Gm.
Potassium Nitrate	250	Gm.
Hot Distilled Water	500	cc.
Oil of Lavender	2.5	cc.
To make	1000	Gm.

Moisten the drugs, previously cut, with a solution of the potassium nitrate in the hot distilled water and dry the mixture at about 40° C. Mix in thoroughly the oil of lavender.

This specie is used by inhaling the smoke from the burning powder.

SPECIES OF PEPPERMINT, MATRICARIA, THYME, ROSEMARY AND SAGE

Species pro Balneo

Badekräuter, Bath Species

(D.M.)

Peppermint, in coarse powder	200 Gm.
Matricaria, in coarse powder	200 Gm.
Thyme, in coarse powder	200 Gm.
Rosemary, in coarse powder	200 Gm.
Sage, in coarse powder	200 Gm
Alcohol	500 cc.
To make	1000 Gm.

Moisten the herbs with the alcohol and permit the alcohol to evaporate.

For a bath, use 200 to 500 Gm.

SPECIES OF ABSINTHIUM, BITTER ORANGE PEEL, CENTAURY, CALAMUS, GENTIAN, MENYANTHES AND CINNAMON
Species Amaræ

Bittertee, Bitter Species
(Ph. Aust.)

Absinthium	210 Gm.
Bitter Orange Peel	210 Gm.
Centaury	210 Gm.
Calamus	105 Gm.
Gentian	105 Gm.
Menyanthes	105 Gm.
Cinnamon	55 Gm.
To make	1000 Gm.

Cut or bruise and mix intimately.

AVERAGE DOSE—2 teaspoonfuls made into an infusion with 8 fluidounces of boiling water and strained.

SPECIES OF CINNAMON, PEPPERMINT AND CENTAURY

Stomachic Species, Magentee
(Ph. Aust.)

Cinnamon	250 Gm.
Peppermint	250 Gm.
Centaury	500 Gm.
To make	1000 Gm.

Cut or bruise and mix intimately.

AVERAGE DOSE—2 teaspoonfuls made into an infusion with 8 fluidounces of boiling water and strained.

SPECIES OF ALTHEA, GLYCYRRHIZA, LINSEED AND FENNEL
Species Demulcentes

Demulcent Tea
(Ph. Dan.)

Althea	400 Gm.
Glycyrrhiza	100 Gm.
Linseed	400 Gm.
Fennel	100 Gm.
To make	1000 Gm.

Cut or bruise and mix intimately.

AVERAGE DOSE—2 teaspoonfuls made into an infusion with 8 fluidounces of boiling water and strained.

SPECIES OF TILIA FLOWERS, SAMBUCUS AND MULLEIN FLOWERS

Species Diaphoreticæ

Muenchen, Diaphoretic Tea

Tilia Flowers (Linden Flowers),
Sambucus,
Mullein Flowers, of each, an equal weight.

Cut or bruise and mix intimately.

AVERAGE DOSE—2 teaspoonfuls made into an infusion with 8 fluidounces of boiling water and strained.

SPECIES OF LINSEED, MATRICARIA AND ALTHEA LEAVES

Species ad Enema

Kräuter zum Klistier, Enema Species

(D.M.)

Linseed.	250 Gm.
Matricaria.	250 Gm.
Althea Leaves	500 Gm.
To make	1000 Gm.

.Cut or bruise and mix intimately.

AVERAGE DOSE—For enema, use 2 teaspoonfuls made into an infusion with 8 fluidounces of boiling water and strained.

SPECIES OF CARAWAY, BITTER ORANGE PEEL AND FRANGULA

Species Anglicæ

English Species

(D.M.)

Caraway	125 Gm.
Bitter Orange Peel.	125 Gm.
Frangula	750 Gm.
To make	1000 Gm.

Cut or bruise and mix intimately.

AVERAGE DOSE—2 teaspoonfuls made into an infusion with 8 fluidounces of boiling water and strained.

SPECIES OF CELERY ROOT, ASPARAGUS ROOT, FENNEL ROOT, PARSLEY ROOT AND BUTCHER'S BROOM ROOT

Five Roots Tea
(R.B. I)

Celery Root,
Asparagus Root,
Fennel Root,
Parsley Root,
Butcher's Broom Root,* of each, an equal weight.

Cut or bruise and mix intimately.

AVERAGE DOSE—2 teaspoonfuls made into an infusion with 8 fluidounces of boiling water and strained.

SPECIES OF HUMULUS, LAVENDER FLOWERS, WILD THYME, ROSEMARY AND MATRICARIA

Species ad Fomentum

Blähungskräuter, Foment Species
(D.M.)

Humulus, in coarse powder.	400 Gm.
Lavender Flowers, in coarse powder	150 Gm.
Wild Thyme, in coarse powder.	150 Gm.
Rosemary, in coarse powder.	150 Gm.
Matricaria, in coarse powder.	150 Gm.
To make	1000 Gm.

Mix intimately.

This specie is used in the form of an infusion as a hot application.

SPECIES OF SENNA, MANNA, CORIANDER AND TARTARIC ACID

Species Hamburgenses

Hamburger Tea
(E.B. IV)

Senna, cut	555 Gm.
Manna, in coarse powder	280 Gm.
Coriander, bruised	140 Gm.
Tartaric Acid, in powder	25 Gm.
To make	1000 Gm.

Mix intimately.

AVERAGE DOSE—2 teaspoonfuls made into an infusion with 8 fluidounces of boiling water and strained.

---

* Rhizome of *Ruscus aculeatus.*

SPECIES OF SENNA, FRANGULA, MILFOIL AND TRITICUM

Martin's Tea

(E.B. III)

Senna,
Frangula,
Milfoil,
Triticum, of each, an equal weight.

Cut or bruise and mix intimately.

AVERAGE DOSE—2 teaspoonfuls made into an infusion with 8 fluidounces of boiling water and strained.

COMPOUND SPECIES OF MELISSA AND WILD MARJORAM

(E.B. III)

Melissa Leaves, in coarse powder	350 Gm.
Wild Marjoram, in coarse powder	350 Gm.
Lavender Flowers, in coarse powder	100 Gm.
Sambucus, in coarse powder	100 Gm.
Matricaria, in coarse powder	100 Gm.
To make	1000 Gm.

Mix intimately.

This specie is moistened with hot water and used as a poultice.

SPECIES OF SENNA, SAMBUCUS, FENNEL, ANISE AND POTASSIUM BITARTRATE

St. Germain Tea

Senna, cut	400 Gm.
Sambucus	250 Gm.
Fennel, bruised	125 Gm.
Anise, bruised	125 Gm.
Potassium Bitartrate, in fine powder	100 Gm.
To make	1000 Gm.

Moisten the senna with a small quantity of water, then sprinkle the potassium bitartrate over it as uniformly as possible. When the senna so treated has become dry, mix it lightly and uniformly with the other ingredients.

AVERAGE DOSE—2 teaspoonfuls made into an infusion with 8 fluidounces of boiling water and strained.

SPECIES OF SARSAPARILLA, SASSAFRAS, GUAIAC WOOD AND CHINA ROOT
Species Sudorificæ
Espéces Sudorfiques, Sudorific Tea
(Cod. Fr., 1884)

Sarsaparilla,
Sassafras,
Guaiac Wood,
China Root,* of each, an equal weight.
Cut or bruise and mix intimately.
AVERAGE DOSE—2 teaspoonfuls made into an infusion with 8 fluidounces of boiling water and strained.

SPECIES OF REST HARROW ROOT, GUAIAC WOOD, GLYCYRRHIZA AND SASSAFRAS
Species Lignorum
Holztee, Wood Species

Rest Harrow Root**	300 Gm.
Guaiac Wood	500 Gm.
Glycyrrhiza	100 Gm.
Sassafras	100 Gm.
To make	1000 Gm.

Cut or bruise and mix intimately.

AVERAGE DOSE—2 teaspoonfuls made into an infusion with 8 fluidounces of boiling water and strained.

SPIRITS

AROMATIC SPIRIT
Spiritus Aromaticus
Aromatic Essence
(E.B. III)

Coriander, in coarse powder	50 Gm.
Myristica, in coarse powder	25 Gm.
Cinnamon, in coarse powder	25 Gm.
Marjoram, in coarse powder	25 Gm.
Clove, in coarse powder	25 Gm.
Alcohol	710 cc.
Distilled Water	895 cc.
To make	1000 cc.

* Rhizome of *Smilax China.*
** Root of *Ononis spinosa.*

Macerate the drugs with the mixture of alcohol and distilled water for 24 hours, with occasional agitation. Place the mixture in a suitable apparatus and distil until 1000 cc. of distillate is obtained.

AVERAGE DOSE—Metric, 2 cc.—Apothecaries, 30 minims.

SPIRIT OF BITTER ALMOND
Spiritus Amygdalæ Amaræ
Spirit of Almond
(N.F. VI)

Oil of Bitter Almond	10 cc.
Alcohol	800 cc.
Distilled Water, a sufficient quantity,	
To make	1000 cc.

Dissolve the oil in the alcohol, and add enough distilled water to make the product measure 1000 cc.

AVERAGE DOSE—Metric, 0.5 cc.—Apothecaries, 8 minims.

One average metric dose contains 0.005 cc. of Oil of Bitter Almond.

NOTE—This Spirit is intended for medicinal use and it must not be used for flavoring foods.

ETHEREAL SPIRIT OF CAMPHOR
Spiritus Camphoræ Æthereus
(B.P.C. 1923)

Camphor	100 Gm.
Ethyl Oxide, a sufficient quantity,	
To make	1000 cc.

Dissolve.

RUBINI'S SPIRIT OF CAMPHOR
(P.F.)

Camphor	446 Gm.
Dehydrated Alcohol, a sufficient quantity,	
To make	1000 cc.

Dissolve.

SPIRIT OF CURAÇAO
Spiritus Curassao
(N.F. III)

Oil of Bitter Almond	1 cc.
Oil of Bitter Orange	165 cc.
Oil of Fennel	3 cc.
Alcohol, a sufficient quantity,	
To make	1000 cc.

Mix.

Keep in completely filled and well-stoppered bottles, in a cool, dark place.

NOTE—The oils must be *absolutely free* from any terebinthinate odor or taste.

COMPOUND SPIRIT OF MENTHOL
(B.P.C. 1934)

Camphor	100 Gm.
Menthol	100 Gm.
Terebene	100 cc.
Eucalyptol	100 cc.
Alcohol, a sufficient quantity,	
To make	1000 cc.

Dissolve the ingredients in the alcohol.

AVERAGE DOSE—10 drops by inhalation.

SPIRIT OF PHOSPHORUS
Tincture of Phosphorus
(R.B. II)

Phosphorus	1.2 Gm.
Dehydrated Alcohol, a sufficient quantity,	
To make	1000 cc.

Weigh the phosphorus in a tared capsule containing water, dry it carefully and quickly with blotting paper and introduce it into a flask containing 1000 cc. of dehydrated alcohol. Into the neck of the flask insert a perforated cork stopper bearing a long (about 50 cm.) glass tube, to serve as a condenser. Place the flask in a water bath and heat it so that the alcohol may be kept gently boiling, until the phosphorus is dissolved. Allow the liquid to cool and add sufficient dehydrated alcohol to make the product measure 1000 cc.

Keep in small, dark amber-colored bottles, securely stoppered, in a cool, dark place.

AVERAGE DOSE—Metric, 0.5 cc.—Apothecaries, 8 minims.

SPIRIT OF COCHLEARIA

Spirit of Scurvy Grass

(R.B. I)

Oil of Cochlearia. . . . .   8 cc.

Alcohol, a sufficient quantity,

To make . . . .   1000 cc.

Dissolve.

SPIRIT OF TANNIC ACID

Tincture of Tannin

(R.B. I)

Tannic Acid . . . .   200 Gm.

Sucrose. . . . .   100 Gm.

Water . . . .   300 cc.

Alcohol, a sufficient quantity,

To make . . . .   1000 cc.

Dissolve the tannic acid and sucrose in the water, and add sufficient alcohol to make the product measure 1000 cc.

AVERAGE DOSE—Metric, 4 cc.—Apothecaries, 1 fluidrachm.

SPRAYS

NOTE—Sprays should be filtered if not clear. The continued or excessive use of sprays containing liquid petrolatum may cause lung injury. Their use for infants and small children should be avoided unless under the supervision of a physician.

BENZEDRINE NASAL SPRAY

(B.N.Y.)

Benzedrine . . . .   10 cc.

Light Liquid Petrolatum, a sufficient quantity,

To make . . . .   1000 cc.

Dissolve.

CAMPHOR, EUCALYPTOL AND MENTHOL NASAL SPRAY

(B.N.Y.)

Camphor . . . .   20 Gm.

Menthol . . . .   10 Gm.

Eucalyptol . . . .   10 cc.

Light Liquid Petrolatum, a sufficient quantity,

To make . . . .   1000 cc.

Triturate the menthol, camphor and eucalyptol until liquefied, and add sufficient liquid petrolatum to make the product measure 1000 cc.

CAMPHOR, MENTHOL AND EUCALYPTOL NASAL SPRAY WITH PINE OIL
(N.H.H.F.)

Camphor	10 Gm.
Menthol	10 Gm.
Eucalyptol	10 cc.
Oil of Dwarf Pine Needles	10 cc.
Light Liquid Petrolatum, a sufficient quantity,	
To make	1000 cc.

Triturate the camphor, menthol, eucalyptol and oil of dwarf pine needles together until liquefied, and add sufficient light liquid petrolatum to make the product measure 1000 cc.

DOUGLAS' NASAL SPRAY
(N.Y.P.G.H.)

Thymol	5 Gm.
Eucalyptol	10 cc.
Menthol	16.5 Gm.
Oil of Cubeb	16.5 cc.
Light Liquid Petrolatum, a sufficient quantity,	
To make	1000 cc.

Dissolve the thymol and menthol in the eucalyptol and oil of cubeb, and add sufficient light liquid petrolatum to make the product measure 1000 cc.

ISOTONIC EPHEDRINE-DEXTROSE NASAL DROPS or SPRAY

Menthol	0.1 Gm.
Chlorobutanol	0.5 Gm.
Ephedrine Hydrochloride	1 Gm.
Alcohol	2 cc.
Dextrose	5.0 Gm.
Distilled Water, a sufficient quantity,	
To make	100 cc.

Dissolve the menthol and chlorobutanol in the alcohol; dissolve the dextrose and ephedrine hydrochloride in the distilled water, and gradually add the alcoholic solution to the aqueous solution.

EUCALYPTOL SPRAY
Nebula Eucalyptolis
(N.F. V)

Eucalyptol	50 cc.
Light Liquid Petrolatum	950 cc.
To make	1000 cc.

Mix.

COMPOUND IODINE SPRAY
(R.B. I)

Iodine . . . . 0.6 Gm.
Menthol . . . . 10 Gm.
Light Liquid Petrolatum, a sufficient quantity,

To make . . . . 1000 cc.

Triturate the iodine very finely, add the menthol and triturate until well mixed. Add gradually a portion of the liquid petrolatum, previously warmed, pouring off the dissolved portions and adding more warmed petrolatum until all the iodine and menthol are dissolved and the product measures 1000 cc.

MENTHOL SPRAY
Nebula Mentholis
(N.F. V)

Menthol . . . . 20 Gm.
Light Liquid Petrolatum, a sufficient quantity,

To make . . . . 1000 cc.

Dissolve the menthol in the liquid petrolatum which has been warmed to about 70° C., and filter if necessary.

MENTHOL AND EUCALYPTOL SPRAY
(N.Y.P.G.H.)

Menthol . . . . 4 Gm.
Eucalyptol . . . . 4 cc.
Light Liquid Petrolatum, a sufficient quantity,

To make . . . . 1000 cc.

Dissolve the menthol in the eucalyptol and add sufficient liquid petrolatum to make the product measure 1000 cc.

COMPOUND PINE OIL NASAL SPRAY
Nebula Olei Pini
(N.Y.P.G.H.)

Oil of Dwarf Pine Needles . . . . 20 cc.
Oil of Cinnamon . . . . 2 cc.
Camphor . . . . 10 Gm.
Menthol . . . . 10 Gm.
Light Liquid Petrolatum, a sufficient quantity,

To make . . . . 1000 cc.

Triturate the camphor and menthol together until liquefied, add the volatile oils and sufficient liquid petrolatum to make the product measure 1000 cc.

COMPOUND THYMOL NASAL SPRAY
Nebula Thymolis Composita
(P.H.N.Y.)

Thymol.	0.5 Gm.
Menthol	4 Gm.
Eucalyptol	10 Gm.
Light Liquid Petrolatum, a sufficient quantity,	
To make	1000 cc.

Triturate the menthol and thymol, add the eucalyptol, and finally, sufficient liquid petrolatum to make the product measure 1000 cc.

SUPPOSITORIES

ASTRINGENT SUPPOSITORIES
Suppositoria Adstringentia
(Lux. F.)

Bismuth Iodotannate	3.75 Gm.
Bismuth, Resorcinated.	3.75 Gm.
Zinc Oxide.	6 Gm.
Peruvian Balsam	1.50 Gm.
Theobroma Oil, grated	19 Gm.
Cerate.	2.50 Gm.
To make.	12 Suppositories

Mix intimately and prepare, by the process of cold compression, 12 rectal suppositories, weighing about 3 Gm. each.

BISMUTH, ZINC AND RESORCINOL SUPPOSITORIES
(E.B. III)

Bismuth Subiodide	1.20 Gm.
Bismuth Subgallate	1.20 Gm.
Zinc Oxide.	1.20 Gm.
Resorcinol	0.12 Gm.
Peruvian Balsam	0.60 Gm.
Theobroma Oil, grated	31.68 Gm.
To make.	12 Suppositories

Mix intimately and prepare, by the process of cold compression, 12 rectal suppositories, weighing 3 Gm. each.

METHYLROSANILINE SUPPOSITORIES
(N.Y.H.F.)

Methylrosaniline Chloride . . . .   1.56 Gm.
Theobroma Oil   72   Gm.

To make . . . . 12 Suppositories

Dissolve the methylrosaniline in a small quantity of alcohol and mix the solution with the theobroma oil. The alcohol is then allowed to evaporate leaving the gentian violet well dispersed. Prepare, by the process of cold compression, 12 vaginal suppositories, weighing 6 Gm. each.

NOTE—These suppositories are intended for vaginal use only.

TANNIN SUPPOSITORIES
Suppositoria Acidi Tannici
(B.P. 1932)

Tannic Acid . . . .   2.4 Gm.
Theobroma Oil, grated, a sufficient quantity,

To make . . . . 12 Suppositories

Mix intimately and prepare, by the process of cold compression, 12 rectal suppositories, weighing about 2 Gm. each.

WITCH HAZEL SUPPOSITORIES
Suppositoria Hamamelidis
Hamamelis Suppositories
(E.B. III)

Fluidextract of Hamamelis Leaf . . . .   60 cc.
Theobroma Oil, grated, a sufficient quantity,

To make . . . . 12 Suppositories

Evaporate the fluidextract on a water bath to a semi-fluid consistence and incorporate with sufficient theobroma oil to make the product weigh 24 Gm. Prepare, by the process of cold compression, 12 rectal suppositories, weighing 2 Gm. each.

SUSPENSIONS

SUSPENSION OF HYDRATED BISMUTH OXIDE
Suspension d'Oxyde de Bismuth Hydraté
(Cod. Fr.)

Hydrated Bismuth Oxide . . . .   93 Gm.
Wool Fat . . . .   60 Gm.
Olive Oil . . . .   986 cc.

To make . . . .   1000 cc.

Mix the melted wool fat and olive oil.   Filter and sterilize by heating in a conical flask of Bohemian glass at 120° C. for 20 minutes or in a hermetically sealed flask in an autoclave at 120° C. for 20 minutes.   Place some alcohol in a mortar, ignite it and pass the pestle through the flame.   When the flame is extinguished and the mortar cool, introduce the hydrated bismuth oxide and mix it with a sufficient quantity of the cooled mixture of wool fat and olive oil, triturating until a homogeneous mixture is obtained.   Add a sufficient quantity of the wool fat in oil to produce a liquid mixture, and transfer to a wide-mouthed glass-stoppered flask of 1500 cc. capacity, graduated at 1000 cc. and previously sterilized at 180° C.   Rinse the mortar and the pestle several times with small amounts of the oil mixture and transfer to the graduated flask.   These operations should be performed with the most rigorous aseptic precautions.   Make up to 1000 cc. by the addition of the requisite amount of wool fat in oil, close the flask and shake vigorously.   Fill into 1-cc. or 2-cc. ampuls, previously sterilized at 180° C., and sterilize by Process E (see N.F. VII, page 36).

One cc. of the suspension contains 0.093 Gm. of hydrated bismuth oxide, corresponding to 0.08 Gm. of bismuth.

SUSPENSION OF PHENYL SALICYLATE
(R.B. I)

Phenyl Salicylate, in fine powder.	50 Gm.
Tragacanth, in fine powder	15 Gm.
Acacia, in fine powder	40 Gm.
Distilled Water, a sufficient quantity,	
To make	1000 cc.

Mix the phenyl salicylate intimately with the acacia and tragacanth.   Triturate the mixture with distilled water to produce a thin paste, then add sufficient distilled water to make the product measure 1000 cc.

AVERAGE DOSE—Metric, 4 cc.—Apothecaries, 1 fluidrachm.

SUSPENSION OF SILVER IODIDE
(R.B. I)

Silver Nitrate	22 Gm.
Potassium Iodide	22 Gm.
Mucilage of Chondrus	500 cc.
Distilled Water, a sufficient quantity,	
To make	1000 cc.

Dissolve the potassium iodide and the silver nitrate separately, each in 200 cc. of distilled water.   Add the mucilage of chondrus to the potassium iodide solution and to this mixture add, in a thin stream and with vigorous agitation, the solution of silver nitrate.   Add sufficient distilled water to make the product measure 1000 cc.

SUSPENSION OF SULFUR
(R.B. I)

Precipitated Sulfur, in extremely fine powder	360 Gm.
Distilled Water	360 cc.
Glycerin	180 cc.
Alcohol, a sufficient quantity,	
To make	1000 cc.

Triturate the precipitated sulfur with the glycerin, add the distilled water, and finally sufficient alcohol to make the product measure 1000 cc.

SYRUPS

SYRUP OF ACACIA (UNFLAVORED)
(U.S.P. IX)

Acacia, in selected pieces	100 Gm.
Sucrose	800 Gm.
Distilled Water, a sufficient quantity,	
To make	1000 cc.

Place the acacia in an enameled or porcelain dish, add 430 cc. of distilled water and stir occasionally until the acacia is dissolved; then having added the sucrose, place the dish on a water bath and apply heat, gradually increasing the temperature until the water in the water bath boils. Maintain the temperature for 15 minutes and stir the syrup from time to time until the sucrose is dissolved. Strain the syrup while hot, add sufficient distilled water, recently boiled, to make the product measure 1000 cc., and transfer it, while yet hot, into small bottles which have been rinsed with boiling water and heated in an oven at 160° C. for from 15 to 30 minutes. Close the bottles tightly with rubber stoppers which have been just previously boiled in water for 30 minutes and cap them with paper.

NOTE—This syrup should be freshly prepared.

SYRUP OF ACETYLSALICYLIC ACID

Acetylsalicylic Acid	30 Gm.
Potassium Citrate	90 Gm.
Sucrose	246 Gm.
Tincture of Lemon	10 cc.
Distilled Water	225 cc.
Glycerin, a sufficient quantity,	
To make	1000 cc.

Dissolve the acetylsalicylic acid and potassium citrate in the distilled water. Percolate the sucrose with the solution and return it, if necessary, until the sucrose has been dissolved. Add the tincture of lemon and sufficient glycerin to make the product measure 1000 cc.

AVERAGE DOSE—Metric, 15 cc.—Apothecaries, ½ fluidounce.

NOTE—This syrup should be freshly prepared.

SYRUP OF AMMONIUM CHLORIDE
(U.C.H.)

Ammonium Chloride . . . .   **84 Gm.**
Syrup of Citric Acid . . . .   **500 cc.**
Syrup of Tolu Balsam, a sufficient quantity,
               To make . . . .   **1000 cc.**

Dissolve the ammonium chloride in the mixture of syrups with the aid of gentle heat if necessary.

AVERAGE DOSE—Metric, 4 cc.—Apothecaries, 1 fluidrachm.

SYRUP OF ANISE
(B.P.C. 1934)

Sucrose. . . . .   **850 Gm.**
Anise Water, a sufficient quantity,
               To make . . . .   **1000 cc.**

Place the sucrose in a large funnel or percolator. Pour gradually over this sufficient anise water to dissolve the sucrose and make the product measure 1000 cc.

Syrups of Fennel, Peppermint, Spearmint and Wintergreen may be prepared according to the above formula.

SYRUP OF BLACKBERRY BARK
Syrupus Rubi
Syrup of Rubus
(N.F. V)

Fluidextract of Rubus, R.B. . . . .   **250 cc.**
Syrup, a sufficient quantity,
               To make . . . .   **1000 cc.**

Mix.

AVERAGE DOSE—Metric, 4 cc.—Apothecaries, 1 fluidrachm.

SYRUP OF BLACKBERRY FRUIT
Syrupus Rubi Fructus
(N.F. IV)

Fresh, Ripe Blackberries,
Sucrose,
Benzoic Acid, of each, a sufficient quantity.

Garble the blackberries, wash the fruit in a colander with water, drain and crush to a pulp. Strain this pulp, with pressure, and to every 1000 cc. of expressed juice add 1 Gm. of benzoic acid and 2000 Gm. of sucrose. Heat the mixture at once, with stirring, and when the sucrose has dissolved continue the heat until the syrup just boils. Strain it while hot into suitable bottles which have been thoroughly cleaned and, just before filling, rinsed with boiling water, and, when the bottles are filled to the neck, immediately insert, to a point at least 5 mm. below the lip of the bottles, well-fitting corks which have been soaked in boiling water. Finally seal the bottles with melted paraffin.

Keep in a cool, dark place.

SYRUP OF BUCKTHORN BARK (For Human Use)

Syrup of Rhamnus Frangula

Fluidextract of Buckthorn Bark	200 cc.
Syrup of Orange	400 cc.
Syrup, a sufficient quantity,	
To make	1000 cc.

Mix the three liquids and filter, if necessary.

NOTE—This syrup should not be confused with the Syrup of Buckthorn Berries (for animals) on page 322 of the Recipe Book III.

SYRUP OF CALCIUM BROMIDE

Sirop de Bromide de Calcium
(Cod. Fr.)

Calcium Bromide	32 Gm.
Distilled Water	20 cc.
Syrup of Orange Flowers	200 cc.
Syrup, a sufficient quantity,	
To make	1000 cc.

Dissolve the calcium bromide in the distilled water, add the syrup of orange flowers and sufficient syrup to make the product measure 1000 cc.

AVERAGE DOSE—Metric, 15 cc.—Apothecaries, 4 fluidrachms.

ACID SYRUP OF CALCIUM PHOSPHATE
Syrupus Calcii Hydrochlorophosphatis

Syrupus Calcii Chlorhydrophosphatis
(N.F. IV)

Precipitated Calcium Phosphate	17 Gm.
Tincture of Lemon	20 cc.
Distilled Water	60 cc.
Hydrochloric Acid, the required quantity,	
Syrup, a sufficient quantity,	
To make	1000 cc.

Triturate the precipitated calcium phosphate with 30 cc. of distilled water, and dissolve it with the aid of hydrochloric acid, avoiding an excess. Then add the tincture of lemon, filter the liquid, and wash the filter with a mixture of 30 cc. each of distilled water and of syrup. Lastly, add sufficient syrup to the filtrate to make the product measure 1000 cc.

AVERAGE DOSE—Metric, 4 cc.—Apothecaries, 1 fluidrachm.

AROMATIC SYRUP OF CASCARA
(B.P.C. 1934)

Aromatic Fluidextract of Cascara Sagrada.	400 cc.
Tincture of Sweet Orange Peel	100 cc.
Cinnamon Water.	150 cc.
Syrup, a sufficient quantity,	
To make	1000 cc.

Mix the aromatic fluidextract of cascara sagrada, tincture of sweet orange peel, and cinnamon water, and add sufficient syrup to make the product measure 1000 cc.

AVERAGE DOSE—Metric, 4 cc.—Apothecaries, 1 fluidrachm.

SYRUP OF CHLORAL
Syrupus Chloralis
(B.P.C. 1934)

Chloral Hydrate	200 Gm.
Distilled Water	200 cc.
Syrup, a sufficient quantity,	
To make	1000 cc.

Dissolve the chloral hydrate in the distilled water and add sufficient syrup to make the product measure 1000 cc.

AVERAGE DOSE—Metric, 4 cc.—Apothecaries, 1 fluidrachm.

COMPOUND SYRUP OF CIMICIFUGA
Syrupus Cimicifugæ Compositus

Syrupus Actææ Compositus, Compound Syrup of Actæa
(N.F. IV)

Fluidextract of Cimicifuga.	40 cc.
Fluidextract of Glycyrrhiza	20 cc.
Fluidextract of Senega	20 cc.
Fluidextract of Ipecac	10 cc.
Wild Cherry, in moderately fine powder.	40 Gm.
Purified Talc	15 Gm.
Sucrose.	650 Gm.
Distilled Water, a sufficient quantity,	
To make	1000 cc.

Mix the wild cherry with 375 cc. of distilled water and allow it to macerate for 1 hour. Then add the fluidextracts and purified talc and stir or agitate the mixture frequently and thoroughly for about 15 minutes. Transfer it to a wetted filter, and, when the liquid ceases to drop from the funnel, wash the contents of the filter with sufficient distilled water to obtain 500 cc. of filtrate. Dissolve the sucrose in this liquid by agitation and add sufficient distilled water to make the product measure 1000 cc.

AVERAGE DOSE—Metric, 4 cc.—Apothecaries, 1 fluidrachm.

SYRUP OF CODEINE
Syrupus Codeinæ
(N.F. IV)

Codeine Sulfate	2 Gm.
Syrup, a sufficient quantity,	
To make	1000 cc.

Dissolve the codeine sulfate in 15 cc. of warm distilled water and add to the syrup with agitation.

AVERAGE DOSE—Metric, 4 cc.—Apothecaries, 1 fluidrachm.

COMPOUND SYRUP OF CODEINE
Syrupus Codeinæ Compositus
(P.F.)

Codeine Sulfate	2 Gm.
Terpin Hydrate	20 Gm.
Fluidextract of Ipecac	4 cc.
Fluidextract of Eucalyptus, R.B.	10 cc.
Fluidextract of Squill.	14 cc.
Tincture of Cudbear	16 cc.
Glycerin	40 cc.
Sucrose.	750 Gm.
Distilled Water, a sufficient quantity,	
To make	1000 cc.

Dissolve the finely powdered terpin hydrate in the mixed fluidextracts, tincture and glycerin. Pour this into 400 cc. of distilled water in which the codeine sulfate has been previously dissolved. Filter this liquid through a wetted filter into a properly prepared percolator containing the sucrose, and pass sufficient distilled water through the percolator to make the percolate measure 1000 cc.

AVERAGE DOSE—Metric, 4 cc.—Apothecaries, 1 fluidrachm.

SYRUP OF COFFEE
(N.F. III)

Coffee, freshly roasted and powdered.	250 Gm.
Sucrose	800 Gm.
Distilled Water, a sufficient quantity,	
To make	1000 cc.

Place the coffee in a container and pour upon it 500 cc. of boiling water, cover the container and boil for 5 minutes. Cool, strain and pass enough water through the strainer to make the volume to 500 cc. Dissolve the sucrose in this solution by agitation without heat. Strain the syrup through muslin and pass enough distilled water through the strainer to make the product measure 1000 cc.

AVERAGE DOSE—Metric, 8 cc.—Apothecaries, 2 fluidrachms.

HUNTER'S EXPECTORANT SYRUP
(R.B. I)

Potassium Bromide.	25 Gm.
Ammonium Bromide	25 Gm.
Potassium Chlorate.	25 Gm.
Tincture of Belladonna	25 cc.
Camphorated Tincture of Opium.	25 cc.
Tincture of Ipecac	25 cc.
Fluidextract of Glycyrrhiza	50 cc.
Syrup of Tolu Balsam.	400 cc.
Syrup of Wild Cherry, a sufficient quantity,	
To make	1000 cc.

Dissolve the salts in the mixture of the liquid ingredients with gentle heat if necessary.

AVERAGE DOSE—Metric, 4 cc.—Apothecaries, 1 fluidrachm.

SYRUP OF FERRIC HYPOPHOSPHITE
Syrupus Ferri Hypophosphitis
(N.F. IV)

Ferric Hypophosphite.	17 Gm.
Potassium Citrate	25 Gm.
Sucrose.	850 Gm.
Orange Flower Water.	90 cc.
Distilled Water, a sufficient quantity,	
To make	1000 cc.

Dissolve the ferric hypophosphite and the potassium citrate in 225 cc. of distilled water with the aid of heat, and filter.   Mix the filtrate with the orange flower water, add sufficient distilled water to make the solution measure 450 cc. and dissolve the sucrose in this liquid with the aid of gentle heat.   Finally add sufficient distilled water to make the product measure 1000 cc.

AVERAGE DOSE—Metric, 4 cc.—Apothecaries, 1 fluidrachm.

SYRUP OF FERROUS CHLORIDE
Syrupus Ferri Protochloridi
Syrup of Protochloride of Iron
(N.F. IV)

Solution of Ferrous Chloride, R.B..	50 cc.
Glycerin	125 cc.
Orange Flower Water.	125 cc.
Syrup, a sufficient quantity,	
To make	1000 cc.

Mix the solution of ferrous chloride with the glycerin and orange flower water, and add sufficient syrup to make the product measure 1000 cc.

AVERAGE DOSE—Metric, 4 cc.—Apothecaries, 1 fluidrachm.

NOTE—This syrup should be freshly prepared.

SYRUP OF FERROUS SULFATE

Elixir of Ferrous Sulfate
(Clark)
(N.Y.H.F.)

Ferrous Sulfate, granular . . . .   46 Gm.
Citric Acid . . . .   2 Gm.
Spirit of Peppermint . . . .   2 cc.
Syrup, a sufficient quantity,

To make . . . .   1000 cc.

Powder the citric acid in a mortar, add the ferrous sulfate and a small amount of syrup and triturate vigorously until the powders are in a very fine state of subdivision. Pour into a suitable bottle, rinse out the mortar with portions of syrup and add these rinsings to the material in the bottle.   Add the spirit of peppermint and enough syrup to make 1000 cc. and shake well.   When the salt is dissolved, strain through 2 or 3 thicknesses of gauze.

AVERAGE DOSE—Metric 4 cc.—Apothecaries, 1 fluidrachm.

NOTE—This syrup should be freshly prepared.

COMPOUND SYRUP OF IRON MALATE WITH RHUBARB

(Ph. Helv. IV)

Ferrated Extract of Apples, R.B.. . . . .   10 Gm.
Cinnamon Water. . . . .   40 cc.
Syrup of Orange. . . . .   200 cc.
Tincture of Cinnamon . . . .   10 cc.
Glycerin . . . .   240 cc.
Syrup of Rhubarb, a sufficient quantity,

To make . . . .   1000 cc.

Incorporate the ferrated extract of apples with the cinnamon water.   Add the other ingredients in order, shaking vigorously.   Finally add sufficient syrup of rhubarb to make the product measure 1000 cc.

AVERAGE DOSE—Metric, 4 to 6 cc.—Apothecaries, 1 to 1½ fluidrachms.

COMPOUND SYRUP OF IRON PHOSPHATE

Syrupus Ferri Phosphatis Compositus

(N.Y.P.G.H.)

Soluble Ferric Phosphate . . . .   37.5 Gm.
Quinine Sulfate . . . .   37.5 Gm.
Strychnine Sulfate . . . .   0.5 Gm.
Diluted Phosphoric Acid   250   cc.
Syrup, a sufficient quantity,

To make   1000   cc.

Dissolve the soluble ferric phosphate, quinine sulfate and strychnine sulfate in the diluted phosphoric acid, then add sufficient syrup to make the product measure 1000 cc.

AVERAGE DOSE—Metric, 4 cc.—Apothecaries, 1 fluidrachm.

SYRUP OF IRON PYROPHOSPHATE
(U.C.H.)

Iron Pyrophosphate	100 Gm.
Syrup of Cherry, a sufficient quantity,	
To make	1000 cc.

Dissolve.

AVERAGE DOSE—Metric, 4 cc.—Apothecaries, 1 fluidrachm.

SYRUP OF IRON AND MANGANESE IODIDE
Syrupus Ferri et Mangani Iodidi
(N.F. IV)

Iodine	81 Gm.
Iron Wire, in fine, bright wire	28 Gm.
Manganese Sulfate	26 Gm.
Sodium Iodide	35 Gm.
Sucrose	800 Gm.
Diluted Alcohol	100 cc.
Distilled Water, a sufficient quantity,	
To make	1000 cc.

Add the iodine to the iron and 200 cc. of distilled water in a flask, and prepare a solution of ferrous iodide, in the usual manner, aiding the process, if necessary, by heating the contents of the flask, at first gently, and finally to boiling. Filter the liquid through a small filter directly upon the sucrose contained in a suitable bottle graduated to 1000 cc. and rinse the flask and filter with two portions, of 20 cc. each, of distilled water, adding the rinsings to the filtrate in the bottle. Dissolve the manganese sulfate in 100 cc. of distilled water, and the sodium iodide in the diluted alcohol, mix the two solutions and filter the mixture, collecting the filtrate in the bottle which contains the sucrose and the iron iodide solution. Wash the filter with 25 cc. of distilled water, receiving the washings in the same bottle. Agitate the mixture until the sucrose has dissolved, then add sufficient distilled water to make the product measure 1000 cc. and filter.

AVERAGE DOSE—Metric, 1 cc.—Apothecaries, 15 minims.

SYRUP OF LACTUCARIUM
Syrupus Lactucarii
(U.S.P. IX)

Tincture of Lactucarium, R.B.	100 cc.
Glycerin	200 cc.
Citric Acid	1 Gm.
Orange Flower Water	25 cc.
Syrup, a sufficient quantity,	
To make	1000 cc.

Mix the tincture of lactucarium with the glycerin, add the orange flower water in which the citric acid has been previously dissolved and filter if necessary. Finally, add sufficient syrup to make the product measure 1000 cc. Mix thoroughly.

AVERAGE DOSE—Metric, 10 cc.—Apothecaries, 2½ fluidrachms.

LAXATIVE SYRUP
(R.B. I)

Aromatic Fluidextract of Cascara Sagrada.	250 cc.
Potassium and Sodium Tartrate	165 Gm.
Syrup, a sufficient quantity,	
To make	1000 cc.

Heat the fluidextract on a water bath until the alcohol is evaporated. Dissolve the potassium and sodium tartrate in 500 cc. of syrup. Mix this solution with the concentrated fluidextract, then add sufficient syrup to make the product measure 1000 cc.

AVERAGE DOSE—Metric, 4 cc.—Apothecaries, 1 fluidrachm.

SYRUP OF MANNA
Syrupus Mannæ
(N.F. V)

Manna, in flakes.	125 Gm.
Sucrose.	775 Gm.
Alcohol	65 cc.
Distilled Water, a sufficient quantity,	
To make	1000 cc.

Dissolve the manna in 400 cc. of hot distilled water, add the alcohol, set the liquid aside for 12 hours in a moderately warm place, and then filter. Dissolve the sucrose in the filtrate, with the aid of gentle heat, allow the syrup to cool, and add sufficient distilled water, passed through the filter previously used, to make the product measure 1000 cc.

AVERAGE DOSE—Metric, 8 cc.—Apothecaries, 2 fluidrachms.

NOTE—This syrup should be freshly prepared.

SYRUP OF MORPHINE AND ACACIA
Syrupus Morphinæ et Acaciæ

Jackson's Pectoral Syrup
(N.F. IV)

Morphine Hydrochloride	0.5 Gm.
Oil of Sassafras	0.5 cc.
Syrup of Acacia, a sufficient quantity,	
To make	1000 cc.

Dissolve the morphine hydrochloride in about 62 cc. of the syrup of acacia, add the oil of sassafras and sufficient syrup of acacia to make the product measure 1000 cc.

AVERAGE DOSE—Metric, 4 cc.—Apothecaries, 1 fluidrachm.

SYRUP OF PINEAPPLE
Syrup of Bromelia
(Fantus)

Pineapple,
Sucrose,
Alcohol,
Benzoic Acid, of each, a sufficient quantity.

Crush the pineapple in a grinder.   Dissolve about 0.1 per cent of benzoic acid in this mixture of crushed pineapple and allow the mixture to stand at room temperature until a small portion of the filtered juice produces a clear solution when it is mixed with one-half its volume of alcohol.   Press the juice from the mixture and filter; add the sucrose to the filtered juice in the proportion of 850 Gm. of sucrose to every 450 cc. of filtered juice.   Dissolve the sucrose by heating on a water bath. Cool and remove the scum.   Add 20 cc. of alcohol for each 1000 cc. of syrup.

NOTE—Canned pineapple may be used in the above formula.   Keep in well-closed containers.   This syrup should be freshly prepared.

This syrup is useful for mixtures containing citrates as other available and generally employed colored syrups are not suitable because they change in color when used in combination with citrates.

SYRUP OF POPPY
Syrupus Papaveris
(N.F. IV)

Poppy Capsules, deprived of seeds and in No. 20 powder	**100 Gm.**
Sucrose.	**850 Gm.**
Distilled Water, a sufficient quantity,	
To make	**1000 cc.**

Pack the powder loosely in a suitable metallic percolator and percolate it with boiling distilled water until it is practically exhausted.   Heat the percolate to boiling for 2 minutes, then concentrate it on a water bath to 450 cc., filter and dissolve the sucrose in the concentrated percolate.   Finally add sufficient distilled water to make the product measure 1000 cc., strain and bottle the syrup while warm.

Keep in small, completely filled bottles, in a cool place.

AVERAGE DOSE—Metric, 4 cc.—Apothecaries, 1 fluidrachm.

SYRUP OF QUININE
Syrupus Quininæ Compositus
Compound Syrup of Quinine
(N.Y.H.F.)

Quinine Sulfate	**80 Gm.**
Aromatic Syrup of Eriodictyon, a sufficient quantity,	
To make	**1000 cc.**

Triturate the quinine sulfate thoroughly and add gradually the aromatic syrup of eriodictyon.

Dispense with a "shake well" label.

AVERAGE DOSE—Metric, 4 cc.—Apothecaries, 1 fluidrachm.

SYRUP OF SANGUINARIA
Syrupus Sanguinariæ
Syrup of Bloodroot
(N.F. IV)

Sanguinaria, in No. 20 powder.	225 Gm.
Acetic Acid	125 cc.
Sucrose.	800 Gm.
Distilled Water, a sufficient quantity,	
To make	1000 cc.

Mix the acetic acid with 375 cc. of distilled water, moisten the sanguinaria with a sufficient quantity of this menstruum and allow it to macerate for 2 hours. Then pack it in a glass percolator, and percolate in the usual manner, first with the remainder of the menstruum and afterwards with distilled water until the percolate measures 750 cc., or until the sanguinaria is practically exhausted. Evaporate the percolate, at a moderate heat, to 480 cc., filter, and dissolve the sucrose in this filtrate, with the aid of gentle heat. Finally add sufficient distilled water to make the product measure 1000 cc.

AVERAGE DOSE—Metric, 2 cc.—Apothecaries, 30 minims.

SYRUP OF SASSAFRAS
(Hager)

Sassafras	100 Gm.
Alcohol	50 cc.
Distilled Water	500 cc.
Sucrose, a sufficient quantity.	

Add the sassafras to the mixture of alcohol and distilled water and allow to macerate for a period of 24 hours; press and filter the liquid and add 60 Gm. of sucrose for every 40 cc. of filtered liquid obtained.

SYRUP OF SENNA AND MANNA
I
(R.B. I)

Syrup of Senna,
Syrup of Manna, R.B., of each, an equal volume.

Mix.

AVERAGE DOSE—Metric, 8 to 15 cc.—Apothecaries, 2 to 4 fluidrachms.

II

Senna, cut	100 Gm.
Star Anise Fruit, in coarse powder	1 Gm.
Manna	130 Gm.
Sucrose	156 Gm.
Magnesium Carbonate	8 Gm.
Distilled Water, a sufficient quantity,	
To make	1000 cc.

Macerate the senna and star anise fruit with 830 cc. of distilled water for 12 hours, shaking frequently. Strain and add the manna, sucrose and magnesium carbonate. Heat to boiling, filter, and to the cooled filtrate add sufficient distilled water to make the product measure 1000 cc.

AVERAGE DOSE—Metric, 2 cc.—Apothecaries, 30 minims.

NOTE—This preparation is intended for administration to children. This syrup should be freshly prepared.

SYRUP OF SODIUM HYPOPHOSPHITE
Syrupus Sodii Hypophosphitis
(N.F. IV)

Sodium Hypophosphite	35 Gm
Hypophosphorous Acid	2 cc.
Sucrose	800 Gm.
Distilled Water, a sufficient quantity,	
To make	1000 cc.

Dissolve the sodium hypophosphite in 450 cc. of distilled water, add the hypophosphorous acid and filter the solution. Dissolve the sucrose in this liquid by agitation and add sufficient distilled water to make the product measure 1000 cc.

AVERAGE DOSE—Metric, 4 cc.—Apothecaries, 1 fluidrachm.

SYRUP OF STRAWBERRY
(R.B. I)

Ripe Strawberries,
Sucrose,
Benzoic Acid, of each, a sufficient quantity.

Press the juice from fully ripe strawberries through a flannel cloth. Dissolve in the juice 0.1 per cent of benzoic acid and set aside at room temperature until a small quantity of the filtered juice produces a clear solution with half its volume of alcohol. Clarify the juice by straining through flannel, or paper if necessary, and add to each .450 cc. of the clarified juice 850 Gm. of sucrose. Dissolve by heating on a water bath, cool and remove the scum.

Keep in well-stoppered bottles in a dark place.

AROMATIC SYRUP OF TEREBENE
(Fenner's Form.)

Terebene	40 cc.
Acacia	28 cc.
Syrup of Orange, a sufficient quantity,	
To make	1000 cc.

Triturate the terebene with the acacia and gradually add the syrup of orange and mix well.

AVERAGE DOSE—Metric, 4 to 8 cc.—Apothecaries, 1 to 2 fluidrachms.

NOTE—This syrup should be dispensed with a "shake well" label.

COMPOUND SYRUP OF TRIFOLIUM
Syrupus Trifolii Compositus
(N.F. VI)

Compound Fluidextract of Trifolium	300	cc.
Tragacanth, powdered	1	Gm.
Oil of Sassafras	0.4	cc.
Oil of Anise	0.2	cc.
Methyl Salicylate	0.2	cc.
Sucrose	650	Gm.
Distilled Water, a sufficient quantity,		
To make	1000	cc.

Mix the powdered tragacanth intimately with the fluidextract, add the oils, methyl salicylate and 250 cc. of distilled water; then add the sucrose, and agitate until it is dissolved. Add sufficient distilled water to make the product measure 1000 cc. and mix thoroughly.

AVERAGE DOSE—Metric, 8 cc.—Apothecaries, 2 fluidrachms.

SYRUP OF YERBA SANTA
Syrupus Eriodictyi
(R.B. I)

Fluidextract of Eriodictyon	60 cc.
Potassium Carbonate	12 Gm.
Distilled Water	30 cc.
Syrup, a sufficient quantity,	
To make	1000 cc.

Dissolve the potassium carbonate in the distilled water and mix the solution with the fluidextract. Add sufficient syrup to make the product measure 1000 cc.

AVERAGE DOSE—Metric, 8 cc.—Apothecaries, 2 fluidrachms.

NOTE—This syrup should not be confused with Aromatic Syrup of Eriodictyon, N.F. VII, which contains less eriodictyon, and which is employed as a vehicle for bitter medicines.

TABLETS

A.A.C. TABLETS
(N.Y.H.F.)

Acetylsalicylic Acid	22.8 Gm.
Acetophenetidin	15 Gm.
Citrated Caffeine	1.5 Gm.
To make	100 Tablets

Mix intimately and compress into 100 tablets.

AVERAGE DOSE—1 tablet.

ACETANILID, CAFFEINE, POTASSIUM BROMIDE AND SODIUM BICARBONATE TABLETS
(P.H.N.Y.)

Potassium Bromide	30 Gm.
Citrated Caffeine	3 Gm.
Acetanilid	12 Gm.
Sodium Bicarbonate	30 Gm.
To make	100 Tablets

Mix intimately and compress into 100 tablets.

AVERAGE DOSE—1 tablet.

ALKALINE WASH TABLETS

Cinnamol Tablets

Wilbert's Tablets
(R.B. I)

Sodium Bicarbonate	25 Gm.
Sodium Borate	25 Gm.
Sodium Chloride	25 Gm.
Sodium Phenolsulfonate	25 Gm.
Oil of Cinnamon	0.5 cc.
To make	100 Tablets

Mix intimately and compress into 100 tablets.

For use, dissolve 1 tablet in a half a glass of water.

DACOSTA'S TABLETS
(R.B. I)

Tincture of Digitalis	12 cc.
Tincture of Strophanthus	12 cc.
Tincture of Belladonna	1.5 cc.
Spirit of Glyceryl Trinitrate	6 cc.
Lactose, a sufficient quantity,	
To make	100 Tablets

Evaporate the mixed tinctures on a water bath or by gentle heat to about 10 cc. Add the spirit of glyceryl trinitrate. Incorporate this mixture intimately with a sufficient quantity of lactose and compress into 100 tablets.

AVERAGE DOSE—1 tablet.

DELAFIELD'S TABLETS
(V.C.N.Y.)

Powdered Extract of Belladonna	0.16 Gm.
Ipecac, in fine powder	0.30 Gm.
Powder of Ipecac and Opium	0.65 Gm.
Quinine Sulfate	1.60 Gm.
Lactose	10 Gm.
To make	100 Tablets

Mix intimately. Moisten with diluted alcohol and compress into 100 tablets.

AVERAGE DOSE—1 tablet.

MERCURIC SALICYLATE TABLETS
(R.B. I)

Mercuric Salicylate	2 Gm.
Lactose	28 Gm.
Diluted Alcohol, a sufficient quantity,	
To make	100 Tablets

Mix intimately, moisten with diluted alcohol and compress into 100 tablets.

AVERAGE DOSE—1 tablet.

Each tablet contains about 0.02 Gm. (⅓ grain) of mercuric salicylate.

SPARTEINE SULFATE TABLETS
(R.B. I)

Sparteine Sulfate	1.5 Gm.
Lactose	8 Gm.
Alcohol, Ethyl Oxide, of each, an equal volume } a sufficient quantity,	
To make	100 Tablets

Mix the powders intimately and moisten with sufficient of the alcohol and ethyl oxide mixture; dry the mixture and compress into 100 tablets.

AVERAGE DOSE—1 tablet.

Each tablet contains about 0.015 Gm. (¼ grain) of sparteine sulfate.

SWEET TABLETS
(R.B. I)

Formulas for Sweet Tablets, originated by Dr. Bernard Fantus, of Chicago, for administration to children, require the use of special preparations, Cacao Sugar Tablet Base, Solution of Tolu Balsam and Saccharin and Alcoholic Solution of Saccharin, the formulas for which follow.

CACAO SUGAR TABLET BASE

Spirit of Cinnamon	0.5	cc.
Cacao, in fine powder	20	Gm.
Sucrose, in fine powder	80	Gm.
To make	100	Gm.

Mix intimately by trituration in a mortar.

Keep in a well-stoppered bottle.

Difficulty in the compression of these tablets may be overcome by the addition of a small amount of heavy liquid petrolatum.

SOLUTION OF TOLU BALSAM AND SACCHARIN

Tolu Balsam	2 Gm.
Saccharin	2 Gm.
Alcohol, a sufficient quantity,	
To make	100 cc.

Dissolve.

ALCOHOLIC SOLUTION OF SACCHARIN

Saccharin	3 Gm.
Alcohol, a sufficient quantity,	
To make	100 cc.

Dissolve.

SWEET TABLETS OF ACETOPHENETIDIN
Tabellæ Acetophenetidini Dulces
Sweet Tablets of Phenacetin

Acetophenetidin	6 Gm.
Alcoholic Solution of Saccharin, R.B.	2 cc.
Cacao Sugar Tablet Base, R.B.	24 Gm.
To make	100 Tablets

Mix the acetophenetidin with the alcoholic solution of saccharin and triturate until the alcohol has evaporated. Then add the cacao sugar tablet base and continue the trituration until an intimate mixture is obtained. Compress in a tablet machine, using ⅜-inch die and punches, to make 100 tablets of 0.3 Gm. each.

AVERAGE DOSE—Child: 1 tablet.

SWEET TABLETS OF ALBUMIN TANNATE

Albumin Tannate	6 Gm.
Cacao Sugar Tablet Base, R.B.	19 Gm.
To make	100 Tablets

Mix intimately by thorough trituration in a mortar, and compress in a tablet machine, using ⅜-inch die and punches, to make 100 tablets of 0.25 Gm. each.

AVERAGE DOSE—Child: 1 tablet.

SWEET TABLETS OF QUININE ETHYLCARBONATE
Tabellæ Aristochinæ Dulces
Sweet Tablets of Euquinine

Quinine Ethylcarbonate	6 Gm.
Alcoholic Solution of Saccharin, R.B.	3 cc.
Sodium Bicarbonate	1 Gm.
Cacao Sugar Tablet Base, R.B.	23 Gm.
To make	100 Tablets

Triturate the quinine ethylcarbonate with the alcoholic solution of saccharin until the alcohol has evaporated. Then add the cacao sugar tablet base and sodium bicarbonate and mix by thorough trituration. Compress in a tablet machine, using ⅜-inch die and punches, to make 100 tablets of 0.3 Gm. each.

AVERAGE DOSE—1 to 2 tablets.

SWEET TABLETS OF ATROPINE
Tabellæ Atropinæ Dulces

Atropine Sulfate	0.03 Gm.
Cacao Sugar Tablet Base, R.B.	30 Gm.
To make	100 Tablets

Mix intimately by thorough trituration in a mortar, and compress in a tablet machine, using ⅜-inch die and punches, to make 100 tablets of 0.3 Gm. each.

AVERAGE DOSE—1 tablet.

Each tablet contains about 0.0003 Gm. (1/200 grain) of atropine sulfate.

SWEET TABLETS OF CALCIUM IODOBEHENATE
Tabellæ Calcii Iodobehenatis Dulces

Calcium Iodobehenate	6 Gm.
Cacao Sugar Tablet Base, R.B.	24 Gm.
To make	100 Tablets

Mix intimately by trituration in a mortar, and compress in a tablet machine using ⅜-inch die and punches, to make 100 tablets of 0.3 Gm. each.

AVERAGE DOSE—Child: 1 tablet.

Each tablet contains about 0.06 Gm. (1 grain) of calcium iodobehenate.

SWEET TABLETS OF DIGITALIS
Tabellæ Digitalis Dulces

Digitalis, in No. 40 powder . . . .   **0.8 Gm.**
Solution of Tolu Balsam and Saccharin, R.B. . . . .   **1.6 cc.**
Cacao Sugar Tablet Base, R.B. . . . .   **29.2 Gm.**

To make . . . .   **100   Tablets**

Moisten the digitalis thoroughly with the liquid.   Place the cacao sugar tablet base upon a No. 20 sieve, add the moistened powder, and pass it through the sieve repeatedly to secure thorough admixture.   Compress the powder in a tablet machine, using ⅜-inch die and punches, to make 100 tablets of 0.3 Gm. each.

Average dose—Child: 1 tablet.

Each tablet contains about 0.008 Gm. (⅛ grain) of digitalis.

SWEET TABLETS OF IPECAC
Tabellæ Ipecacuanhæ Dulces

Ipecac, in No. 40 powder . . . .   **3 Gm.**
Solution of Tolu Balsam and Saccharin, R.B. . . . .   **3 cc.**
Cacao Sugar Tablet Base, R.B. . . . .   **27 Gm.**

To make . . . .   **100 Tablets**

Moisten the ipecac thoroughly with the liquid.   Place the cacao sugar tablet base upon a No. 20 sieve, add the moistened powder, and pass it through the sieve repeatedly to secure thorough admixture.   Compress the powder in a tablet machine, using ⅜-inch die and punches, to make 100 tablets.

Average dose—Child: 1 tablet.

Each tablet contains 0.03 Gm. (½ grain) of ipecac.

SWEET TABLETS OF IRON
Tabellæ Ferri Dulces

Saccharated Ferrous Carbonate . . . .   **13   Gm.**
Cacao Sugar Tablet Base, R.B. . . . .   **17.5 Gm.**

To make . . . .   **100   Tablets**

Mix intimately by trituration in a mortar, and compress in a tablet machine using ⅜-inch die and punches, to make 100 tablets.

Average dose—Child: 1 tablet.

Each tablet contains 0.13 Gm. (2 grains) of saccharated ferrous carbonate.

SWEET TABLETS OF IRON AND ARSENIC
Tabellæ Ferri et Arseni Dulces

Arsenic Trioxide.	0.06 Gm.
Saccharated Ferrous Carbonate	13 Gm.
Cacao Sugar Tablet Base, R.B.	17.50 Gm.
To make	100 Tablets

Mix intimately by trituration in a mortar, and compress in a tablet machine, using ⅜-inch die and punches, to make 100 tablets of 0.3 Gm. each.

AVERAGE DOSE—Child: 1 tablet.

Each tablet contains about 0.0006 Gm. ($\frac{1}{100}$ grain) of arsenic trioxide and 0.13 Gm. (2 grains) of saccharated ferrous carbonate.

SWEET TABLETS OF METHENAMINE
Tabellæ Methenaminæ Dulces

Methenamine	3 Gm.
Cacao Sugar Tablet Base, R.B.	27 Gm.
To make	100 Tablets

Mix intimately by trituration in a mortar, and compress in a tablet machine, using ⅜-inch die and punches, to make 100 tablets.

AVERAGE DOSE—Child: 1 tablet.

Each tablet contains about 0.03 Gm. ($\frac{1}{2}$ grain) of methenamine.

SWEET TABLETS OF TERPIN HYDRATE
Tabellæ Terpini Hydratis Dulces

Terpin Hydrate	3 Gm.
Cacao Sugar Tablet Base, R.B.	27 Gm.
To make	100 Tablets

Mix intimately by trituration in a mortar, and compress in a tablet machine, using ⅜-inch die and punches, to make 100 tablets of 0.3 Gm. each.

AVERAGE DOSE—Child: 1 tablet.

Each tablet contains about 0.0375 Gm. ($\frac{1}{2}$ grain) of terpin hydrate.

TINCTURES

Tinctures are alcoholic or hydro-alcoholic solutions of established strength, containing the active principles and extractives of vegetable or animal drugs, or, in a few instances, crystalline chemicals. Tinctures are made either by percolation or maceration according to the directions of the N.F. VII, page 439.

COMPOUND TINCTURE OF ALOE
Tinctura Aloes Composita
(D.A.B. V)

Aloe, in fine powder	30 Gm.
Zedoary, in fine powder.	5 Gm.
Crocus, in fine powder	5 Gm.
Rhubarb, in fine powder	5 Gm.
Gentian, in fine powder.	5 Gm.
Alcohol,	
Water, of each, a sufficient quantity,	
To make about	1000 cc.

Prepare the Tincture by Process M (see N.F. VII, page 439), using a mixture of 7 volumes of alcohol and 3 volumes of water as the menstruum.

AVERAGE DOSE—Metric, 8 cc.—Apothecaries, 2 fluidrachms.

NOTE—The following synonyms are applied to this preparation or to slight variations of it: Elixir Sacrum, Elixir Succicum, Elixir Jernitzii, Lebenselixir, Lebenessenz Lebenstropfen, Magentropfen and Quintropfen.

TINCTURE OF ANGELICA ROOT
Tinctura Angelicæ Radicis
(D.A.B. V)

Angelica Root, cut	200 Gm.
Alcohol,	
Water, of each, a sufficient quantity,	
To make	1000 cc.

Prepare the Tincture by Process M (see N.F. VII, page 439), using a mixture of 2 volumes of alcohol and 1 volume of water as the menstruum.

AVERAGE DOSE—Metric, 4 cc.—Apothecaries, 1 fluidrachm.

ANTIPERIODIC TINCTURE
Tinctura Antiperiodica
Warburg's Tincture
(N.F. V)

Rhubarb, in moderately coarse powder	8	Gm.
Angelica Fruit, in moderately coarse powder	8	Gm.
Inula, in moderately coarse powder	4	Gm.
Crocus, in moderately coarse powder	4	Gm.
Fennel, in moderately coarse powder	4	Gm.
Gentian, in moderately coarse powder	2	Gm.
Zedoary, in moderately coarse powder	2	Gm.
Cubeb, in moderately coarse powder	2	Gm.
Myrrh, in coarse powder	2	Gm.
Camphor, in coarse powder	2	Gm.
Agaric, in moderately coarse powder	2	Gm.
Pepper, in moderately coarse powder	0.35	Gm.
Cinnamon, in moderately coarse powder	0.75	Gm.
Ginger, in moderately coarse powder	0.75	Gm.
Quinine Hydrochloride	15	Gm.
Aloe	35	Gm.
Alcohol,		
Water, of each, a sufficient quantity,		
To make	1000	cc.

Mix alcohol and water in the proportion of 3 volumes of alcohol and 2 volumes of water. Saturate the mixed drugs with the menstruum and having macerated them for 24 hours, percolate according to Process P (see N.F. VII, page 439) until the Tincture measures 960 cc. In this dissolve the quinine hydrochloride and aloe by the aid of gentle heat, and add sufficient menstruum to make the product measure 1000 cc. Finally filter the Tincture through paper.

DOSE—The dosage of Warburg's Tincture depends on the intended purpose, and varies from 4 cc. (1 fluidrachm) to 15 cc. (4 fluidrachms). The larger quantity is given when Dr. Warburg's original directions are followed for administering the remedy in remittent fevers. These directions were as follows: "One-half ounce to be given alone, without dilution, after the bowels have been evacuated by any convenient purgative, all liquids being withheld. After 3 hours, another half ounce is to be given."

AROMATIC TINCTURE
Tinctura Aromatica
(N.F. V)

Cinnamon, in moderately coarse powder	100 Gm.
Ginger, in moderately coarse powder	40 Gm.
Galangal, in moderately coarse powder	20 Gm.
Clove, in coarse powder	20 Gm.
Cardamom Seed, in coarse powder	20 Gm.
Alcohol,	
Water, of each a sufficient quantity,	
To make	1000 cc.

Prepare the Tincture by Process P (N.F. VII, page 439), using a mixture of 2 volumes of alcohol and 1 volume of water as the menstruum.

AVERAGE DOSE—Metric, 2 cc.—Apothecaries, 30 minims.

ACID AROMATIC TINCTURE
Tinctura Acida Aromatica
I
(R.B. I)

Aromatic Tincture, R.B.	980 cc.
Sulfuric Acid, a sufficient quantity,	
To make	1000 cc.

Add the acid gradually to the tincture, keeping the mixture cooled below 50° C.

AVERAGE DOSE—Metric, 4 cc.—Apothecaries, 1 fluidrachm.

II
Elixir Vitrioli Mynsichti
(E.B. III)

Cinnamon, in fine powder.	100 Gm.
Ginger, in fine powder	40 Gm.
Galangal, in fine powder	20 Gm.
Cardamom Seed, in fine powder	20 Gm.
Clove, in fine powder.	20 Gm.
Hydrochloric Acid,	
Water,	
Alcohol, of each, a sufficient quantity,	
To make	1000 cc.

Prepare the Tincture by Process P (see N.F. VII, page 439), using a mixture of 1 volume of hydrochloric acid, 7 volumes of water and 20 volumes of alcohol as the menstruum.

AVERAGE DOSE—Metric, 8 cc.—Apothecaries, 2 fluidrachms.

AROMATIC TINCTURE WITH PEPPERMINT AND ETHYL ACETATE
(P.F.)

Oil of Peppermint	20 cc.
Aromatic Tincture, R.B.	800 cc.
Ethyl Acetate	180 cc.
To make	1000 cc.

Mix.

AVERAGE DOSE—Metric, 4 cc.—Apothecaries, 1 fluidrachm.

BASTLER'S TINCTURE
(P.F.)

Oil of Anise.	120 cc.
Oil of Cajuput.	120 cc.
Oil of Juniper.	120 cc.
Spirit of Ether.	240 cc.
Tincture of Vitriol, R.B.	30 cc.
Tincture of Cinnamon, a sufficient quantity,	
To make	1000 cc.

Mix.

AVERAGE DOSE—Metric, 4 cc.—Apothecaries, 1 fluidrachm.

BITTER TINCTURE
Tinctura Amara

Stomach Drops
(N.F. V)

Gentian, in moderately coarse powder	60 Gm.
Centaury, in moderately coarse powder	60 Gm.
Bitter Orange Peel, in moderately coarse powder	60 Gm.
Zedoary, in moderately coarse powder	20 Gm.
Alcohol,	
Water, of each, a sufficient quantity,	
To make	1000 cc.

Prepare the Tincture by Process P (see N.F. VII, page 439), using a mixture of 2 volumes of alcohol and 1 volume of water as the menstruum.

AVERAGE DOSE—Metric, 2 cc.—Apothecaries, 30 minims.

AROMATIC BITTER TINCTURE
Tinctura Aromatica Amara
(E.B. III)

Aromatic Tincture, R.B.,
Bitter Tincture, R.B., of each, an equal volume.

Mix.

AVERAGE DOSE—Metric, 2 cc.—Apothecaries, 30 minims.

TINCTURE OF CALAMUS
Tinctura Calami
(D.A.B. V)

Calamus, in moderately coarse powder	200 Gm.
Alcohol,	
Water, of each, a sufficient quantity,	
To make	1000 cc.

Prepare the Tincture by Process P (see N.F. VII, page 439), using a mixture of 7 volumes of alcohol and 3 volumes of water as the menstruum.

AVERAGE DOSE—Metric, 4 cc.—Apothecaries, 1 fluidrachm.

STRONGER TINCTURE OF CAPSICUM
Tinctura Capsici Fortior
Turnbull's Tincture of Capsicum
(B.P.C. 1934)

Capsicum, in moderately coarse powder.	333 Gm.
Alcohol,	
Water, of each, a sufficient quantity,	
To make	1000 cc.

Prepare the Tincture by Process P (see N.F. VII, page 439), using a mixture of 2 volumes of alcohol and 1 volume of water as the menstruum.

TINCTURE OF CARAMEL
Tinctura Caramellis
(N.F. IV)

Caramel	100 Gm.
Alcohol	250 cc.
Water, a sufficient quantity,	
To make	1000 cc.

Dissolve the caramel in 500 cc. of water, with the aid of heat if necessary add the alcohol and sufficient water to make the product measure 1000 cc., and filter.

TINCTURE OF CARDAMOM
Tinctura Cardamomi
(U.S.P. X)

Cardamom Seed, in moderately coarse powder.	200 Gm.
Diluted Alcohol, a sufficient quantity,	
To make	1000 cc.

Prepare the Tincture by Process P (see N.F. VII, page 439), using diluted alcohol as the menstruum.

AVERAGE DOSE—Metric, 2 cc.—Apothecaries, 30 minims.

CARMINATIVE TINCTURE
Tinctura Carminativa
Tinctura Calami Composita
(E.B. III)

Zedoary, cut	80 Gm.
Calamus, cut	40 Gm.
Galangal, cut	40 Gm.
Anthemis, in coarse powder	20 Gm.
Caraway, in coarse powder	20 Gm.
Anise, in coarse powder	20 Gm.
Laurel Berries,* in coarse powder	15 Gm.
Clove, in coarse powder	15 Gm.
Mace, in coarse powder	15 Gm.
Bitter Orange Peel, in coarse powder	5 Gm.
Alcohol,	
Peppermint Water, of each, a sufficient quantity,	
To make	1000 cc.

Prepare the Tincture by Process M (see N.F. VII, page 439), using equal volumes of alcohol and peppermint water as the menstruum.

NOTE—Before dispensing add to every 9 cc. of this tincture 1 cc. of spirit of ethyl nitrite.

AVERAGE DOSE—Metric, 4 cc.—Apothecaries, 1 fluidrachm.

TINCTURE OF CASCARILLA
Tinctura Cascarillæ
(B.P.C. 1934)

Cascarilla, in moderately coarse powder	200 Gm.
Alcohol,	
Water, of each, a sufficient quantity,	
To make	1000 cc.

Prepare the Tincture by Process P (see N.F. VII, page 439), using a mixture of 5 volumes of alcohol and 2 volumes of water as the menstruum.

AVERAGE DOSE—Metric, 2 to 4 cc.—Apothecaries, 30 to 60 minims.

TINCTURE OF CASTOR
Tinctura Castorei
(E.B. III)

Castor, in coarse powder	100 Gm.
Alcohol,	
Water, of each, a sufficient quantity,	
To make	1000 cc.

* Dried ripe fruit of *Laurus nobilis*, Linné.

Prepare the Tincture by Process M (see N.F. VII, page 439), using a mixture of 19 volumes of alcohol and 1 volume of water as the menstruum.

AVERAGE DOSE—Metric, 4 cc.—Apothecaries, 1 fluidrachm.

ETHEREAL TINCTURE OF CASTOR
Tinctura Castorei Ætherea
(E.B. III)

Castor, in coarse powder . . . .   80 Gm.
Ethyl Oxide,
Alcohol, of each, a sufficient quantity,
                                    To make . . . .   1000 cc.

Prepare the Tincture by Process M (see N.F. VII, page 439), using a mixture of 3 volumes of alcohol and 1 volume of ethyl oxide as the menstruum.

AVERAGE DOSE—Metric, 4 cc.—Apothecaries, 1 fluidrachm.

TINCTURE OF CHLOROFORM AND MORPHINE WITH ETHYL OXIDE
Tinctura Chloroformi et Morphinæ
Chlorodyne
(B.P.C. 1934)

Chloroform 125   cc.
Ethyl Oxide. . . . . 31.25 cc.
Alcohol 125   cc.
Morphine Hydrochloride . . . .   2.29 Gm.
Diluted Hydrocyanic Acid. . . . . 62.50 cc.
Oil of Peppermint . . . . 1.04 cc.
Fluidextract of Glycyrrhiza 125   cc.
Molasses 125   cc.
Syrup, a sufficient quantity,
                                    To make 1000   cc.

Dissolve the morphine hydrochloride and the oil of peppermint in the alcohol and add the chloroform and ethyl oxide. Mix the fluidextract of glycyrrhiza and molasses with 400 cc. of syrup and add this to the first solution. Mix thoroughly, add the diluted hydrocyanic acid and sufficient syrup to make the product measure 1000 cc.

AVERAGE DOSE—Metric, 0.3 to 0.6 cc.—Apothecaries, 5 to 10 minims.

NOTE—This preparation must be dispensed on prescription only.

TINCTURE OF CINCHONA
Tinctura Cinchonæ
(U.S.P. X)

Cinchona, in moderately coarse powder. . . . .   **200 Gm.**
Glycerin . . . .   **75 cc.**
Alcohol,
Water, of each, a sufficient quantity,
To make . . . . 1000 cc.

Prepare the Tincture by Process P, as modified for assayed tinctures (see N.F. VII, page 439). Use a mixture of the glycerin, 675 cc. of alcohol and 250 cc. of water as the first menstruum, and complete the percolation with a mixture of 2 volumes of alcohol and 1 volume of water.

Adjust the Tincture to make each 100 cc. of the finished product contain 0.9 Gm. of the alkaloids of cinchona, using the second menstruum for dilution, if necessary.

AVERAGE DOSE—Metric, 4 cc.—Apothecaries, 1 fluidrachm.

TINCTURE OF COCHINEAL
Tinctura Cocci
(E.B. III)

Cochineal, in coarse powder. . . . .   **100 Gm.**
Alcohol,
Water, of each, a sufficient quantity,
To make . . . . 1000 cc.

Prepare the Tincture by Process M (see N.F. VII, page 439), using a mixture of 7 volumes of alcohol and 3 volumes of water as the menstruum.

AVERAGE DOSE—Metric, 4 to 6 cc.—Apothecaries, 1 to 1½ fluidrachms

TINCTURE OF COLOCYNTH
Tinctura Colocynthidis
Tincture of Bitter Apple
(D.A.B. V)

Colocynth, deprived of seeds and cut . . . .   **100 Gm.**
Alcohol,
Water, of each, a sufficient quantity,
To make . . . . 1000 cc.

Prepare the Tincture by Process P (see N.F. VII, page 439), using a mixture of 19 volumes of alcohol and 1 volume of water as the menstruum.

AVERAGE DOSE—Metric, 1 cc.—Apothecaries, 15 minims.

TINCTURE OF CONDURANGO
Tinctura Condurango
(E.B. III)

Condurango, in coarse or moderately coarse powder . . . .   100 Gm.
Alcohol,
Water, of each, a sufficient quantity,
                              To make . . . .   1000 cc.

Prepare the Tincture by Process P (see N.F. VII, page 439), using a mixture of 7 volumes of alcohol and 3 volumes of water as the menstruum.

AVERAGE DOSE—Metric, 4 cc.—Apothecaries, 1 fluidrachm.

EPISCOPAL TINCTURE
Tinctura Episcopalis
Essentia Episcopalis
Bischoff-Essenz

Tincture of Cinnamon   200   cc.
Oil of Clove . . . .   0.50 cc.
Oil of Lemon . . . .   1.25 cc.
Oil of Orange   5   cc.
Tincture of Bitter Orange Peel, a sufficient quantity,
                              To make   1000   cc.

Mix and filter.
AVERAGE DOSE—Metric, 4 cc.—Apothecaries, 1 fluidrachm.

AMMONIATED TINCTURE OF ERGOT
Tinctura Ergotæ Ammoniata
(N.F. IV)

Ergot, in coarse powder. . . . .   250 Gm.
Diluted Solution of Ammonia . . . .   100 cc.
Alcohol,
Water, of each, a sufficient quantity,
                              To make . . . .   1000 cc.

Mix the diluted solution of ammonia with 600 cc. of alcohol and 200 cc. of water. Saturate the powder with this menstruum and, after macerating for 24 hours, percolate it, in the usual manner, first with the remainder of the above menstruum and afterward with a mixture of 2 volumes of alcohol and 1 volume of water, until the product measures 1000 cc.

AVERAGE DOSE—Metric, 4 cc.—Apothecaries, 1 fluidrachm.

TINCTURE OF EUCALYPTUS
Tinctura Eucalypti
(B.P.C. 1934)

Eucalyptus, in coarse powder . . . . 200 Gm.
Alcohol,
Water, of each, a sufficient quantity,

To make . . . . 1000 cc.

Prepare the Tincture by Process P (see N.F. VII, page 439), using a mixture of 6 volumes of alcohol and 4 volumes of water as the menstruum.

AVERAGE DOSE—Metric, 2 to 8 cc.—Apothecaries, ½ to 2 fluidrachms.

TINCTURE OF FENNEL
Tinctura Fœniculi

Romershausen's Augenessenz
(E.B. III)

Fennel, bruised . . . . 175 Gm.
Oil of Fennel . . . . 1.8 cc.
Alcohol,
Water, of each, a sufficient quantity,

To make . . . . 1000 cc.

Macerate the fennel in 1000 cc. of a mixture of 7 volumes of alcohol and 3 volumes of water for 3 days at a temperature of 15° to 20° C. Filter, add the oil and pass sufficient of the menstruum through the filter to make the product measure 1000 cc.

This tincture, diluted with 5 volumes of water, is used as an eye wash, which is known as Romershausen's Eye Water (see R.B., page 86).

TINCTURE OF FERRATED EXTRACT OF APPLE
Tinctura Ferri Pomata

Tinctura Ferri Malatis Crudi, Tincture of Crude Malate of Iron
(N.F. V)

Ferrated Extract of Apple, R.B. . . . . 100 Gm.
Alcohol . . . . 100 cc.
Cinnamon Water, a sufficient quantity,

To make . . . . 1000 cc.

Dissolve the ferrated extract of apple in 750 cc. of cinnamon water, add the alcohol, filter and pass sufficient cinnamon water through the filter to make the product measure 1000 cc.

AVERAGE DOSE—Metric, 4 cc.—Apothecaries, 1 fluidrachm.

TINCTURE OF GALANGAL
Tinctura Galangæ
(E.B. III)

Galangal, in coarse powder . . . .   200 Gm.
Alcohol,
Water, of each, a sufficient quantity,
                              To make . . . .   1000 cc.

Prepare the Tincture by Process P (see N.F. VII, page 439), using a mixture of 7 volumes of alcohol and 3 volumes of water as the menstruum.

AVERAGE DOSE—Metric, 4 cc.—Apothecaries, 1 fluidrachm.

TINCTURE OF GAMBIR
Tinctura Catechu
Tincture of Catechu
(B.P.)

Gambir, crushed. . . . .   200 Gm.
Cinnamon, bruised. . . . .   50 Gm.
Alcohol,
Water, of each, a sufficient quantity,
                              To make . . . .   1000 cc.

Prepare the Tincture by Process M (see N.F. VII, page 439), using a mixture of 1 volume of alcohol and 1 volume of water as the menstruum.

AVERAGE DOSE—Metric, 2 to 4 cc.—Apothecaries, 30 to 60 minims.

TINCTURE OF GENTIAN
Tinctura Gentianæ
(B.P.C.)

Gentian, in coarse powder. . . . .   100 Gm.
Alcohol,
Water, of each, a sufficient quantity,
                              To make . . . .   1000 cc.

Prepare the Tincture by Process M (see N.F. VII, page 439), using a mixture of 7 volumes of alcohol and 3 volumes of water as the menstruum.

AVERAGE DOSE—Metric, 4 cc.—Apothecaries, 1 fluidrachm.

TINCTURE OF IGNATIA
Tinctura Ignatiæ
(N.F. V)

Ignatia, in fine powder . . . .   100 Gm.
Alcohol,
Water, of each, a sufficient quantity,
                              To make . . . .   1000 cc.

Prepare the Tincture by Process P as modified for assayed tinctures (see N.F. VII, page 439), using a mixture of 8 volumes of alcohol and 1 volume of water as the menstruum, and adjusting the volume of the finished Tincture so that each 100 cc. contains 0.2 Gm. of the alkaloids of ignatia.

AVERAGE DOSE—Metric, 0.6 cc.—Apothecaries, 10 minims.

OILY TINCTURE OF IODINE
Tinctura Iodi Oleosa
Liquor Iodi Oleosus; Oily Solution of Iodine
(B.P.C. 1934)

Iodine	80	Gm.
Castor Oil	162.5	cc.
Alcohol, a sufficient quantity,		
To make	1000	cc.

Dissolve the iodine in 800 cc. of the alcohol by the aid of gentle heat; add the castor oil and sufficient alcohol to make the product measure 1000 cc.

AROMATIC TINCTURE OF IRON
Tinctura Ferri Aromatica
(E.B. III)

Solution of Ferric Oxychloride, R.B.	60	cc.
Syrup	230	cc.
Sodium Hydroxide	0.6	Gm.
Alcohol	185	cc.
Tincture of Sweet Orange Peel	3	cc.
Aromatic Spirit, R.B.	1.5	cc.
Tincture of Vanilla	1.5	cc.
Ethyl Acetate	0.3	cc.
Distilled Water, a sufficient quantity,		
To make	1000	cc.

Mix the solution of ferric oxychloride and syrup and add at once the sodium hydroxide dissolved in 35 cc. of distilled water. Agitate briskly and add the remainder of the distilled water (484 cc.) and the other ingredients, previously mixed.

AVERAGE DOSE—Metric, 4 cc.—Apothecaries, 1 fluidrachm.

COMPOUND TINCTURE OF IRON
Tinctura Ferri Composita
(G.H.N.Y.)

Tincture of Nux Vomica.	376 cc.
Fluidextract of Rhubarb.	25 cc.
Tincture of Bitter Orange Peel	30 cc.
Tincture of Cardamom, R.B.	25 cc.
Sucrose.	40 Gm.
Tincture of Ferrated Extract of Apple, R.B.	312 cc.
Sherry Wine, a sufficient quantity,	
To make	1000 cc.

Dissolve the sucrose in the mixed liquids by agitation.

AVERAGE DOSE—Metric, 4 cc.—Apothecaries, 1 fluidrachm.

ETHEREAL TINCTURE OF IRON ACETATE
Tinctura Ferri Acetatis Ætherea

Tinctura Martis, Klaprothii; Klaproth's Tincture of Iron
(D.A.B. III)

Solution of Ferric Acetate, R.B.	490 cc.
Ethyl Acetate	115 cc.
Alcohol	115 cc.
Distilled Water, a sufficient quantity,	
To make	1000 cc.

Mix the ethyl acetate and alcohol and add gradually to the solution of ferric acetate.   Finally, add sufficient distilled water to make the product measure 1000 cc.

Keep in well-stoppered bottles in a cool place, protected from light.

AVERAGE DOSE—Metric, 4 cc.—Apothecaries, 1 fluidrachm.

COMPOUND TINCTURE OF KINO AND OPIUM
Tinctura Kino et Opii Composita

Tinctura Kino Composita; Compound Tincture of Kino
(N.F. IV)

Tincture of Kino.	200	cc.
Tincture of Opium	100	cc.
Spirit of Camphor	65	cc.
Oil of Clove.	1.5	cc.
Cochineal, in fine powder	8.5	Gm
Aromatic Spirit of Ammonia.	8	cc.
Diluted Alcohol, a sufficient quantity,		
To make	1000	cc.

Triturate the cochineal with the aromatic spirit of ammonia, and add gradually 625 cc. of diluted alcohol. Then add the two tinctures, spirit of camphor, oil of clove and sufficient diluted alcohol to make the product measure 1000 cc. Filter.

AVERAGE DOSE—Metric, 4 cc.—Apothecaries, 1 fluidrachm.

NOTE—This preparation must be dispensed on prescription only.

TINCTURE OF KRAMERIA
Tinctura Krameriæ

Krameria, in moderately coarse powder.	200 Gm.
Glycerin,	
Alcohol, a sufficient quantity,	
To make	1000 cc.

Prepare the Tincture by Process P (see N.F. VII, page 439), using a mixture of 9 volumes of alcohol and 1 volume of glycerin as the menstruum.

AVERAGE DOSE—Metric, 4 cc.—Apothecaries, 1 fluidrachm.

TINCTURE OF KRAMERIA, VALERIAN, CASCARILLA AND OPIUM WITH PEPPERMINT
(E.B. IV)

Oil of Peppermint	20 cc.
Tincture of Cascarilla, R.B.	80 cc.
Tincture of Opium	100 cc.
Tincture of Krameria, R.B.	200 cc.
Ethereal Tincture of Valerian*	300 cc.
Aromatic Tincture, R.B.	300 cc.
To make	1000 cc.

Mix, set aside for 3 days and filter.

AVERAGE DOSE—Metric, 4 cc.—Apothecaries, 1 fluidrachm.

NOTE—This preparation must be dispensed on prescription only.

TINCTURE OF LACTUCARIUM
Tinctura Lactucarii
(U.S.P. IX)

Lactucarium.	500 Gm.
Glycerin	250 cc.
Alcohol,	
Purified Benzin,	
Diluted Alcohol,	
Water, of each, a sufficient quantity,	
To make	1000 cc.

* Prepared according to the general formula for Ethereal Tinctures (see N.F. VII, page 465).

Beat the lactucarium with clean sand, in an iron mortar, to a coarse powder, and then transfer it to a bottle; add 2000 cc. of purified petroleum benzin, stopper the bottle tightly and set it aside for 48 hours, frequently agitating the mixture. Pour the mixture on a double filter, cover the funnel and, when the liquid has passed through the filter, wash the residue gradually with 1500 cc. of purified petroleum benzin, and then allow the lactucarium to dry by exposing it to a current of air. When it is dry and free from the odor of benzin, reduce it to a powder, using more sand, if necessary, and pack it moderately in a conical percolator. Mix the glycerin with 250 cc. of water and 500 cc. of alcohol, and pour this mixture gradually on the powder. When the liquid begins to drop from the percolator, close the lower orifice, and, having covered the percolator tightly, macerate for 24 hours. Then allow the percolation to proceed slowly, adding gradually first the remainder of the menstruum and then diluted alcohol, until the drug is exhausted. Reserve the first 750 cc. of the percolate, evaporate the remainder on a water bath at a temperature not exceeding 70° C. until it measures 250 cc. and mix this with the reserved portion. Filter the mixed liquids and wash the filter with sufficient diluted alcohol to make the product measure 1000 cc.

AVERAGE DOSE—Metric. 2 cc.—Apothecaries, 30 minims.

TINCTURE OF MATRICARIA
Tinctura Chamomillæ
(Ph. Aust.)

Matricaria Flowers.	200 Gm.
Alcohol.	800 cc.
Water	350 cc.
To make about	1000 cc.

Macerate the matricaria flowers in the mixed alcohol and water for 8 days, shaking frequently. Strain, press, set aside for 2 days and filter.

TINCTURE OF OIL OF BIRCH TAR
Tinctura Olei Rusci
(P.F.)

Rectified Oil of Birch Tar.	200 cc.
Ethyl Oxide.	340 cc.
Oil of Lavender.	40 cc.
Oil of Rosemary.	40 cc.
Oil of Rue.	40 cc.
Alcohol, a sufficient quantity,	
To make	1000 cc.

Dissolve the oils in a mixture of the alcohol and ethyl oxide.

COMPOUND TINCTURE OF OPIUM AND GAMBIR

Bateman's Pectoral Drops; Pectoral Drops; Tr. Pectoralis N.F. IV
(N.F. V)

Tincture of Opium	42 cc.
Compound Tincture of Gambir	64 cc.
Spirit of Camphor	40 cc.
Oil of Anise	1 cc.
Caramel	10 cc.
Diluted Alcohol, a sufficient quantity,	
To make	1000 cc.

Mix the ingredients with sufficient diluted alcohol to make the product measure 1000 cc.

AVERAGE DOSE—For infants: Metric, 0.6 cc.—Apothecaries, 10 minims.
Each average dose represents:

> 0.025 cc. or $\frac{2}{5}$ minim of Tincture of Opium
> 0.038 cc. or $\frac{3}{5}$ minim of Comp. Tincture of Gambir
> 0.0024 Gm. or $\frac{1}{27}$ grain of Camphor

NOTE—This preparation must be dispensed on prescription only.

TINCTURE OF OPIUM WITH SAFFRON
Tinctura Opii Crocata

Sydenham's Laudanum
(N.F. V)

Granulated Opium	100 Gm.
Crocus, in coarse powder	25 Gm.
Cinnamon, in fine powder	6 Gm.
Clove, in coarse powder	6 Gm.
Diluted Alcohol, a sufficient quantity,	
To make about	1000 cc.

Mix the drugs with about an equal bulk of clean sand and prepare the Tincture by Process P as modified for assayed tinctures (see N.F. VII, page 439), using diluted alcohol as the menstruum, and adjusting the volume of the finished Tincture so that each 100 cc. will contain 1 Gm. of anhydrous morphine.

AVERAGE DOSE—Metric, 0.6 cc.—Apothecaries, 10 minims.

NOTE—This preparation must be dispensed on prescription only.

TINCTURE OF PARACOTO
Tinctura Paracoto

Tinctura Coto (N.F. III)
(N.F. IV)

Paracoto, in No. 40 powder	125 Gm.
Alcohol, a sufficient quantity,	
To make	1000 cc.

Prepare the Tincture by Process P (see N.F. VII, page 439), using alcohol as the menstruum.

AVERAGE DOSE—Metric, 2 cc.—Apothecaries, 30 minims.

TINCTURE OF PHYSOSTIGMA
Tinctura Physostigmatis
Tincture of Calabar Bean
(U.S.P. IX)

Physostigma, in moderately fine powder. . . . .   100 Gm.
Alcohol, a sufficient quantity,

To make about . . . .   1000 cc.

Prepare the Tincture by Process P, as modified for assayed tinctures (see N.F. VII, page 439), using alcohol as the menstruum.

AVERAGE DOSE—Metric, 1 cc.—Apothecaries, 15 minims.

This tincture is standardized to contain 0.015 Gm. of alkaloids in 100 cc.

TINCTURE OF PIMPINELLA
Tinctura Pimpinellæ
(N.F. IV)

Pimpinella, in No. 40 powder . . . .   200 Gm.
Alcohol,
Water, of each, a sufficient quantity,

To make . . . .   1000 cc.

Prepare the Tincture by Process P (see N.F. VII, page 439), using a mixture of 2 volumes of alcohol and 1 volume of water as the menstruum.

AVERAGE DOSE—Metric, 4 cc.—Apothecaries, 1 fluidrachm.

TINCTURE OF PODOPHYLLUM
Tinctura Podophylli
(B.P.C. 1934)

Resin of Podophyllum . . . .   36.5 Gm.
Alcohol, a sufficient quantity,

To make . . . .   1000 cc.

Macerate the resin of podophyllum for 24 hours in 900 cc. of alcohol. Filter and pass sufficient alcohol through the filter to make the product measure 1000 cc.

AVERAGE DOSE—Metric, 0.3 to 1 cc.—Apothecaries, 5 to 15 minims.

AMMONIATED TINCTURE OF PODOPHYLLUM
Tinctura Podophylli Ammoniata
(B.P.C. 1934)

Resin of Podophyllum . . . .   20 Gm.
Aromatic Spirit of Ammonia, a sufficient quantity,

To make . . . .   1000 cc.

Macerate the resin of podophyllum with 900 cc. of aromatic spirit of ammonia for a period of 24 hours, shaking occasionally. Filter and pass sufficient aromatic spirit of ammonia through the filter to make the product measure 1000 cc.

AVERAGE DOSE—Metric, 0.6 to 1.2 cc.—Apothecaries, 10 to 20 minims.

TINCTURE OF PYRETHRUM
Tinctura Pyrethri

Tincture of Pellitory
(U.S.P. IX)

Pyrethrum, in moderately fine powder . . . .   200 Gm.
Alcohol, a sufficient quantity,

To make . . . .   1000 cc.

Prepare the Tincture by Process P (see N.F. VII, page 439), using alcohol as the menstruum.

AMMONIATED TINCTURE OF QUININE
Liquor Quininæ Ammoniatus
(B.P. 1932)

Quinine Sulfate . . . .   20 Gm.
Diluted Solution of Ammonia . . . .   100 cc.
Alcohol . . . .   570 cc.
Distilled Water, a sufficient quantity,

To make . . . .   1000 cc.

Mix the diluted solution of ammonia and alcohol with 300 cc. of distilled water. Add the quinine sulfate and shake until dissolved. Set aside for 3 days, filter and pass sufficient distilled water through the filter to make the product measure 1000 cc.

AVERAGE DOSE—Metric, 4 cc.—Apothecaries, 1 fluidrachm.

COMPOUND TINCTURE OF QUININE
Tinctura Quininæ Composita
Loomis's Quinine
(P.F.)

Quinine Sulfate	6 Gm.
Salicin	6 Gm.
Cinchona, in coarse powder	10 Gm.
Bitter Orange Peel, in coarse powder	10 Gm.
Water	100 cc.
Alcohol, a sufficient quantity,	
To make	1000 cc.

Macerate the cinchona and bitter orange peel in a mixture of the water and 900 cc. of alcohol for 3 days. Filter and pass sufficient alcohol through the filter to make the product measure 1000 cc. Dissolve the quinine sulfate and salicin in the filtrate.

AVERAGE DOSE—Metric, 4 cc.—Apothecaries, 1 fluidrachm.

TINCTURE OF RED SAUNDERS
Tinctura Santali Rubri
(E.B. III)

Red Saunders, in coarse powder	200 Gm.
Alcohol,	
Water, of each, a sufficient quantity,	
To make	1000 cc.

Prepare the Tincture by Process P (see N.F. VII, page 439), using a mixture of 19 volumes of alcohol and 1 volume of water as the menstruum.

AQUEOUS TINCTURE OF RHUBARB
Tinctura Rhei Aquosa
(N.F. V)

Rhubarb	100 Gm.
Potassium Carbonate.	10 Gm.
Cinnamon Water	125 cc.
Alcohol	110 cc.
Water, a sufficient quantity,	
To make	1000 cc.

Dissolve the potassium carbonate in 750 cc. of water and macerate the rhubarb in this solution during 24 hours, having first cut it into thin slices or broken it into small pieces and freed it from adhering fine powder. Strain this mixture through muslin, heat the strained liquid to boiling, add the cinnamon water and alcohol, stir it well and, while warm, filter it in a covered funnel. To the cold filtrate add sufficient water to make the product measure 1000 cc.

AVERAGE DOSE—Metric, 4 cc.—Apothecaries, 1 fluidrachm.

RUGGLES' TINCTURE

Tincture of Iodine . . . . 193 cc.
Spirit of Camphor . . . . 807 cc.
To make . . . . 1000 cc.

Mix.

TINCTURE OF SAFFRON
Tinctura Croci
(N.F. V)

Crocus . . . . 100 Gm.
Diluted Alcohol, a sufficient quantity,
To make . . . . 1000 cc.

Prepare the Tincture by Process P (see N.F. VII, page 439), using diluted alcohol as the menstruum.

TINCTURE OF STAR ANISE
Tinctura Anisi Stellati
Teinture de Badiane
(R.B. I)

Star Anise, in moderately fine powder . . . . 200 Gm.
Alcohol,
Water, of each, a sufficient quantity,
To make . . . . 1000 cc.

Prepare the Tincture by Process M (see N.F. VII, page 439), using a mixture of 5 volumes of alcohol and 1 volume of water as the menstruum.

AVERAGE DOSE—Metric, 4 cc.—Apothecaries, 1 fluidrachm.

TINCTURE OF STAVESACRE
Tinctura Staphisagriæ
(R.B. I)

Stavesacre, in coarse powder. . . . . 200 Gm.
Alcohol, a sufficient quantity,
To make . . . . 1000 cc.

Prepare the Tincture by Process P (see N.F. VII, page 439), using alcohol as the menstruum.

TINCTURE OF VITRIOL
Tinctura Vitriolis
Mistura Sulfurica Acida; Haller's Acid Elixir
(P.F.)

Alcohol	870 cc.
Sulfuric Acid, a sufficient quantity,	
To make	1000 cc.

Add the sulfuric acid very gradually to the alcohol, contained in a flask, agitating after each addition, and taking care that the temperature of the mixture is not allowed to rise above 50° C.

AVERAGE DOSE—Metric, 0.5 cc.—Apothecaries, 8 minims.

BITTER TINCTURE OF ZEDOARY
Tinctura Zedoariæ Amara
Compound Tincture of Zedoary
(N.F. IV)

Zeodary, in moderately coarse powder	250 Gm.
Aloe, in fine powder	125 Gm.
Rhubarb, in moderately coarse powder	62 Gm.
Gentian, in moderately coarse powder	62 Gm.
Agaric, in moderately coarse powder	62 Gm.
Crocus, in moderately coarse powder	62 Gm.
Glycerin	125 cc.
Alcohol,	
Distilled Water, of each, a sufficient quantity,	
To make	1000 cc.

Mix 2 volumes of alcohol with 1 volume of water. Saturate the mixed drugs and percolate in the usual manner, with this menstruum, until the product measures 750 cc. Add the glycerin and set aside. Continue the percolation until the drugs are practically exhausted, evaporate this percolate to about 120 cc., mix it with the reserved portion and then add sufficient menstruum to make the product measure 1000 cc.

AVERAGE DOSE—Metric, 4 cc.—Apothecaries, 1 fluidrachm.

TROCHES

TROCHES OF AMMONIUM CHLORIDE
Trochisci Ammonii Chloridi
(U.S.P. X)

Ammonium Chloride, in fine powder	10 Gm.
Extract of Glycyrrhiza, in fine powder	20 Gm.
Tragacanth, in very fine powder	2 Gm.
Sucrose, in fine powder.	40 Gm.
Syrup of Tolu Balsam, a sufficient quantity,	
To make	100 Troches

Triturate the powders until they are thoroughly mixed; form a mass with syrup of tolu balsam, and divide it into 100 troches.

AVERAGE DOSE—1 troche.

TROCHES OF CHARCOAL
Trochisci Carbonis
(N.F. IV)

Activated Charcoal, in very fine powder	30	Gm.
Tragacanth, in fine powder	4	Gm.
Sucrose, in fine powder	66	Gm.
Vanillin	0.3	Gm.
Water, a sufficient quantity,		
To make	100	Troches

Triturate the vanillin with 20 Gm. of sucrose until reduced to a fine powder, add the remainder of the sucrose and the other ingredients, mix thoroughly and form a mass with water. Divide the mass into 100 troches and dry these in a current of warm air.

AVERAGE DOSE—1 troche.

TROCHES OF CUBEB
Trochisci Cubebæ
(U.S.P. IX)

Oleoresin of Cubeb	2	Gm.
Oil of Sassafras	1	cc.
Extract of Glycyrrhiza, in fine powder	25	Gm.
Acacia, in fine powder	12	Gm.
Syrup of Tolu Balsam, a sufficient quantity,		
To make	100	Troches

Triturate the powders together until they are thoroughly mixed; then add the oleoresin and the oil, and incorporate them with the mixture. Lastly, form a mass with syrup of tolu balsam and divide it into 100 troches. Dry these in a current of warm air.

AVERAGE DOSE—1 troche.

TROCHES OF GAMBIR
Trochisci Gambir
(N.F. IV)

Gambir, in fine powder	6	Gm.
Tragacanth, in fine powder	3	Gm.
Sucrose, in fine powder	91	Gm.
Oil of Cinnamon	0.2	cc.
Water, a sufficient quantity,		
To make	100	Troches

Triturate the powders together until well mixed; then incorporate the oil, and form a mass with water. Divide the mass into 100 troches and dry in a current of warm air.

AVERAGE DOSE—1 troche.

TROCHES OF MENTHOL
(R.B. I)

Sodium Bicarbonate	12	Gm.
Ginger, in fine powder	3	Gm.
Menthol	0.8	Gm.
Sucrose, in fine powder	100	Gm.
Acacia, in fine powder	10	Gm.
Water, a sufficient quantity,		
To make	100 Troches	

Triturate the ingredients together until well mixed, and form a mass with water. Divide the mass into 100 troches and dry in a current of warm air.

AVERAGE DOSE—1 troche.

TROCHES OF PEPPERMINT
Trochisci Menthæ Piperitæ
(N.F. IV)

Oil of Peppermint	1 cc.
Sucrose, in fine powder	100 Gm.
Mucilage of Tragacanth, a sufficient quantity,	
To make	100 Troches

Triturate the oil of peppermint with the sucrose until they are thoroughly mixed, then form a mass with mucilage of tragacanth. Divide the mass into 100 troches and dry in a current of warm air.

AVERAGE DOSE—1 troche.

TROCHES OF PHENOLPHTHALEIN
Trochisci Phenolphthaleini
(N.F. IV)

Phenolphthalein, in fine powder	6	Gm.
Acacia, in fine powder	10	Gm.
Sucrose, in fine powder	84	Gm.
Vanillin	0.3	Gm.
Carmine	0.1	Gm.
Water, a sufficient quantity,		
To make	100 Troches	

Triturate the carmine and vanillin with 20 Gm. of sucrose until uniformly mixed, then add the remainder of the sucrose and the other ingredients, mix thoroughly and form a mass with water. Divide the mass into 100 troches, and dry these in a current of warm air.

AVERAGE DOSE—1 troche.

TROCHES OF POTASSIUM CHLORATE
Trochisci Potassii Chloratis
(U.S.P. IX)

Potassium Chlorate, in fine powder.	15 Gm.
Sucrose, in fine powder.	60 Gm.
Tragacanth, in fine powder	3 Gm.
Water, a sufficient quantity,	
To make	100 Troches

Mix the sucrose with the tragacanth by trituration in a mortar; then transfer the mixture to a sheet of paper, and by means of a bone or wooden spatula mix it with the potassium chlorate, being careful to avoid unnecessary trituration or pressure, which might cause the mixture to ignite or explode. Lastly form a mass with water and divide into 100 troches. Dry in a current of warm air.

AVERAGE DOSE—1 troche.

TROCHES OF QUININE TANNATE
Trochisci Quininæ Tannatis
(N.F. IV)

Quinine Tannate.	6 Gm.
Tragacanth, in fine powder	3 Gm.
Theobroma Oil	5 Gm.
Prepared Cacao, in fine powder	25 Gm.
Sucrose, in fine powder.	60 Gm.
Vanillin.	0.3 Gm.
Soluble Saccharin	0.2 Gm.
Chloroform,	
Water, of each, a sufficient quantity,	
To make	100 Troches

Triturate the soluble saccharin and the vanillin with 20 Gm. of sucrose until uniformly mixed, add the remainder of the sucrose, tragacanth and prepared cacao and mix thoroughly. Triturate the quinine tannate and the theobroma oil in a mortar with sufficient chloroform to produce a thin paste, set aside until the chloroform has evaporated, then incorporate the powdered ingredients and form a mass with water. Divide the mass into 100 troches and dry in a current of warm air.

AVERAGE DOSE—1 troche.

NOTE—Avoid contact with iron utensils or discoloration will take place.

TROCHES OF SANTONIN
Trochisci Santonini
(N.F. IV)

Santonin, in fine powder	3	Gm.
Tragacanth, in fine powder	3	Gm.
Sucrose, in fine powder	54	Gm.
Cacao, in fine powder	40	Gm.
Vanillin, in fine powder	0.1 Gm.	
Water, a sufficient quantity,		
To make	100 Troches	

Triturate the vanillin with the santonin and tragacanth until they are thoroughly mixed; then incorporate the other powders and form a mass with water. Divide the mass into 100 troches and dry in a current of warm air.

AVERAGE DOSE—1 troche.

CAUTION—*Because of the pleasant flavor of these tablets and the possibility of their being mistaken for candy, it is advisable to dispense only a few at a time, preferably not more than three, as 0.13 Gm. of santonin has caused the death of a child.*

COMPOUND TROCHES OF SANTONIN
Trochisci Santonini Compositi
Troches of Santonin and Calomel
(N.F. IV)

Santonin, in fine powder	3	Gm.
Mild Mercurous Chloride	3	Gm.
Tragacanth, in fine powder	3	Gm.
Sucrose, in fine powder	51	Gm.
Cacao, in fine powder	40	Gm.
Vanillin	0.1 Gm.	
Water, a sufficient quantity,		
To make	100 Troches	

Triturate the vanillin, santonin and mild mercurous chloride with 20 Gm. of sucrose until uniformly mixed, then add the remainder of the sucrose and the other ingredients, mix thoroughly and form a mass with water. Divide the mass into 100 troches and dry in a current of warm air.

AVERAGE DOSE—1 troche.

CAUTION—*Because of the pleasant flavor of these tablets and the possibility of their being mistaken for candy, it is advisable to dispense only a few at a time, preferably not more than three, as 0.13 Gm. of santonin has caused the death of a child.*

TROCHES OF SULFUR AND POTASSIUM BITARTRATE
Trochisci Sulfuris et Potassii Bitartratis
Troches of Sulfur and Cream of Tartar
(N.F. IV)

Washed Sulfur.	30	Gm.
Potassium Bitartrate .	6	Gm.
Tragacanth, in fine powder	4	Gm.
Sucrose, in fine powder.	60	Gm.
Oil of Orange .	0.5	cc.
Water, a sufficient quantity,		
To make .	100	Troches

Triturate the powdered ingredients together until uniformly mixed, then incorporate the oil and form a mass with water.   Divide the mass into 100 troches and dry in a current of warm air.

AVERAGE DOSE—1 troche.

TROCHES OF TANNIC ACID
Trochisci Acidi Tannici
(U.S.P. X)

Tannic Acid.	6 Gm.
Sucrose, in fine powder.	65 Gm.
Tragacanth, in very fine powder	2 Gm.
Orange Flower Water, a sufficient quantity,	
To make .	100 Troches

Triturate the powders until they are thoroughly mixed, form a mass with orange flower water and divide it into 100 troches.

AVERAGE DOSE—1 troche.

NOTE—Avoid the use of iron utensils or discoloration will take place.

VEHICLES

(This section has been compiled from information obtained, by permission, from "Essentials of Prescription Writing" by Cary Eggleston, M.D. (through the courtesy of W. B. Saunders Company) and from material received from Bernard Fantus, M.D.)

Vehicles are flavoring and coloring agents for fluid prescriptions.   They are used to disguise disagreeable tastes of some drugs in solution or suspension.   They may be classified according to the purposes for which they are suitable; the following classification is based on that made by Eggleston:

A.   Flavoring Agents

    1.   Aqueous Vehicles

        (a)   Aromatic Waters, for water-soluble salts and for preparations which are not intensely disagreeable in taste.
        Aromatic Waters of the U.S.P. XII and N.F. VII.

(b) Syrups, when aqueous solvents and flavors are required.

Syrup
Syrup of Acacia
Syrup of Anise, R.B.
Syrup of Blackberry Fruit, R.B.
Syrup of Cherry
Syrup of Cinnamon
Syrup of Cacao
Syrup of Fennel, R.B.
Syrup of Peppermint, R.B.
Syrup of Pineapple, R.B.
Syrup of Raspberry
Syrup of Sassafras, R.B.
Syrup of Spearmint, R.B.
Syrup of Strawberry, R.B.
Syrup of Tolu Balsam
Syrup of Wild Cherry
Syrup of Wintergreen, R.B.

Syrup of Citric Acid } For alkaline salts of the organic acids. Not to
Syrup of Orange   } be used with alkaline carbonates.

Syrup of Ginger   } Particularly suitable for children's
Syrup of Glycyrrhiza   } tastes.
Aromatic Syrup of Rhubarb }

Aromatic Syrup of Eriodictyon { For concealing the taste of quinine, which should be suspended in the syrup; a "shake well" label should be used.

Compound Syrup of Sarsaparilla { Especially for halides and salts of mercury.

Extract of Malt { For suspensions and emulsions.

(c) Mucilages, for water-soluble substances; used in the preparation of emulsions and suspensions.

Mucilage of Acacia   { Incompatible with strong alcohol.
Mucilage of Tragacanth { Miscible with alcoholic preparations.

2. Hydro-alcoholic Vehicles, for substances soluble in either water or dilute alcohol.

Elixir of Almond, R.B.
Elixir Aqueous, R.B.
Aromatic Elixir
Red Aromatic Elixir
Compound Elixir of Almond
Compound Elixir of Pepsin
Glycerinated Elixir of Gentian

Elixir of Glycyrrhiza { For bitter and saline drugs. Incompatible with acids and acid salts.

Iso-alcoholic Elixir
{ The alcoholic strength of this is adjusted by a mixture of the low-alcoholic elixir and the high-alcoholic elixir in such proportion as to produce a clear solution of the particular medicine.

3. Alcoholic Vehicles, for substances soluble in rather strong alcohol; also as flavors to be added in small quantities to other vehicles, such as syrups and elixirs.

(a) Elixir of Eriodictyon, R.B. { For strongly alcoholic preparations of alkaloidal drugs.

(b) Tinctures.
Aromatic Tincture, R.B.
Tincture of Calumba
Tincture of Cardamom, R.B.
Compound Tincture of Cardamom
Tincture of Cinnamon
Compound Tincture of Gentian
Tincture of Ginger
Compound Tincture of Lavender
Tincture of Lemon
Tincture of Bitter Orange Peel
Tincture of Sweet Orange Peel
Tincture of Vanilla

(c) Spirits.
Spirit of Anise
Spirit of Coriander (prepared according to the general formula for Spirits of Volatile Oils, N.F.)
Spirit of Lavender
Compound Spirit of Orange
Spirit of Peppermint
Spirit of Spearmint

4. Certain cordials, e. g., Fruit Cordials, both non-alcoholic and alcoholic, and Liqueurs, may also be used as vehicles.

B. Coloring Agents

Solution of Amaranth
Tincture of Caramel, R.B.
Compound Tincture of Cardamom
Solution of Cochineal
Tincture of Cudbear
Compound Tincture of Cudbear
Tincture of Saffron, R.B.
} For aqueous and alcoholic solutions; acid, alkaline and neutral.

Solution of Carmine { For aqueous and alcoholic solutions; neutral and alkaline. Not with acids or acid salts.

Tincture of Hydrastis
Compound Tincture of Lavender
{ For alcoholic and hydro-alcoholic solutions; acid, alkaline and neutral. Precipitated by water.

VINEGARS

AROMATIC VINEGAR

Acetum Aromaticum
(N.F. V)

Oil of Lavender	0.5 cc.
Oil of Rosemary	0.5 cc.
Oil of Juniper	0.5 cc.
Oil of Peppermint	0.5 cc.
Oil of Cinnamon	0.5 cc.
Oil of Lemon	1 cc.
Oil of Clove	1 cc.
Alcohol	250 cc.
Acetic Acid	260 cc.
Distilled Water, a sufficient quantity,	
To make	1000 cc.

Dissolve the oils in the alcohol, add the acetic acid and sufficient distilled water to make the product measure 1000 cc. Set the mixture aside for 8 days, occasionally agitating it, and filter.

CAMPHORATED VINEGAR

Acetum Camphoratum
(E.B. III)

Camphor	10 Gm.
Alcohol	100 cc.
Diluted Acetic Acid, a sufficient quantity,	
To make	1000 cc.

Dissolve the camphor in the alcohol and add sufficient diluted acetic acid to make the product measure 1000 cc. Set aside for 24 hours and filter.

VINEGAR OF CANTHARIDES

Acetum Cantharidis
(B.P.C. 1934)

Cantharides, bruised	100 Gm.
Glacial Acetic Acid,	
Distilled Water, of each, a sufficient quantity,	
To make	1000 cc.

Macerate the cantharides with 900 cc. of a mixture of equal volumes of glacial acetic acid and water for 24 hours. Transfer to a percolator and, when the liquid ceases to pass, pour sufficient of the same menstruum in successive portions through the contents of the percolator to make the product measure 1000 cc.

VINEGAR OF CANTHARIDIN
Acetum Cantharidini
(B.P.C. 1934)

Cantharidin . . . . 0.5 Gm.
Glacial Acetic Acid . . . . 100 cc.
Acetic Acid, a sufficient quantity,
To make . . . . 1000 cc.

Dissolve the cantharidin in the glacial acetic acid with the aid of gentle heat; cool and add sufficient acetic acid to make the product measure 1000 cc.

VINEGAR OF OPIUM
Acetum Opii
(N.F. IV)

Granulated Opium . . . . 100 Gm.
Myristica, in No. 40 powder . . . . 30 Gm.
Sucrose . . . . 200 Gm.
Diluted Acetic Acid, a sufficient quantity,
To make . . . . 1000 cc.

Macerate the opium, myristica and sucrose in 500 cc. of diluted acetic acid for 7 days, shaking the mixture frequently, then transfer it to a cylindrical percolator in the neck of which a pledget of purified cotton has been placed. Allow the percolation to proceed slowly until the liquid has entirely disappeared from the surface, then gradually pour on diluted acetic acid and continue the percolation until the product measures 1000 cc.

AVERAGE DOSE—Metric, 0.5 cc.—Apothecaries, 8 minims.

NOTE—This preparation must be dispensed on prescription only.

WASHES

ALIBOUR WATER
Eau d'Alibour Forte; Aqua Cupro-Zincica
(Cod. Fr.)

Copper Sulfate . . . . 10 Gm.
Zinc Sulfate . . . . 35 Gm.
Camphor . . . . 1 Gm.
Alcohol . . . . 9 cc.
Tincture of Saffron . . . . 1 cc.
Distilled Water, a sufficient quantity,
To make . . . . 1000 cc.

Dissolve the camphor in the alcohol; dissolve the copper sulfate and zinc sulfate in a portion of the distilled water, add the tincture of saffron and the alcoholic solution of camphor and sufficient distilled water to make the product measure 1000 cc. Shake the solution, set aside for 24 hours and filter.

NOTE—This solution *must* be diluted with 5 or 6 times its volume of water before using as a wet dressing.

ALUM AND NUTGALL WASH
(R.B. I)

Alum . . . .   100 Gm.
Tincture of Nutgall. . . . .   100 cc.
Distilled Water, a sufficient quantity,

To make . . . .   1000 cc.

Dissolve the alum in 800 cc. of distilled water.   Add the tincture of nutgall and sufficient distilled water to make the product measure 1000 cc.

Dispense with a "shake well" label.

BORAX WASH
Lotio Boracina
(R.B. II)

Borax . . . .   40 Gm.
Rose Water . . . .   880 cc.
Alcohol . . . .   40 cc.
Glycerin, a sufficient quantity,

To make . . . . : . . . . . .   1000 cc.

Dissolve the borax in the rose water.   Add 40 cc. of alcohol and enough glycerin to make 1000 cc.

CARBOLIC WASH
Lotio Carbolica
(R.B. II)

Liquefied Phenol . . . .   10 cc.
Glycerin . . . .   75 cc.
Alcohol . . . .   75 cc.
Distilled Water . . . .   840 cc.

To make about . . . .   1000 cc.

Dissolve the phenol in 500 cc. of distilled water, add the glycerin and alcohol. Then add the distilled water.

HEMOSTATIC WASH
Aqua Hæmostatica
Pagliari's Solution
(Ital. Ph. V) (Belg. Ph. IV) (Ext. Ph.)

Potassium Alum	80 Gm.
Tincture of Benzoin	10 cc.
Benzoic Acid	2 Gm.
Distilled Water, a sufficient quantity,	
To make	1000 cc.

Dissolve the alum in the distilled water and the benzoic acid in the tincture of benzoin; mix the 2 solutions, allow to precipitate completely and filter.

NOTE—This solution if made with 10 per cent of sodium chloride is known as Pollacci's Modification of Pagliari's Solution.

RED WASH—RED SOLUTION
(King's College Hospital)
(P.F.)

Boric Acid	22 Gm.
Zinc Sulfate.	2 Gm.
Spirit of Rosemary	18 cc.
Tincture of Lavender	18 cc.
Distilled Water, a sufficient quantity,	
To make	1000 cc.

Dissolve the boric acid and zinc sulfate in 700 cc. of distilled water and gradually add the spirit and tincture. Finally add sufficient distilled water to make the product measure 1000 cc.

RESORCINOL WASH
(V.C.N.Y.)

Resorcinol.	195 Gm.
Glycerin	21 cc.
Diluted Alcohol, a sufficient quantity,	
To make	1000 cc.

Dissolve the resorcinol in 500 cc. of the diluted alcohol, add the glycerin and then sufficient diluted alcohol to make the product measure 1000 cc.

STYPTIC WATER
Aqua Styptica

Alum. . . . . 30 Gm.
Zinc Sulfate. . . . . 30 Gm.
Rose Water, a sufficient quantity,
               To make . . . . 1000 cc.

Triturate the salts together and dissolve in the rose water, allow to stand for 2 days and filter.

WATERS

AROMATIC SPIRIT WATER
Aqua Aromatica Spirituosa
(P.F.)

Oil of Clove . . . . 2 cc.
Oil of Cinnamon. . . . . 2 cc.
Oil of Lemon . . . . 2 cc.
Oil of Fennel . . . . 1 cc.
Oil of Lavender . . . . 1 cc.
Oil of Mace. . . . . 1 cc.
Oil of Peppermint . . . . 1 cc.
Oil of Rosemary . . . . 1 cc.
Oil of Sage . . . . 1 cc.
Alcohol . . . . 600 cc.
Distilled Water, a sufficient quantity,
               To make . . . . 1000 cc.

Dissolve the oils in 600 cc. of alcohol. To this solution add distilled water in small portions to make 1000 cc., agitating after each addition. Filter, with the aid of purified talc if necessary, and pass sufficient distilled water through the filter to make the product measure 1000 cc.

AVERAGE DOSE—Metric, 30 cc.—Apothecaries, 1 fluidounce.

NOTE—This preparation is not to be confused with Aromatic Spirit on page 228.

BITTER WATER
Aqua Amara
(P.F.)

Magnesium Sulfate . . . . 75 Gm.
Sodium Sulfate . . . . 63 Gm.
Potassium Sulfate . . . . 4 Gm.
Sodium Chloride. . . . . 6 Gm.
Sodium Bicarbonate . . . . 2.75 Gm.
Distilled Water, a sufficient quantity,
               To make . . . . 1000 cc.

Dissolve and filter if necessary.

SEDATIVE BITTER WATER
Aqua Amara Sedativa
(R.B. I)

Sodium Bicarbonate	30 Gm.
Potassium Bromide	60 Gm.
Spirit of Chloroform	30 cc.
Tincture of Cardamom, R.B.	30 cc.
Tincture of Quassia	120 cc.
Peppermint Water	240 cc.
Distilled Water, a sufficient quantity,	
To make	1000 cc.

Dissolve the salts in a mixture of the liquids, adding sufficient distilled water to make the product measure 1000 cc.

AVERAGE DOSE—Metric, 8 cc.—Apothecaries, 2 fluidrachms.

CARMINATIVE WATER
Aqua Carminativa
(R.B. I)

Oil of Orange	1 cc.
Oil of Caraway.	1 cc.
Oil of Fennel	1 cc.
Oil of Coriander	1 cc.
Oil of Lemon	1 cc.
Oil of Spearmint.	1 cc.
Oil of Matricaria.	2 cc.
Alcohol	100 cc.
Distilled Water, a sufficient quantity,	
To make	1000 cc.

Dissolve the oils in the alcohol and add sufficient distilled water to make the product measure 1000 cc. Filter, using purified talc if necessary.

AVERAGE DOSE—Metric, 30 cc.—Apothecaries, 1 fluidounce.

CREOSOTE WATER
Aqua Creosoti
(U.S.P. IX)

Creosote	10 cc.
Distilled Water, recently boiled	990 cc.
To make	1000 cc.

Agitate the creosote vigorously with the distilled water and filter, returning the filtrate to the filter until it is perfectly clear.

AVERAGE DOSE—Metric, 10 cc.—Apothecaries, 2½ fluidrachms.

NOTE—This water should be freshly prepared.

IMPERIAL DRINK
Potus Imperialis
Haustus Imperialis
(B.P.C. 1934)

Potassium Bitartrate	4.6 Gm.
Citric Acid	0.8 Gm.
Sucrose	50 Gm.
Oil of Lemon	0.3 cc.
Tincture of Lemon	5.2 cc.
Distilled Water, a sufficient quantity,	
To make	1000 cc.

Dissolve the potassium bitartrate, citric acid and sucrose in 900 cc. of boiling distilled water; allow to cool, add the oil of lemon previously dissolved in the tincture of lemon, and then add sufficient distilled water to make the product measure 1000 cc.

AVERAGE DOSE—Metric, 1 to 4 Gm.—Apothecaries, ¼ to 1 drachm.

PURGATIVE SALINE WATER
Aqua Salina Purgans
(Cod. Fr.)

Sodium Sulfate	100 Gm.
Magnesium Sulfate	120 Gm.
Distilled Water, a sufficient quantity,	
To make	1000 cc.

Dissolve.

AVERAGE DOSE—Metric, 15 cc.—Apothecaries, 4 fluidrachms.

WINES

BITTER WINE OF IRON
Vinum Ferri Amarum
(N.F. IV)

Iron and Quinine Citrate	50 Gm.
Tincture of Sweet Orange Peel	60 cc.
Syrup	300 cc.
Sherry Wine, a sufficient quantity,	
To make	1000 cc.

Dissolve the iron and quinine citrate in 500 cc. of sherry wine. Add to this the tincture of sweet orange peel and the syrup, and lastly, sufficient sherry wine to make the product measure 1000 cc. Set the mixture aside for 2 days and filter.

AVERAGE DOSE—Metric, 8 cc.—Apothecaries, 2 fluidrachms.

WINE OF IRON CITRATE
Vinum Ferri
(N.F. IV)

Iron and Ammonium Citrates	40 Gm.
Tincture of Sweet Orange Peel	60 cc.
Syrup	100 cc.
Sherry Wine, a sufficient quantity,	
To make	1000 cc.

Dissolve the iron and ammonium citrates in 700 cc. of sherry wine; add this solution to the tincture of sweet orange peel and syrup. Lastly, add sufficient sherry wine to make the product measure 1000 cc. Set the mixture aside for 2 days and filter.

AVERAGE DOSE—Metric, 8 cc.—Apothecaries, 2 fluidrachms.

MISCELLANEOUS PREPARATIONS

EUCALYPTOL COMPOUND
(R.B. I)

Menthol	32 Gm.
Thymol.	48 Gm.
Eucalyptol, a sufficient quantity,	
To make	1000 cc.

Triturate the menthol and thymol until liquefied, then add sufficient eucalyptol to make the product measure 1000 cc.

HONEY OF SODIUM BORATE
Mel Sodii Boratis
Mel Boracis; Honey and Borax
(N.F. V)

Sodium Borate, in fine powder.	10 Gm.
Glycerin	5 Gm.
Honey	85 Gm.
To make	100 Gm.

Mix the sodium borate with the glycerin, add the honey and stir until solution is effected.

AROMATIZED IODOFORM
Iodoformum Aromatisatum
(N.F. V)

Iodoform, in fine powder	96 Gm.
Coumarin, in fine powder	4 Gm.
To make	100 Gm.

Mix intimately by trituration.

OXYMEL OF SQUILL
Oxymel Scillæ
(N.F. V)

Vinegar of Squill.	50 Gm.
Honey	100 Gm.
To make	100 Gm.

Mix the honey and the vinegar of squill in a tared porcelain dish or enameled iron vessel, and heat on a water bath until the mixture has been reduced to a weight of 100 Gm. Then strain the preparation, allow it to cool and transfer it to bottles, which should be well stoppered.

AVERAGE DOSE—Metric, 4 cc.—Apothecaries, 1 fluidrachm.

PARAFFIN DRESSING
Curatio Paraffini
(N.F. VI)

Resorcinol	1 Gm.
Oil of Eucalyptus	2 Gm.
Olive Oil or Peanut Oil	3 Gm.
White Petrolatum	12 Gm.
Paraffin	82 Gm.
To make	100 Gm.

Melt the paraffin, add the white petrolatum and olive oil, and stir, continuing the heat if necessary, until a uniform liquid is obtained. Dissolve the resorcinol in the oil of eucalyptus, add to the warm paraffin mixture and mix well. Stir the mixture frequently until it begins to congeal.

SURGICAL PARAFFIN
(R.B. I)

Eucalyptol	0.5 cc.
Asphalt.	4.5 Gm.
Paraffin.	95 Gm.
To make	100 Gm.

Melt the paraffin with the aid of gentle heat, add the asphalt and incorporate thoroughly. Stir in the eucalyptol just before the mixture congeals.

PHENOL COMPOUND
(R.B. I)

Menthol	80 Gm.
Thymol.	160 Gm.
Liquefied Phenol	760 Gm.
To make	1000 Gm.

Triturate the menthol and thymol until liquefied, then add the liquefied phenol.

POTASSA WITH LIME
Potassa cum Calce
(N.F. IV)

Potassium Hydroxide,
Calcium Oxide, of each, an equal weight.

Triturate the ingredients together in a warm mortar, so as to form a powder.

Keep in well-closed containers.

SANDARAC COATING FOR PILLS
Sandarac Varnish; Sandarac Solution
(Cooper and Dyer)

Sandarac . . . .   20 Gm.
Ethyl Oxide . . . .   40 cc.
Dehydrated Alcohol . . . .   40 cc.

Dissolve the sandarac in the ethyl oxide-alcohol mixture by shaking; pour off the supernatant liquid and filter if necessary.

NOTE—To color pills black, a certified black dye (alcohol soluble) may be used. To completely coat the pills, it is usually necessary to apply a minimum of 2 coats of varnish.

SALOL VARNISH FOR PILLS
(B.P.C. 1923)

Phenyl Salicylate . . . .   20 Gm.
Amber Shellac. . . . .   30 Gm.
Dehydrated Alcohol . . . .   30 cc.
Ethyl Oxide, a sufficient quantity,
                          To make . . . .   100 cc.

Dissolve the phenyl salicylate and shellac in a mixture of the alcohol and ethyl oxide.

SODIUM BORO-BENZOATE
Sodii Boro-Benzoas
(N.F. IV)

Sodium Borate, in fine powder. . . . .   43 Gm.
Sodium Benzoate, in fine powder . . . .   57 Gm.
                          To make . . . .   100 Gm.

Mix intimately.

AVERAGE DOSE—Metric, 2 Gm.—Apothecaries, 30 grains.

PART I—B

PREPARATIONS FOR USE BY DIABETIC PERSONS

SUGAR-FREE COMPOUND ELIXIR OF ALMOND

Vanillin	1	Gm.
Soluble Saccharin	0.75	Gm.
Oil of Bitter Almond or Benzaldehyde	0.5	cc.
Alcohol	50	cc.
Orange Flower Water	150	cc.
Distilled Water, a sufficient quantity,		
To make	1000	cc.

Dissolve the vanillin, soluble saccharin and oil in the alcohol; add the orange flower water and sufficient distilled water to make the product measure 1000 cc.; then filter the product until clear.

SUGAR-FREE AQUEOUS ELIXIR

Vanillin	1	Gm.
Soluble Saccharin	0.75	Gm.
Oil of Bitter Almond or Benzaldehyde	0.3	cc.
Oil of Fennel	0.6	cc.
Chloroform	0.6	cc.
Glycerin	50	cc.
Orange Flower Water	200	cc.
Purified Talc	10	Gm.
Distilled Water, a sufficient quantity,		
To make	1000	cc.

Dissolve the soluble saccharin and the vanillin in the orange flower water and add the glycerin in which the oils and the chloroform have been mixed. Then add sufficient distilled water to make the product measure 1000 cc. Shake well, add the purified talc, set aside for about 6 hours and then filter.

SUGAR-FREE AROMATIC ELIXIR

Compound Spirit of Orange	12	cc.
Soluble Saccharin	0.6	Gm.
Purified Talc	30	Gm.
Alcohol	250	cc.
Glycerin	250	cc.
Distilled Water, a sufficient quantity,		
To make	1000	cc.

To the compound spirit of orange add the alcohol in which the soluble saccharin has been dissolved, add the glycerin and enough distilled water to make the product measure 1000 cc. Mix the purified talc intimately with the liquid, and filter through a wetted filter, returning the first portions until a clear liquid is obtained.

SUGAR-FREE ELIXIR OF BITTER ORANGE

Oil of Bitter Orange	1	cc.
Tincture of Bitter Orange Peel	20	cc.
Soluble Saccharin	0.75	Gm.
Orange Flower Water	20	cc.
Alcohol	300	cc.
Distilled Water, a sufficient quantity,		
To make	1000	cc.

Mix the oil of bitter orange and the tincture of bitter orange peel with the alcohol in which the soluble saccharin has been dissolved, add the orange flower water and sufficient distilled water, in several portions, shaking the mixture after each addition, to make the product measure 1000 cc. Let it stand 24 hours, and then filter, using 10 Gm. of purified talc, if necessary, to clarify the product.

SUGAR-FREE COMPOUND ELIXIR OF CARDAMOM

Compound Spirit of Cardamom	10	cc.
Soluble Saccharin	0.75	Gm.
Alcohol	90	cc.
Distilled Water, a sufficient quantity,		
To make	1000	cc.

Mix the compound spirit of cardamom with the alcohol in which the soluble saccharin has been dissolved, add sufficient distilled water in several portions to make the product measure 1000 cc.; let it stand 24 hours, shaking occasionally, then filter, using 10 Gm. of purified talc, if necessary, to clarify the product.

SUGAR-FREE ISO-ALCOHOLIC ELIXIR, HIGH

Compound Spirit of Orange	4	cc.
Saccharin	0.75	Gm.
Glycerin	200	cc.
Alcohol, a sufficient quantity,		
To make	1000	cc.

Dissolve the compound spirit of orange and the saccharin in 700 cc. of alcohol, add the glycerin and sufficient alcohol to make the product measure 1000 cc., mix well and filter.

SUGAR-FREE ISO-ALCOHOLIC ELIXIR, LOW

Compound Spirit of Orange 10   cc.
Soluble Saccharin . . . . 0.75 Gm.
Alcohol 100   cc.
Glycerin 200   cc.
Distilled Water, a sufficient quantity,

           To make 1000   cc.

Dissolve the soluble saccharin in the alcohol and mix with the glycerin and compound spirit of orange, and add sufficient distilled water to make the product measure 1000 cc. Let stand 24 hours and filter through a hard paper filter, returning, if necessary, the first portions of the filtrate until it filters clear.

SUGAR-FREE ELIXIR OF THREE BROMIDES

Ammonium Bromide . . . . 80 Gm.
Potassium Bromide . . . . 80 Gm.
Sodium Bromide . . . . 80 Gm.
Glycerin . . . . 200 cc.
Solution of Amaranth . . . . 3 cc.
Cinnamon Water, a sufficient quantity,

           To make . . . . 1000 cc.

Dissolve the bromides in 700 cc. of cinnamon water, add the glycerin and solution of amaranth, and sufficient cinnamon water to make the product measure 1000 cc. and filter if necessary.

AVERAGE DOSE—Metric, 4 cc.—Apothecaries, 1 fluidrachm.

One average metric dose contains about 0.32 Gm. (5 grains) each of ammonium bromide, potassium bromide and sodium bromide.

SUGAR-FREE ELIXIR OF TERPIN HYDRATE

Terpin Hydrate 17   Gm.
Tincture of Sweet Orange Peel 20   cc.
Spirit of Benzaldehyde 5   cc.
Saccharin . . . . 0.2 Gm.
Alcohol 425   cc.
Glycerin 400   cc.
Distilled Water, a sufficient quantity,

           To make 1000   cc.

Dissolve the terpin hydrate and saccharin in the alcohol, add successively the tincture, the spirit, the glycerin, and sufficient distilled water to make the product measure 1000 cc., mix well and filter until the product is clear.

AVERAGE DOSE—Metric, 4 cc.—Apothecaries, 1 fluidrachm.

One average metric dose, contains about 0.07 Gm. of terpin hydrate.

MAYONNAISE (For Use by Diabetic Persons)

Egg Yolks	6 yolks
Heavy Liquid Petrolatum	900 cc.
Sodium Chloride	6 Gm.
Mustard, powdered	3 Gm.
Lemon Juice	60 cc.
Diluted Acetic Acid	45 cc.

Beat the egg yolks in a mechanical mixer. Add the lemon juice, the mustard, and the sodium chloride, continue the beating and incorporate the liquid petrolatum gradually, beating the mixture thoroughly throughout the addition of the oil. Finally add the diluted acetic acid and mix well. The finished product should be smooth and thick.

NOTE—The amount of diluted acetic acid may be varied to suit the individual taste.

OINTMENT OF BORIC ACID AND SULFUR

Boric Acid	105 Gm.
Precipitated Sulfur	105 Gm.
Phenol Ointment	790 Gm.
To make	1000 Gm.

Incorporate the boric acid and precipitated sulfur in the phenol ointment and triturate until a uniform ointment results.

OINTMENT OF SALICYLIC ACID AND SULFUR

Ointment 2230

Salicylic Acid	60 Gm.
Precipitated Sulfur	60 Gm.
Petrolatum	880 Gm.
To make	1000 Gm.

Incorporate the salicylic acid and sulfur in the petrolatum.
To be applied to the feet.

COMPOUND OINTMENT OF UREA

Urea	120 Gm.
Pectin Paste	440 Gm.
Sulfonated and Hydrogenated Castor Oil	440 Gm.
To make	1000 Gm.

Triturate the urea with the pectin paste and sulfonated and hydrogenated castor oil until a uniform ointment results.

For use, apply to diabetic ulcers and wounds for healing.

FOOT POWDER OF SALICYLIC AND BENZOIC ACIDS
Foot Powder No. 1923

Salicylic Acid	10 Gm.
Benzoic Acid	10 Gm.
Purified Talc	980 Gm.
To make	1000 Gm.

Mix intimately the purified talc and mixed acids until a uniform powder results. Use as a dusting powder for the feet.

DIABETIC—SOLUTION OF MERCUROCHROME (10 per cent)

Mercurochrome	10 Gm.
Distilled Water, a sufficient quantity,	
To make	100 cc.

Dissolve. Use as a medicated paint.

SOLUTION OF AMMONIUM CHLORIDE WITH CODEINE

Codeine Phosphate	1.1 Gm.
Ammonium Chloride	35 Gm.
Glycerin	375 cc.
Solution of Amaranth	3 cc.
Wintergreen Water, a sufficient quantity,	
To make	1000 cc.

Dissolve the salts in the wintergreen water, add the glycerin and solution of amaranth and sufficient wintergreen water to make the product measure 1000 cc.

AVERAGE DOSE—Metric, 4 to 8 cc.—Apothecaries, 1 to 2 fluidrachms.

SUGAR-FREE SYRUP OF CODEINE WITH CHLOROFORM
Diabetic Cough Syrup
(U.C.H.)

Codeine Phosphate	2 Gm.
Chloroform	5 cc.
Citric Acid	12 Gm.
Sodium Citrate	41 Gm.
Cherry Fruit Essence	17 cc.
Saccharin	0.6 Gm.
Distilled Water, a sufficient quantity,	
To make	1000 cc.

Dissolve the codeine phosphate, citric acid and sodium citrate in the water; dissolve the saccharin in the cherry fruit essence and mix the two solutions, add the chloroform and sufficient distilled water to make the product measure 1000 cc.

AVERAGE DOSE—Metric, 4 cc.—Apothecaries, 1 fluidrachm.

PART I—C

DENTAL FORMULAS

TOOTH PASTES

TOOTH PASTE BASE

Precipitated Calcium Carbonate	552	Gm.
Hard Soap, in fine powder	60	Gm.
Soluble Saccharin	0.5	Gm.
Heavy Liquid Petrolatum	14	Gm.
Distilled Water	25	cc.
Glycerin	348.5	Gm.
To make about	1000	Gm.

Mix the hard soap and glycerin and warm until dissolved. Dissolve the saccharin in the distilled water and add to the glycerin-soap mixture. While constantly stirring, slowly sift in the precipitated calcium carbonate and lastly add the oil and mix to form a uniform paste. Remix the following day and add the flavor.

This may be flavored with Oil of Peppermint, 10 cc., or Tooth Paste Flavoring, R.B., 30 cc., if desired.

Flavor to suit taste and add enough water to produce the desired consistency.

TOOTH PASTE FLAVORING

Benzoic Acid	65 Gm.
Thymol	65 Gm.
Oil of Eucalyptus	400 cc.
Oil of Peppermint, a sufficient quantity,	
To make	1000 cc.

Dissolve the benzoic acid and thymol in the oils, previously mixed.

Three cc. of this flavoring is sufficient for 100 Gm. of tooth paste base.

CARBONATE TOOTH PASTE

Magnesium Carbonate	40	Gm.
Hard Soap, in fine powder	45	Gm.
Tragacanth, in fine powder	12	Gm.
Soluble Saccharin	0.5	Gm.
Glycerin	425	Gm.
Distilled Water	15	cc.
Heavy Liquid Petrolatum	13.50	Gm.
Oil of Spearmint	4.50	cc.
Oil of Peppermint	8.50	cc.
Precipitated Calcium Carbonate	436	Gm.
To make about	1000	Gm.

299

Pass the hard soap, tragacanth, magnesium and calcium carbonates through a No. 60 sieve. Dissolve the soluble saccharin in the distilled water and mix with the glycerin. Add the oils to the liquid petrolatum. Incorporate the liquids into the powder, mixing thoroughly.

TOOTH PASTE

Tragacanth, in fine powder	5 Gm.
Hard Soap, in fine powder	50 Gm.
Oil of Peppermint	10 cc.
Precipitated Calcium Carbonate	535 Gm.
Distilled Water	200 cc.
Glycerin	200 Gm.
To make about	1000 Gm.

Mix together the tragacanth, hard soap and precipitated calcium carbonate, incorporate the oil of peppermint, and make into a paste with the glycerin and distilled water.

TOOTH POWDERS

ALKALINE TOOTH POWDER

I
(P.H.N.Y.)
Saponaceous

Precipitated Calcium Carbonate	710 Gm.
Hard Soap, in fine powder	120 Gm.
Monohydrated Sodium Carbonate	150 Gm.
Methyl Salicylate	20 cc.
To make about	1000 Gm.

Mix the dry ingredients, then incorporate the methyl salicylate.

NOTE—This powder is to be dispensed only on the dentist's prescription.

II
Pink

Carmine	0.1 Gm.
Methyl Salicylate	6.5 cc.
Oil of Clove	6.5 cc.
Sodium Bicarbonate	987 Gm.
To make about	1000 Gm.

Triturate the carmine with a small quantity of the sodium bicarbonate until the color is thoroughly distributed, then add to the rest of the sodium bicarbonate and mix until a uniform color results. Finally incorporate the oils.

BORATED TOOTH POWDER
(U.C.H.)

Potassium Bicarbonate	475 Gm.
Sodium Borate	475 Gm.
Thymol.	10 Gm.
Eucalyptol	24 cc.
Methyl Salicylate	16 cc.
To make about	1000 Gm.

Triturate the powders together until uniformly mixed and add the eucalyptol and methyl salicylate; continue the trituration until the flavoring oils are uniformly incorporated in the mixed powders.

SODIUM PERBORATE TOOTH POWDER

Sodium Perborate	100 Gm.
Magnesium Carbonate	100 Gm.
Oil of Peppermint	10 cc.
Precipitated Calcium Carbonate	790 Gm.
To make about	1000 Gm.

Triturate the oil of peppermint with the magnesium carbonate, add the sodium perborate and lastly the precipitated calcium carbonate. Mix thoroughly and sift.

MOUTH WASHES

COLORS FOR MOUTH WASHES AND OTHER PHARMACEUTICAL PREPARATIONS

Bright Red	Solution of Cochineal
	Tincture of Cudbear
Reddish Brown	Compound Tincture of Cudbear
Brown	Caramel
	Tincture of Caramel, R.B.
Golden-Yellow	Tincture of Saffron, R.B.

Additional colors for mouth washes and other pharmaceutical preparations, namely, Coal Tar Dyes Permitted for Foods, Drugs and Cosmetics may be found on page 341 of the Recipe Book.

LIQUID DENTIFRICE

Hard Soap, powdered	60 Gm.
Soluble Saccharin	2 Gm.
Solution of Amaranth	8 cc.
Oil of Cinnamon	5 cc.
Oil of Peppermint	5 cc.
Oil of Clove	10 cc.
Alcohol	750 cc.
Distilled Water, a sufficient quantity,	
To make	1000 cc.

Dissolve the hard soap and volatile oils in the alcohol; add the solution of amaranth, the soluble saccharin and sufficient distilled water to make 1000 cc.

For use, sprinkle on a moistened tooth brush.

MOUTH WASH

Mouth Washes I, II and III are pleasantly flavored solutions intended for the dentist's office atomizer or for the patient's use. They produce a sensation of cleanliness in the oral cavity. Medication may be added to them or they may be used plain, as the dentist desires. They are suitable vehicles for Zinc Chloride 0.1 per cent; Zinc Iodide 1.0 per cent; Zinc Phenolsulfonate 1.0 per cent; Tincture of Myrrh 0.5 per cent. They may be colored if desired.

I

Soluble Saccharin	0.10 Gm.
Solution of Amaranth	8 cc.
Oil of Cinnamon	0.25 cc.
Oil of Peppermint	0.25 cc.
Oil of Clove	0.50 cc.
Alcohol	300 cc.
Purified Talc	10 Gm.
Distilled Water, a sufficient quantity,	
To make	1000 cc.

Dissolve the volatile oils in the alcohol and the soluble saccharin in 650 cc. of distilled water, mix the two solutions and add the purified talc, shake well and filter. Lastly, add the solution of amaranth and sufficient distilled water through the filter to make the product measure 1000 cc.

Use undiluted or dilute with 2 or 3 volumes of water.

II

Soluble Saccharin	0.1 Gm.
Thymol	0.5 Gm.
Menthol	1 Gm.
Oil of Peppermint	3 cc.
Alcohol	300 cc.
Purified Talc	10 Gm
Distilled Water, a sufficient quantity,	
To make	1000 cc.

Dissolve the thymol, menthol and oil of peppermint in the alcohol and add the solution slowly to 650 cc. of distilled water in which the soluble saccharin has been dissolved. Add the purified talc, shake well and filter. Lastly, add sufficient distilled water through the filter to make the product measure 1000 cc.

Use undiluted or dilute with 2 or 3 volumes of water.

III

Soluble Saccharin	0.1 Gm.
Menthol	0.5 Gm.
Thymol	0.5 Gm.
Eucalyptol	2.5 cc.
Methyl Salicylate	0.6 cc.
Purified Talc	10 Gm.
Alcohol	150 cc.
Distilled Water, a sufficient quantity,	
To make	1000 cc.

Dissolve the menthol, thymol, eucalyptol and methyl salicylate in the alcohol and add the solution slowly to 800 cc. of distilled water in which the soluble saccharin has been dissolved. Add the purified talc, shake well and filter. Lastly, add sufficient distilled water through the filter to make the product measure 1000 cc.

Use undiluted or dilute with 2 or 3 volumes of water.

ACID AROMATIC MOUTH WASH
(R.B. I)

Benzoic Acid	8 Gm.
Boric Acid	16 Gm.
Thymol	2 Gm.
Alcohol	180 cc.
Oil of Peppermint	3 cc.
Oil of Eucalyptus	6 cc.
Methyl Salicylate	6 cc.
Purified Talc	5 Gm.
Distilled Water, a sufficient quantity,	
To make	1000 cc.

Dissolve the benzoic acid, thymol and volatile oils in 150 cc. of alcohol. Dissolve the boric acid in 800 cc. of distilled water and mix the solutions. Add the purified talc and filter, returning the first portions until the filtrate is clear. Add 30 cc. of alcohol to the filtrate and then sufficient distilled water to make the product measure 1000 cc.

HOSPITAL MOUTH WASH

Tincture of Myrrh	5 cc.
Alcohol	100 cc.
Glycerin	100 cc.
Boric Acid	10 Gm.
Distilled Water, a sufficient quantity,	
To make	1000 cc.

Dissolve the boric acid in 500 cc. of distilled water. Mix the tincture of myrrh, alcohol and glycerin and add to the boric acid solution. Add sufficient distilled water to make the product measure 1000 cc. Filter if necessary.

SALINE MOUTH WASH

Calcium Oxide	20 Gm.
Phenolphthalein	1 Gm.
Soluble Saccharin	3 Gm.
Oil of Cinnamon	5 cc.
Sodium Chloride, a sufficient quantity,	
To make	1000 Gm.

Triturate the calcium oxide, soluble saccharin and phenolphthalein until a deep red color is produced. Then gradually add the sodium chloride, which has been previously mixed with the oil of cinnamon.

Add a level teaspoonful to a cup of warm water for a saline mouth wash. The acids in the mouth discharge the pink color of the solution.

TANNIN MOUTH WASH

Tannic Acid	64 Gm.
Liquefied Phenol	18 cc.
Glycerin	120 cc.
Distilled Water, a sufficient quantity,	
To make	1000 cc.

Dissolve the tannic acid in 500 cc. of distilled water, and add the glycerin in which the liquified phenol has been previously dissolved. Finally add sufficient distilled water to make the product measure 1000 cc., and filter.

For use, this mouth wash is diluted with 3 or 4 volumes of water.

ZINC CHLORIDE MOUTH WASH

Zinc Chloride	1	Gm.
Menthol	0.5	Gm.
Oil of Cinnamon	1.3	cc.
Oil of Clove	0.5	cc.
Solution of Formaldehyde	0.5	cc.
Soluble Saccharin	0.4	Gm.
Purified Talc	15	Gm.
Alcohol	45	cc.
Solution of Amaranth	8	cc.
Distilled Water, a sufficient quantity,		
To make	1000	cc.

Dissolve the menthol and volatile oils in the alcohol; dissolve the zinc chloride and soluble saccharin in 800 cc. of distilled water and add the solution of amaranth; mix the two solutions, then add the solution of formaldehyde and triturate with 15 Gm. of purified talc. Filter through paper and add sufficient distilled water to the filtrate to make the product measure 1000 cc.

A pleasant, slightly astringent mouth wash.

Use undiluted or dilute with 2 or 3 volumes of water.

GLYCERIN THYMOL COMPOUND
Glycerinum Thymolis Alkalinum, Squire
(B.P.C. 1934)

Sodium Bicarbonate	10	Gm.
Sodium Borate	20	Gm.
Sodium Benzoate	8	Gm.
Sodium Salicylate	5	Gm.
Menthol	0.3	Gm.
Oil of Dwarf Pine Needles	0.5	cc.
Methyl Salicylate	0.3	cc.
Thymol	0.5	Gm.
Eucalyptol	1.3	cc.
Alcohol	25	cc.
Glycerin	100	cc.
Solution of Bordeaux B	10	cc.
Purified Talc	25	Gm.
Distilled Water, a sufficient quantity,		
To make	1000	cc.

Dissolve the salts in 800 cc. of distilled water, and add the glycerin. Dissolve the menthol, thymol, eucalyptol and oils in the alcohol, triturate with the purified talc, add the mixture gradually to the solution of salts, then add the solution of Bordeaux B. Filter and pass sufficient distilled water through the filter to make the product measure 1000 cc.

NOTE—Solution of Bordeaux B is a 1 per cent solution of the dye in chloroform water.

MISCELLANEOUS DENTAL PREPARATIONS

TOOTH SOAP

Precipitated Calcium Carbonate	660	Gm.
Carmine	6	Gm.
Coumarin	0.5	Gm.
Thymol	9	Gm.
Menthol	9	Gm.
Oil of Clove	4.5	cc.
Hard Soap, in powder	177	Gm.
Glycerin	44	Gm.
Alcohol, a sufficient quantity,		
To make about	1000	Gm.

Dissolve the carmine in a few drops of diluted solution of ammonia in a mortar and triturate it with the precipitated calcium carbonate until the color is evenly distributed. Dissolve the coumarin, thymol, menthol and oil of clove in the alcohol, add the glycerin and dissolve the hard soap in this mixture; then incorporate the powder. Press into suitable molds, expose to the air for 24 hours and finally paint the pieces with tincture of benzoin to give them a gloss.

DENTURE ADHESIVE

Tragacanth, in fine powder	730 Gm.
Karaya Gum, in fine powder	250 Gm.
Oil of Sassafras	20 cc.
To make about	1000 Gm·

Mix well.

For use, sprinkle sparingly on the denture before placing it in the mouth.

DENTURE CLEANER

Trisodium Phosphate	98.15 Gm.
Solution of Amaranth	1.6 cc.
Oil of Cinnamon	0.25 cc.
To make about	100 Gm.

Triturate the trisodium phosphate with the solution of amaranth and oil of cinnamon until a uniform powder results.

For use, dissolve ¼ teaspoonful in half a glass of water and use with a brush.

Note—Cellulose acetate type denture is decomposed by alkaline substances. Formaldehyde and phenol-formaldehyde type dentures withstand most chemical agents.

CLEANER FOR "ESTER TYPE" DENTURES
(U.C.H.)

Calcium Carbonate . . . . 75 Gm.
Triisopropanolamine . . . . 250 Gm.
Water, a sufficient quantity to make a paste.

For use, prepare a paste with water and brush thoroughly, finally rinsing well with water.

DENTURE CLEANER
(U.C.H.)

Precipitated Calcium Carbonate . . . . 775 Gm.
Heavy Magnesium Carbonate . . . . 192 Gm.
Sodium Metasilicate, in fine powder . . . . 13 Gm.
Sodium Lauryl Sulfate . . . . 20 Gm.

To make . . . . 1000 Gm.

Mix the powders.

For use, prepare a paste with water and brush thoroughly, finally rinsing well with water.

TROCHES OF ETHYL AMINOBENZOATE

Ethyl Aminobenzoate, in fine powder . . . . 6.30 Gm.
Vanillin . . . . 0.25 Gm.
Sucrose, powdered . . . . 67.7 Gm.
Tragacanth, in fine powder . . . . 2.1 Gm.
Carmine . . . . 0.09 Gm.
Distilled Water, a sufficient quantity,

To make . . . . 100 Troches

Mix the powders intimately until a uniform color is obtained. Form a mass with the distilled water and divide into 100 troches of uniform size.

DOSE—One troche allowed to dissolve on the tongue to prevent gagging.

PREPARATIONS TO BE USED BY THE DENTIST

ABRASIVE PASTE

Pumice, in very fine powder . . . . 40 Gm.
Methyl Salicylate . . . . 1 cc.
Solution of Amaranth . . . . 2 cc.
Glycerite of Starch . . . . 57 Gm.

To make about . . . . 100 Gm.

Mix the methyl salicylate and the pumice, add the solution of amaranth and incorporate the glycerite of starch.

ABRASIVE POWDER

Pumice, in very fine powder 11   Gm.
Starch, in very fine powder 2   Gm.
Methyl Salicylate . . . . 0.50 cc.
Carmine . . . . 0.04 Gm.

Mix and divide into 100 capsules.

For use, moisten the contents of one or more capsules with glycerin or water in a dappan dish.

TOPICAL ANESTHETIC

I

Ethyl Aminobenzoate 10   Gm.
Alcohol 74   cc.
Oil of Cinnamon . . . . 0.25 cc.
Solution of Amaranth . . . . 0.25 cc.
Distilled Water, a sufficient quantity,
                                        To make 100   cc.

Dissolve the ethyl aminobenzoate in the alcohol; add the oil of cinnamon, solution of amaranth and sufficient distilled water to make the product measure 100 cc.

II

Saligenin . . . . 10 Gm.
Alcohol, a sufficient quantity,
                                        To make . . . . 100 cc.

Dissolve the saligenin in the alcohol.

COPAL CAVITY LINING

Copal . . . . 5 Gm.
Chloroform, a sufficient quantity,
                                        To make . . . . 100 cc.

Powder the copal and mix it with an equal weight of washed sand; place in a flask or wide-mouth bottle and add the chloroform, shake the bottle occasionally over a period of 72 hours. Decant the clear portion and add chloroform to make the product measure 100 cc. and filter. Discard the gummy residue in the flask.

Note—Extraction may be made by means of a Soxhlet apparatus if preferred. Keep in well-closed containers and in a cool place.

ROSIN CAVITY LINING

Rosin . . . . 6.70 Gm.
Chloroform, a sufficient quantity,

To make . . . . 100 cc.

Dissolve the rosin in sufficient chloroform to make the product measure 100 cc.

NOTE—Keep in well-closed containers and in a cool place.

CAVITY RINSE

I

Thymol. . . . . 50 Gm.
Chloroform, a sufficient quantity,

To make . . . . 100 cc.

Dissolve the thymol in the chloroform.

NOTE—Keep in a cool place protected from light.

II

Alcohol . . . . 73.5 cc.
Distilled Water, a sufficient quantity,

To make . . . . 100 cc.

Mix.   Alcohol content, approximately 70 per cent.

NOTE—Keep in a cool place.

III

Thymol. . . . . 50 Gm.
Alcohol, a sufficient quantity,

To make . . . . 100 cc.

Dissolve the thymol in sufficient alcohol to make the product measure 100 cc.

NOTE—Keep in a cool place.

OINTMENT—FOR PAINFUL TOOTH SOCKETS

Ethyl Aminobenzoate . . . . 5 Gm.
Chlorobutanol . . . . 5 Gm.
Methyl Salicylate . . . . 1 cc.
White Wax . . . . 10 Gm.
Wool Fat, a sufficient quantity,

To make . . . . 100 Gm.

Melt the white wax, add the wool fat and stir until about to congeal; incorporate a small amount at a time, with the mixture of ethyl aminobenzoate, chlorobutanol and methyl salicylate previously mixed in a mortar.

NOTE—If desired, the consistency may be changed by varying the quantity of white wax.

PULP CAPPING VARNISH

Compound Chloroformic Solution of Mastic
(N.F. V)

Mastic . . . .   30 Gm.
Peruvian Balsam . . . .   30 Gm.
Chloroform, a sufficient quantity,
                              To make . . . .   100 cc.

Dissolve the mastic and peruvian balsam in about 50 cc. of chloroform and add sufficient chloroform to make 100 cc. of solution.

NOTE—Preserve in small tightly-closed containers in a cool place.

CALCIUM PHOSPHATE WITH THYMOL

Thymol. . . . .   20 Gm.
Precipitated Calcium Phosphate . . . .   980 Gm.
Ethyl Oxide. . . . .   40 cc.
                              To make . . . .   1000 Gm.

Dissolve the thymol in the ethyl oxide and pour the solution over the calcium phosphate while triturating. Triturate until the odor of ethyl oxide is no longer perceptible and then pass through a No. 40 sieve.

This powder is used for capping vital pulps by mixing it with sufficient oil of clove to form a paste.

DISCLOSING SOLUTION

Potassium Iodide . . . .   3 Gm.
Iodine . . . .   3 Gm.
Glycerin
Distilled Water, of each, a sufficient quantity,
                              To make . . . .   100 cc.

Mix the potassium iodide and iodine and dissolve in the mixture of glycerin and sufficient distilled water to make the product measure 100 cc.

SOLUTION FOR HYPERSENSITIVE DENTIN

I

Benzyl Alcohol . . . .   30 cc.
Chloroform, a sufficient quantity,
                              To make . . . .   100 cc.

Mix and dissolve.

NOTE—Store in a tightly-closed container in a cool place.

II

Hartman's Solution

Ethyl oxide	20 cc.
Alcohol	10 cc.
Thymol	12.5 Gm.

Dissolve the thymol in the mixture of the alcohol and ethyl oxide.

III

Ethyl Aminobenzoate	11.7 Gm.
Benzyl Alcohol	58.3 cc.
Oil of Clove	30 cc.

Dissolve the oil in the benzyl alcohol and add the ethyl aminobenzoate. Mix until dissolved.

NEOARSPHENAMINE—GLYCERIN SOLUTION

Neoarsphenamine	10 Gm.
Glycerin, a sufficient quantity,	
To make	100 cc.

Mix the neoarsphenamine with the glycerin until dissolved.

NOTE—Keep in a cool place protected from light.

ZINC OXIDE AND THYMOL MIXTURE

Zinc Oxide	67 Gm.
Thymol	33 Gm.
To make	100 Gm.

Melt the thymol in a porcelain evaporating dish on a water bath, add the zinc oxide and rub to a smooth paste and cool. Break into small pieces.

NOTE—Keep in small well-closed containers.

COLD STERILIZING SOLUTION FOR DENTAL INSTRUMENTS

Solution of Formaldehyde	554 cc.
Sodium Borate	62.5 Gm.
Distilled Water, a sufficient quantity,	
To make	1000 cc.

Dissolve the sodium borate in the distilled water and add the solution of formaldehyde.

NOTE—Hypodermic needles should be rinsed with this solution by drawing the solution through the needle while yet attached to the syringe. None of the common sterilizing solutions will penetrate the lumen of the needle just lying in the solution.

PART I—D

CHIROPODY—PODIATRY FORMULAS

ACETIC AND SALICYLIC COLLODION

Salicylic Acid	20 Gm.
Glacial Acetic Acid	100 cc.
Celluloid	50 Gm.
Camphor	50 Gm.
Castor Oil	25 cc.
Acetone, a sufficient quantity,	
To make	1000 cc.

Shred the celluloid and dissolve it in the warmed glacial acetic acid. Dissolve the camphor and salicylic acid in 750 cc. of acetone. Mix the two solutions, then add the castor oil and sufficient acetone to make the product measure 1000 cc.

LACTIC AND SALICYLIC COLLODION

Salicylic Acid	160 Gm.
Lactic Acid	26 cc.
Chlorophyll, alcohol soluble	1 Gm.
Acetone	60 cc.
Flexible Collodion, a sufficient quantity,	
To make	1000 cc.

Incorporate the chlorophyll with the acetone and dissolve the acids in the mixture. Add sufficient flexible collodion to make the product measure 1000 cc.

Keep in a cool place, remote from fire.

LOTION OF CAMPHOR AND CHLORAL

Chloral Hydrate	44 Gm.
Camphor	22 Gm.
Glycerin	325 cc.
Water, a sufficient quantity,	
To make	1000 cc.

Triturate the chloral hydrate and camphor together until liquefied and add the glycerin; gradually add sufficient water to make the product measure 1000 cc., and continue the stirring until a uniform lotion results.

For use, apply freely on itching surfaces.

NOTE—This lotion should be dispensed with a "shake well" label.

312

OIL SOLUTION OF CAMPHOR, CHLORAL AND PHENOL

Camphor . . . . 100 Gm.
Chloral Hydrate . . . . 65 Gm.
Phenol . . . . 130 Gm.
Olive Oil or Peanut Oil, a sufficient quantity,

To make . . . . 1000 cc.

Triturate the camphor with the chloral hydrate and phenol until liquefied and add sufficient olive oil or peanut oil to make the product measure 1000 cc.

For use, apply with a cotton applicator to the matrix and nail bed.

OIL SOLUTION OF GUAIACOL AND TURPENTINE

Guaiacol . . . . 130 cc.
Oil of Turpentine . . . . 425 cc.
Olive Oil or Peanut Oil, a sufficient quantity,

To make . . . . 1000 cc.

Mix the guaiacol and the oil of turpentine and add sufficient olive oil or peanut oil to make the product measure 1000 cc.

For use, massage gently into affected part.

ANODYNE OINTMENT

Camphor . . . . 65 Gm.
Guaiacol . . . . 16 cc.
Methyl Salicylate . . . . 50 cc.
Sulfonated and Hydrogenated Castor Oil, a sufficient quantity,

To make . . . . 1000 Gm.

Incorporate the camphor, guaiacol and methyl salicylate in the sulfonated and hydrogenated castor oil and triturate until a uniform ointment results.

For use, rub a very small amount into the painful area night and morning.

COD LIVER OIL OINTMENT WITH RESORCIN AND TANNIC ACID

Resorcin . . . . 66 Gm.
Tannic Acid . . . . 10 Gm.
Ointment of Cod Liver Oil, R.B. a sufficient quantity,

To make . . . . 1000 Gm.

Triturate the resorcin and tannic acid with the ointment of cod liver oil until a uniform ointment results.

For use, apply daily to ulcerated area.

ICHTHAMMOL AND IODINE OINTMENT

Ichthammol,
Iodine Ointment, of each . . . .   500 Gm.

    Incorporate the ichthammol with the iodine ointment

LEAD OLEATE OINTMENT WITH BORIC AND TANNIC ACIDS
Foot Ointment
(R.B. I)

Boric Acid, powdered . . . .   60 Gm.
Tannic Acid . . . .   20 Gm.
Plaster of Lead Oleate . . . .   480 Gm.
Peanut Oil . . . .   80 Gm.
White Petrolatum . . . .   360 Gm.
Oil of Melissa, as desired,

            To make . . . .   1000 Gm.

    Triturate the tannic and boric acids together and incorporate the peanut oil. Melt the plaster of lead oleate and petrolatum, using gentle heat. To this fused material add the peanut oil mixture and, finally, the oil of melissa, stirring constantly until the ointment is completely cooled.

COMPOUND RESIN ADHESIVE PAINT
(Goldwag)

Guaiac, powdered . . . .   45 Gm.
Myrrh, powdered . . . .   45 Gm.
Mastic, powdered . . . .   90 Gm.
Ethyl Cellulose . . . .   60 Gm.
Isopropyl Alcohol . . . .   250 cc.
Acetone, a sufficient quantity,

            To make . . . .   1000 cc.

    Dissolve the powdered guaiac, myrrh and mastic with the ethyl cellulose in the mixture of isopropyl alcohol and acetone.

    For use, paint on the skin prior to adhesive strapping.

COMPOUND PECTIN PASTE WITH ETHYL AMINOBENZOATE, AMMONIATED MERCURY AND ZINC OXIDE

Ethyl Aminobenzoate . . . .   50 Gm.
Ammoniated Mercury . . . .   20 Gm.
Zinc Oxide . . . .   80 Gm.
Pectin Paste . . . .   740 Gm.

         To make . . . .   1000 Gm.

    Triturate together the ethyl aminobenzoate, ammoniated mercury and zinc oxide and incorporate the mixed powders in the pectin paste.

    For use, apply once daily.

PERUVIAN BALSAM PASTE

Peruvian Balsam	400 Gm.
Sulfonated and Hydrogenated Castor Oil	600 Gm.
To make	1000 Gm.

Incorporate the peruvian balsam in the sulfonated and hydrogenated castor oil. For use, apply once daily to the wounded part.

PYROGALLOL PASTE

Pyrogallol	300 Gm.
Wool Fat	350 Gm.
Sulfonated and Hydrogenated Castor Oil	350 Gm.
To make	1000 Gm.

Triturate the pyrogallol with the wool fat and incorporate in the sulfonated and hydrogenated castor oil. Continue the trituration until a uniform paste results.

NOTE—To be applied by the podiatrist.

CAUSTIC SALICYLIC ACID PASTE WITH CAMPHOR AND CHLORAL HYDRATE

Salicylic Acid	600 Gm.
Camphor	130 Gm.
Chloral Hydrate	130 Gm.
Wool Fat	140 Gm.
To make	1000 Gm.

Triturate the camphor with the chloral hydrate and salicylic acid and incorporate in the wool fat, continuing the trituration until a uniform paste results.

NOTE—To be applied by the podiatrist.

COMPOUND ZINC OXIDE PASTE

Phenol	5 Gm.
Bismuth Subnitrate	10 Gm.
Boric Acid	10 Gm.
Zinc Oxide	70 Gm.
Starch	70 Gm.
Oil of Rose	1 cc.
Sulfonated and Hydrogenated Castor Oil	835 Gm.
To make about	1000 Gm.

Triturate the phenol with the other powders and incorporate in the sulfonated and hydrogenated castor oil; add the oil of rose and mix until a uniform paste results.

For use, apply once daily.

ASTRINGENT FOOT POWDER

I
(P.F.)

Alum, in fine powder	600 Gm.
Tannic Acid, in fine powder	50 Gm.
Salicylic Acid, in fine powder	20 Gm.
Orris, in fine powder	330 Gm.
To make	1000 Gm.

Mix thoroughly and pass through a No. 80 sieve.

II

Thymol, powdered	8 Gm.
Salicylic Acid, powdered	33 Gm.
Alum, powdered	125 Gm.
Boric Acid, powdered	210 Gm.
Tannic Acid	160 Gm.
Bentonite	464 Gm.
To make	1000 Gm.

Mix thoroughly and pass through a No. 60 sieve.

BORIC ACID AND ZINC OXIDE FOOT POWDER
(R.B. I)

Boric Acid, powdered	750 Gm.
Zinc Oxide	50 Gm.
Purified Talc	200 Gm.
Oil of Eucalyptus or Oil of Thyme	2 cc.
To make about	1000 Gm.

Mix intimately and pass through a No. 60 sieve.

MEDICATED FOOT DUSTING POWDER

Menthol	5.5 Gm.
Phenol	3.8 Gm.
Alcohol	15 cc.
Zinc Stearate	330 Gm.
Boric Acid, powdered	650 Gm.
To make about	1000 Gm.

Dissolve the menthol and phenol in the alcohol and mix the solution with the zinc stearate, triturate until the alcohol is all evaporated and then add the boric acid, triturating until a uniform powder results and pass through a No. 60 sieve.

For use, apply freely on itching surfaces.

MODIFIED WHITFIELD'S FOOT POWDER

Salicylic Acid	16 Gm.
Benzoic Acid	11 Gm.
Thymol	5 Gm.
Menthol	5 Gm.
Boric Acid	250 Gm.
Bentonite	713 Gm.
To make	1000 Gm.

Triturate the thymol and menthol together until liquefied and add the boric acid, mixing until the thymol-menthol mixture is uniformly dispersed in the boric acid. Mix the salicylic and benzoic acids with the bentonite and add this mixture of powders to the mixture of boric acid, triturating until a uniform powder results and pass through a No. 60 sieve.

For use, dust between the toes daily, for excess perspiration.

ZINC PEROXIDE FOOT POWDER WITH BORIC ACID AND SODIUM PERBORATE

Zinc Peroxide	100 Gm.
Sodium Perborate	150 Gm.
Boric Acid	250 Gm.
Bentonite	500 Gm.
To make	1000 Gm.

Mix thoroughly and pass through a No. 60 sieve.
For use, dust on foot and between the toes, for foul odors.

COMPOUND SOLUTION OF ALUMINUM CHLORIDE

Aluminum Chloride	100 Gm.
Alcohol	240 cc.
Oil of Lavender	1.2 cc.
Tincture of Cudbear	1.2 cc.
Distilled Water, a sufficient quantity,	
To make	1000 cc.

Dissolve the aluminum chloride in 700 cc. of distilled water, mix the oil and tincture with the alcohol and add to the aqueous solution, and finally add sufficient distilled water to make the product measure 1000 cc.

SOLUTION OF PECTIN

Pectin	20 Gm.
Distilled Water, a sufficient quantity,	
To make	1000 cc.

Dissolve the pectin in sufficient distilled water to make the product measure 1000 cc.

For use, apply to the inflamed and/or infected area of nail root.

COMPOUND SPIRIT OF BENZYL ALCOHOL, BUTYN SULFATE, MENTHOL AND CAMPHOR

Butyn Sulfate	20 Gm.
Menthol	50 Gm.
Camphor	50 Gm.
Benzyl Alcohol	350 cc.
Alcohol	300 cc.
Acetone, a sufficient quantity,	
To make	1000 cc.

Dissolve the butyn sulfate, menthol, camphor and benzyl alcohol in the alcohol and add sufficient acetone to make the product measure 1000 cc.

For use, apply to part for a few minutes for topical anesthesia.

COMPOUND SPIRIT OF MENTHOL AND CAMPHOR

Menthol	8	Gm.
Camphor	8	Gm.
Oil of Lavender	3	cc.
Oil of Bergamot	3	cc.
Oil of Orange Flowers	0.6	cc.
Alcohol.	735	cc.
Distilled Water, a sufficient quantity,		
To make	1000	cc.

Dissolve the menthol, camphor and oils in the alcohol, add sufficient distilled water to make the product measure 1000 cc. and mix well.

SPIRIT OF RESORCINOL, SALICYLIC AND BENZOIC ACIDS

Salicylic Acid	50 Gm.
Benzoic Acid	33 Gm.
Resorcinol	30 Gm.
Acetone	450 cc.
Alcohol, a sufficient quantity,	
To make	1000 cc.

Dissolve the acids and resorcinol in the mixture of acetone, and sufficient alcohol to make the product measure 1000 cc.

For use, apply locally twice daily on the infected area.

COMPOUND SPIRIT OF THYMOL WITH BENZOIC AND SALICYLIC ACIDS

Benzoic Acid	16	Gm.
Salicylic Acid	16	Gm.
Thymol	10	Gm.
Methylthionine Chloride	0.24	Gm.
Oil of Orange Flowers	0.6	cc.
Alcohol	735	cc.
Distilled Water, a sufficient quantity,		
To make	1000	cc.

Dissolve the acids, thymol and oil in 500 cc. of alcohol and the methylthionine chloride in the remainder. Mix the solutions and add sufficient distilled water to make the product measure 1000 cc. Mix well.

SPIRIT OF SALICYLATED IODINE WITH THYMOL

Iodine	11 Gm.
Thymol	11 Gm.
Salicylic Acid	33 Gm.
Alcohol, a sufficient quantity,	
To make	1000 cc.

Dissolve the iodine, thymol and salicylic acid in sufficient alcohol to make the product measure 1000 cc.

For use, apply locally twice daily on the infected area.

WET DRESSING OF BENZYL ALCOHOL AND ETHYL AMINOBENZOATE

Benzyl Alcohol	40 cc.
Ethyl Aminobenzoate	10 Gm.
Water, a sufficient quantity,	
To make	1000 cc.

Dissolve the ethyl aminobenzoate in the benzyl alcohol and gradually add sufficient water to make 1000 cc.

For use, apply as an anodyne wet dressing to affected part.

Dispense with a "shake well" label.

WET DRESSING OF UREA

Urea	20 Gm.
Distilled Water, a sufficient quantity,	
To make	1000 cc.

Dissolve the urea in sufficient distilled water to make the product measure 1000 cc.

For use, apply as a wet dressing to affected part.

PART I—E
VETERINARY FORMULAS

PREPARATIONS FOR BIRDS
BIRD SEED

Hemp Seed	417 Gm.
Canary Seed	334 Gm.
Millet Seed	83 Gm.
Rape Seed	83 Gm.
Poppy Seed	83 Gm.
To make	1000 Gm.

Mix.

CANARY FEED

Egg Yolk, dried	200 Gm.
Cuttlefish Bone, in powder	100 Gm.
Sucrose, in powder	100 Gm.
Fenugreek, in powder	100 Gm.
Capsicum, in powder	400 Gm.
Poppy Seed, bruised	100 Gm.
To make	1000 Gm.

Mix.

FOOD FOR MOCKING BIRDS

Corn Meal	449 Gm.
Rice, in coarse powder	100 Gm.
Broken Crackers, in coarse powder	400 Gm.
Hemp Seed, in coarse powder	50 Gm.
Capsicum, in powder	1 Gm.
To make	1000 Gm.

Mix.

PREPARATIONS FOR CATTLE
CRUDE OIL EMULSION FOR DIPPING CATTLE

Rosin	380 Gm.
Sodium Hydroxide	50 Gm.
Crude Oil	35 liters
Water, a sufficient quantity,	
To make	100 liters

Dissolve the sodium hydroxide in 3 liters of water; add the rosin and boil until dissolved. Place 2 liters of crude oil in a 50-liter vessel, add the hot rosin solution and agitate the mixture briskly until it becomes as thick as jelly. Add a liter or more of crude oil and 250 cc. of water and mix by agitation. Continue adding oil and water until sufficient have been added to make 50 liters of emulsion. This is a 35 per cent solution of crude oil in the form of a homogeneous emulsion, which is emptied into the dipping vat and reduced to a 24 per cent solution by adding 50 liters of water.

EVERY DAY LINIMENT FOR CATTLE

Strong Solution of Ammonia	15 cc.
Oleic Acid	30 cc.
Ammonium Chloride	4 Gm.
Methyl Salicylate	30 cc.
Oil of Turpentine	90 cc.
Water, a sufficient quantity,	
To make	1000 cc.

Place the strong solution of ammonia in a liter bottle, add 125 cc. of lukewarm water, mix, add the oleic acid, shake well, then add another 125 cc. of warm water and then the ammonium chloride dissolved in 125 cc. of water. Mix in the methyl salicylate, and a further 125 cc. portion of water, shake again, then add the oil of turpentine, make up to 1000 cc. with warm water and mix and shake well. Set aside for a week.

COMPOUND OINTMENT OF PHYTOLACCA

Extract of Phytolacca	100	Gm.
Camphor	20	Gm.
Eucalyptol	10	cc.
Oil of Turpentine	10	cc.
Menthol	0.25	Gm.
Wool Fat	700	Gm.
Petrolatum	160	Gm.
To make about	1000	Gm.

Triturate together the camphor and menthol with the oil of turpentine and eucalyptol and mix with 500 Gm. of wool fat, mix the extract of phytolacca with the remainder of the wool fat and the petrolatum. Mix the two ointments until a uniform product results.

This ointment is used for inflammation of the mammary glands and other glandular enlargements.

OINTMENT FOR UDDER

Pilular Extract of Belladonna	7.5 Gm.
Fluidextract of Phytolacca	30 cc.
Potassium Iodide	10 Gm.
Distilled Water	10 cc.
Wool Fat, a sufficient quantity,	
To make	100 Gm.

Evaporate the fluidextract of phytolacca to a semi-solid mass and mix with the extract of belladonna and 50 Gm. of wool fat. Dissolve the potassium iodide in the distilled water and incorporate the remainder of the wool fat. Mix the two ointments.

PURGE FOR CATTLE

Ginger, powdered	70 Gm.
Sodium Chloride	175 Gm.
Nux Vomica, powdered	5 Gm.
Magnesium Sulfate	750 Gm.
To make	1000 Gm.

Mix.

Dissolve 500 Gm. in at least 3 quarts of warm water and administer in 1 dose.

LOUSE SPRAY

Sodium Fluoride	4 Gm.
Water, a sufficient quantity,	
To make	1000 cc.

Dissolve the sodium fluoride in sufficient water to make the product measure 1000 cc.

Use as a spray for lice on cattle.

PREPARATIONS FOR DOGS

LAXATIVES FOR DOGS

I

SYRUP OF RHAMNUS CATHARTICA

Fluidextract of Rhamnus Cathartica	200 cc.
Oil of Fennel	0.2 cc.
Oil of Cinnamon	0.2 cc.
Syrup, a sufficient quantity,	
To make	1000 cc.

Add the oils to the fluidextract and mix this with sufficient syrup to make the product measure 1000 cc.

AVERAGE DOSE—30 cc. for large dogs, 15 cc. for smaller dogs.

II
CALOMEL POWDER

Calomel	0.1 Gm.
Sucrose, powdered	1 Gm.
To make	1 Dose

Mix.

III
COMPOUND POWDER OF SENNA AND FRANGULA

Senna, in powder.	30 Gm.
Glycyrrhiza, in powder	3 Gm.
Extract of Glycyrrhiza, in powder	3 Gm.
Fluidextract of Frangula	15 cc.
Sucrose, powdered	60 Gm.
Oil of Anise.	3 cc.
To make	100 Powders

Mix the powdered ingredients, incorporate the fluidextract and oil, and divide into 100 powders.

AVERAGE DOSE—1 powder, given on an empty stomach in the morning. Bones should be withheld from the diet.

RHEUMATIC LINIMENT FOR DOGS

Tincture of Aconite	125 cc.
Methyl Salicylate	125 cc.
Chloroform	125 cc.
Camphor and Soap Liniment, a sufficient quantity,	
To make	1000 cc.

Mix. Dispense with a "shake well" label.

To be applied to affected parts three times a day.

MIXTURE FOR ASTHMA IN DOGS

Fluidextract of Stramonium	33 cc.
Fluidextract of Gelsemium	65 cc.
Fluidextract of Lobelia	100 cc.
Syrup of Orange	250 cc.
Water, a sufficient quantity,	
To make	1000 cc.

Mix. Dispense with a "shake well" label.

AVERAGE DOSE—Metric, 4 cc.—Apothecaries, 1 fluidrachm. To be given every hour or two until relieved.

ASTRINGENT MIXTURE FOR DOGS

Zinc Sulfocarbolate	2.5 Gm.
Pepsin	11 Gm.
Salol	6.5 Gm.
Acacia	25 Gm.
Bismuth Subsalicylate	16.5 Gm.
Aromatic Elixir, a sufficient quantity,	
To make	1000 cc.

Mix the zinc sulfocarbolate, salol and bismuth subsalicylate with about 25 Gm. of acacia, dissolve the pepsin in a small amount of warm water and add to the aromatic elixir. Gradually add the liquid to the mixture of acacia and powders to make a suspension.

AVERAGE DOSE—Metric, 4 to 8 cc.—Apothecaries, 1 to 2 fluidrachms.

NOTE—This mixture should be dispensed with a "shake well" label.

MIXTURE FOR DIARRHEA

Phenyl Salicylate	18 Gm.
Camphorated Tincture of Opium	100 cc.
Bismuth Subcarbonate	88 Gm.
Compound Elixir of Pepsin	330 cc.
Compound Chalk Mixture, a sufficient quantity,	
To make	1000 cc.

Dissolve the phenyl salicylate in the camphorated tincture of opium and add the elixir of lactated pepsin; make a paste of the bismuth subcarbonate with a portion of the compound chalk mixture and gradually add the remainder of the chalk mixture, and lastly add the mixture of the phenyl salicylate in the camphorated tincture of opium and elixir.

AVERAGE DOSE—Metric, 4 cc.—Apothecaries, 1 fluidrachm to be administered every 3 hours.

NOTE—Dispense this mixture with a "shake well" label.

POWDERS FOR DIARRHEA

Phenyl Salicylate	33.3 Gm.
Bismuth Subnitrate	66 6 Gm.
Prepared Chalk	50 Gm.
Oil of Peppermint	6 cc.
To make	100 powders

Triturate the powders together in a mortar and incorporate the oil of peppermint.

AVERAGE DOSE—1 powder every 4 hours.

MIXTURE FOR DISTEMPER BRONCHITIS

Menthol . . . . 0.6 Gm.
Ammonium Chloride . . . . 33.3 Gm.
Codeine Sulfate . . . . 2.1 Gm.
Syrup of Wild Cherry, a sufficient quantity,

To make . . . . 1000 cc.

Dissolve the codeine sulfate in part of the syrup of wild cherry, incorporate the remaining ingredients, and add sufficient syrup of wild cherry to make the product measure 1000 cc.

AVERAGE DOSE—Metric, 4 cc.—Apothecaries, 1 fluidrachm, to be administered every 4 hours.

TONIC MIXTURE FOR DISTEMPER IN DOGS

Tincture of Nux Vomica . . . . 65 cc.
Elixir of Pepsin Compound . . . . 650 cc.
Solution of Potassium Arsenite . . . . 65 cc.
Compound Mixture of Rhubarb, a sufficient quantity,

To make . . . . 1000 cc.

Mix well with vigorous shaking. Dispense with a "shake well" label.

AVERAGE DOSE—Metric, 2 to 4 cc.—Apothecaries, ½ to 1 fluidrachm three times a day depending on the weight of the dog.

OINTMENT FOR MOIST ECZEMA

Phenol . . . . 0.6 Gm.
Coal Tar . . . . 1 Gm.
Carbon Tetrachloride . . . . 2 cc.
Zinc Oxide . . . . 6.6 Gm.
Starch . . . . 6.6 Gm.
Ointment of Rose Water, a sufficient quantity,

To make . . . . 100 Gm.

Mix the phenol, coal tar and carbon tetrachloride, and incorporate the mixed powders and the ointment of rose water and triturate until a uniform ointment results.

Apply to affected parts 2 or 3 times a day.

MANGE OR RINGWORM OINTMENT

Peruvian Balsam . . . . 12 Gm
Sulfur Ointment . . . . 88 Gm.

To make . . . . 100 Gm.

Mix.
To be applied 3 times daily.

SULFUR AND TAR OINTMENT FOR DOGS

Precipitated Sulfur.	25 Gm.
Pine Tar	25 Gm.
Zinc Oxide Ointment.	50 Gm.
To make	100 Gm.

Mix thoroughly by trituration.

This ointment should be rubbed well into the skin and used in small quantity, on not more than one quarter of the body at a time.

PILLS OF ALOIN AND ASAFETIDA FOR CONSTIPATION IN DOGS

Aloin	1.3 Gm.
Asafetida	15.0 Gm.
To make	100 Pills

Mix and divide into 100 pills.

AVERAGE DOSE—1 or 2 pills late at night.

IRON, ARSENIC AND STRYCHNINE PILLS FOR DOGS

Mass of Ferrous Carbonate	18 Gm.
Arsenic Trioxide.	0.06 Gm.
Strychnine Sulfate	0.06 Gm.
To make	100 Pills

Mix intimately, form a mass and divide it into 100 pills.

AVERAGE DOSE—For puppies and small dogs, 1 pill twice daily before meals. For larger dogs, 1 pill 3 times daily.

FLEA POWDER
I

Boric Acid, in powder.	142 Gm.
Sublimed Sulfur, in powder	142 Gm.
Naphthalene, in powder.	142 Gm.
Oil of Pennyroyal	10 cc.
Pyrethrum Flowers, in powder	564 Gm.
To make about	1000 Gm.

Mix the dry ingredients by trituration, then add the oil, triturate again, and finally pass the mixture through a No. 20 sieve.

II

Derris Root, in powder	20 Gm.
Pyrethrum Flowers, in powder	20 Gm.
Kieselguhr	60 Gm.
To make	100 Gm.

Mix.

KILL-FLEAS

Oil of Wormwood	8 cc.
Oil of Pennyroyal	15 cc.
Oil of Sassafras	15 cc.
Spirit of Camphor	60 cc.
Saponated Solution of Cresol	500 cc.
Acetone, a sufficient quantity,	
To make	1000 cc.

Mix the oils and the spirit with 300 cc. of acetone, add gradually the saponated solution of cresol with agitation, and lastly add sufficient acetone to make the product measure 1000 cc.

This solution is to be diluted with water, about 4 fluidrachms to 1 pint, and then applied to the dog.

CAUTION—*This liquid is inflammable.*

SARCOPTIC MANGE SOLUTION FOR DOGS

Coal Tar	150 Gm.
Soft Soap	150 Gm.
Oil of Turpentine	150 cc.
Juniper Tar	150 cc.
Purified Benzin, a sufficient quantity,	
To make	1000 cc.

Triturate the tar with the soft soap, incorporate the juniper tar and the oil of turpentine, and finally add sufficient purified benzin to make the product measure 1000 cc.

To be rubbed in once daily over the area involved.

CAUTION—*This liquid is inflammable.*

PHENOLATED GLYCERIN

Phenol	3 Gm.
Glycerin, a sufficient quantity,	
To make	100 cc.

Dissolve.

Place 5 drops in the infected ear 3 times a day.

TABLETS FOR LARGE ROUND WORMS AND WHIP WORMS IN DOGS

Santonin	0.6 Gm.
Mild Mercurous Chloride	0.6 Gm.
Lactose	28.8 Gm.
Diluted Alcohol, a sufficient quantity,	
To make	100 Tablets

Mix intimately, moisten with diluted alcohol and compress into tablets of 0.3 Gm. each.

AVERAGE DOSE—For puppies and small dogs, 1 tablet in the morning on an empty stomach after feeding lightly the night before. Give castor oil 2 hours later. Repeat the dose every morning for a week. For larger dogs, 2 tablets.

PREPARATIONS FOR HORSES

EYE WASH FOR HORSES

I

Arnica Flowers	50 Gm.
Chamomile Flowers	50 Gm.
Water, boiling, a sufficient quantity,	
To make	1000 cc.

Infuse the flowers in the hot water. Filter when cool. Add sufficient water to make 1000 cc.

II

Zinc Sulfate	16 Gm.
Boric Acid	40 Gm.
Rose Water	720 cc.
Distilled Water, a sufficient quantity,	
To make	1000 cc.

Dissolve the zinc sulfate in the distilled water and the boric acid in the rose water. Mix the solutions and filter.

COMPOUND ACONITE LINIMENT

Tincture of Aconite	125 cc.
Chloroform	125 cc.
Tincture of Iodine	125 cc.
Diluted Solution of Ammonia	125 cc.
Camphor and Soap Liniment, a sufficient quantity,	
To make	1000 cc.

Mix by agitation.

LINIMENT FOR HORSES

Tincture of Iodine . . . . 85 cc.
Alcohol. . . . . 350 cc.
Oil of Turpentine . . . . 350 cc.
Camphor . . . . 45 Gm.
Heavy Liquid Petrolatum, a sufficient quantity,

To make . . . . 1000 cc.

Dissolve the camphor in the alcohol, add the tincture of iodine, the oil of turpentine and the liquid petrolatum and mix.

STIMULATING LINIMENT

Tincture of Capsicum . . . . 16 cc.
Tincture of Cantharides . . . . 16 cc.
Camphor and Soap Liniment . . . . 125 cc.
Alcohol . . . . 250 cc.
Water, a sufficient quantity,

To make . . . . 1000 cc.

Mix the tinctures with the alcohol and add to the camphor and soap liniment and
water which have previously been mixed, and shake.

NOTE—Dispense with a "shake well" label.

LOTION FOR HORSES

Solution of Lead Subacetate. . . . . 30 cc.
Oil of Eucalyptus. . . . . 120 cc.
Diluted Acetic Acid . . . . 210 cc.
Sesame Oil . . . . 600 cc.
Yolks of Two Fresh Eggs

To make about . . . . 1000 cc.

Triturate the yolks in a mortar and add gradually the sesame oil previously mixed
with the oil of eucalyptus. Then incorporate the diluted acetic acid and finally the
solution of lead subacetate.

Alkanet may be added as a coloring agent if desired.

MIXTURE FOR "HEAVES" IN HORSES

Solution of Potassium Arsenite . . . . : . . . 60 cc.
Fluidextract of Belladonna . . . . 120 cc.
Fluidextract of Stramonium . . . . 120 cc.
Sodium Iodide . . . . 120 Gm.
Fluidextract of Grindelia . . . . 90 cc.
Water, a sufficient quantity,

To make . . . . 1000 cc.

Dissolve the sodium iodide in about 200 cc. of water and add the solution of potassium arsenite; mix the fluidextracts and add gradually to the aqueous solution, and lastly add sufficient water to make the product measure 1000 cc., and shake well.

NOTE—Dispense with a "shake well" label.

AVERAGE DOSE—Metric, 15 cc.—Apothecaries, ½ fluidounce after each feed.

BLACK OIL
Oleum Nigrum
Farrier's Oil; Currier's Oil; Fuming Oil

Oil of Turpentine	485 cc.
Linseed Oil	485 cc.
Sulfuric Acid	30 cc.
To make	1000 cc.

Mix the oils and add gradually the sulfuric acid, stirring constantly. Great care must be used when the sulfuric acid is added, and the operation is best conducted in an open vessel.

This preparation is used as a liniment in veterinary practice. The quantity of sulfuric acid is increased or decreased according to the desired counterirritant effect.

SARCOPTIC MANGE OINTMENT FOR HORSES

Ammoniated Mercury	18.5 Gm.
Sublimed Sulfur	185 Gm.
Phenol	23 Gm.
Lard	773.5 Gm.
To make	1000 Gm.

Mix thoroughly.

Clip the body and limbs all over and rub the ointment into the affected parts. On the following day brush the body vigorously. Repeat the grooming in 2 days, then apply the ointment again and continue treatment as before.

OINTMENT FOR "SCRATCHES" IN HORSES

Zinc Carbonate	65 Gm.
Alum	45 Gm.
Precipitated Calcium Carbonate	300 Gm.
Creosote	45 cc.
Yellow Wax	45 Gm.
Benzoinated Lard, a sufficient quantity,	
To make	1000 Gm.

Melt the yellow wax and benzoinated lard and incorporate the other ingredients in the cooled mixture of wax and lard, triturating until a smooth ointment results.

DUSTING POWDER FOR SUPERFICIAL WOUNDS AND RAW SURFACES

Bismuth Subnitrate . . . . 275 Gm.
Tannic Acid . . . . 140 Gm.
Iodoform . . . . 80 Gm.
Activated Charcoal, a sufficient quantity,
                 To make . . . . 1000 Gm.

Mix.

Use as a dusting powder.

CAMPHOR, POTASSIUM CHLORATE AND BELLADONNA POWDER

Camphor, in powder . . . . 2 Gm.
Potassium Chlorate, in powder . . . . 1 Gm.
Belladonna Leaf, in fine powder . . . . 1 Gm.
Anise, in powder. . . . . 1.3 Gm.
                 To make . . . . 1 Powder

Mix well the camphor, belladonna leaf and anise and gradually and carefully add the potassium chlorate with gentle stirring or an explosion may ensue.

AVERAGE DOSE—1 powder twice a day in food.

IRON, GENTIAN, FENUGREEK AND CHARCOAL POWDER

Activated Charcoal, in powder . . . . 125 Gm.
Fenugreek, in powder. . . . . 125 Gm.
Exsiccated Ferrous Sulfate . . . . 312 Gm.
Gentian, in powder. . . . . 438 Gm.
                 To make . . . . 1000 Gm

Mix.

AVERAGE DOSE—½ ounce in food.

REPELLENT FOR STABLE AND HORSE FLIES

Naphthalene, in powder. 26.5 Gm.
Kerosene. . . . . 100 cc.
Hard Soap . . . . 40 Gm.
Water, a sufficient quantity,
                 To make . . . . 1000 cc.

Dissolve the naphthalene in the kerosene. Shave the hard soap and dissolve it in 800 cc. of boiling water. Allow to cool, add the naphthalene solution and sufficient water to make the product measure 1000 cc.

This is stainless and will not "gum up" on the coat. It may be used in a spray gun or applied in other ways for both horses and cattle.

STOCK FOOD

Fenugreek, in powder	65 Gm.
Anise, in powder	20 Gm.
Sodium Chloride, in powder	40 Gm.
Ferrous Sulfate, in powder	10 Gm.
Ginger, in powder	10 Gm.
Cottonseed Oil Cake, ground	425 Gm.
Miller's Shorts	215 Gm.
St. John's Bread, ground	215 Gm.
To make	1000 Gm.

Mix intimately.

AVERAGE DOSE—1 to 2 tablespoonfuls in food.

PREPARATIONS FOR POULTRY

CHICKEN MASH FOR LAYERS

Wheat Bran, coarse	100 Gm.
Wheat Middlings	100 Gm.
Meat Scraps	650 Gm.
Corn Meal	150 Gm.
To make	1000 Gm.

Mix.

For general hens, the meat scraps may be diminished and ground oats added.

Feed in a self-feeder in unlimited quantity.

COMPOUND POWDER OF CALCIUM CARBONATE AND PHOSPHATE WITH SODIUM CHLORIDE

Sodium Bicarbonate	2 Gm.
Calcium Phosphate	8 Gm.
Calcium Carbonate	34 Gm.
Cottonseed Oil Cake, ground	136 Gm.
Oyster Shells, in powder	270 Gm.
Sodium Chloride	550 Gm.
To make	1000 Gm.

Mix intimately.

AVERAGE DOSE—1 teaspoonful mixed with a quart of food.

POWDER OF CALCIUM HYPOPHOSPHITE WITH IRON AND MAGNESIUM SULFATES AND SODIUM CHLORIDE

Sodium Chloride	25 Gm.
Magnesium Sulfate	75 Gm.
Exsiccated Ferrous Sulfate	290 Gm.
Calcium Hypophosphite	610 Gm.
To make	1000 Gm.

Mix intimately.

AVERAGE DOSE—1 teaspoonful mixed with a quart of food.

IRON, LIME, PEPPER AND CAPSICUM POWDER

Capsicum, in powder	28 Gm.
Black Pepper, in powder	110 Gm.
Red Ferric Oxide	28 Gm.
Calcium Hydroxide	278 Gm.
Oyster Shells, in powder	556 Gm.
To make	1000 Gm.

Mix intimately.

AVERAGE DOSE—1 tablespoonful mixed with food.

COMPOUND POWDER OF IRON AND MAGNESIUM SULFATES

Magnesium Sulfate, in powder	635 Gm.
Magnesium Oxide	73 Gm.
Ferrous Sulfate, in powder	146 Gm.
Ginger, in powder	146 Gm.
To make	1000 Gm.

Mix intimately.

AVERAGE DOSE—1 teaspoonful mixed with a quart of food.

POULTRY POWDER

Ginger, in powder	120 Gm.
Capsicum, in powder	60 Gm.
Sulfur, in powder	60 Gm.
Gentian, in powder	60 Gm.
Calcium Hydroxide	700 Gm.
To make	1000 Gm.

Mix intimately.

AVERAGE DOSE—1 teaspoonful mixed with a quart of food.

PART II

FLAVORING EXTRACTS

The following definitions and excerpts are taken from the circular, "Flavoring Extracts," under the Federal Food, Drug and Cosmetic Act, issued by the Federal Security Agency, Food and Drug Administration (August 15, 1939, and reprinted June, 1941). The standards described are for preparations intended for food purposes and are not to be confounded with similar preparations described in the Pharmacopœia and National Formulary intended for medicinal purposes.

Flavors should contain no ingredients that may render them injurious to health.

Flavor labels should not be false or misleading in any particular. The term "labeling" means all labels and other written, printed or graphic matter upon any article or any of its containers or wrappers, or accompanying such article.

A **flavoring extract** is a solution in ethyl alcohol of proper strength of the sapid and odorous principles derived from an aromatic plant, or parts of the plant, with or without its coloring matter, and conforms in name to the plant used in its preparation.

EXTRACTS, FLAVORS AND MENSTRUA

The vehicle or menstruum of a flavoring extract is ethyl alcohol of proper strength. The terms "extract" and "flavor" are not synonymous. The former implies an alcoholic product. Non-alcoholic flavoring products may be labeled with the term "flavor" provided they contain the same kinds and proportions of flavoring ingredients as are required by the Administration's definitions and standards for extracts, and provided further they are labeled with some term in direct connection with their names to show that the vehicle is not alcohol.

There is no objection to the use of (1) edible **vegetable** oils, such as corn oil and peanut oil, as vehicles for non-alcoholic flavors, provided the oils contain no impurities that might render the products injurious to health and provided suitable labeling is employed, and (2) small quantities of glycerin in food products, provided it is of a purity suitable for food use and provided its presence is plainly declared in the labeling when it is not a normal ingredient of the article (in the case of vanilla extract, etc., glycerin is regarded as a normal ingredient and it is unnecessary to declare its presence in the labeling). The use of mineral oil and so-called "alcoholic substitutes" other than propylene glycol is not allowable.

The Federal Food Drugs and Cosmetic Act does not require a statement of the proportion of alcohol on the label of flavoring extracts used exclusively for food purposes, although certain State laws make this requirement.

IMITATION EXTRACTS AND FLAVORS

An imitation (food product) shall bear on the label the word "imitation" and in addition a clear statement of the principal or essential ingredients of the article.

The word "imitation" will not be regarded as being plainly stated on the package unless it is displayed as prominently as and directly precedes the name of the genuine article, as for example "Imitation Vanilla Extract." The statement "Artificially Flavored and Colored," or an equivalent statement, will be regarded as meeting the second requirement of the law relating to imitation food products. If preferred, however, the important ingredients may be named on the label.

There are no substitutes under the law for the word "imitation." Such words as "synthetic" or "artificial" do not take its place.

The character of imitation extracts and flavors should be such that they will substantially take the place of the products they imitate.

Only colors certified by the Food and Drug Administration as harmless and suitable for such use may be employed. These are certified coal-tar colors. (See R.B., page 341, for a representative list of certified coal-tar colors.)

Any harmless vegetable dye may be used in flavors or other food. There is no system of certification in the case of vegetable colors.

The presence of a chemical preservative must be declared on the label, stating the name and amount of the preservative used.

Almond extract is the flavoring extract prepared from oil of bitter almond, free from hydrocyanic acid, and contains not less than 1 per cent by volume of oil of bitter almond.

Anise extract is the flavoring extract prepared from oil of anise, and contains not less than 3 per cent by volume of oil of anise.

Celery seed extract is the flavoring extract prepared from celery seed or the oil of celery seed, or both, and contains not less than 0.3 per cent by volume of oil of celery seed.

Cinnamon extract, cassia extract, cassia cinnamon extract, is the flavoring extract prepared from oil of cinnamon, and contains not less than 2 per cent by volume of oil of cinnamon.

Ceylon cinnamon extract is the flavoring extract prepared from oil of Ceylon cinnamon, and contains not less than 2 per cent by volume of oil of Ceylon cinnamon.

Clove extract is the flavoring extract prepared from oil of clove, and contains not less than 2 per cent by volume of oil of clove.

Ginger extract is the flavoring extract prepared from ginger, and contains in each 100 cc. the alcohol-soluble matters from not less than 20 Gm. of ginger.

Lemon extract is the flavoring extract prepared from oil of lemon or from lemon peel, or both, and contains not less than 5 per cent by volume of oil of lemon.

Terpeneless extract of lemon is the flavoring extract prepared by shaking oil of lemon with diluted alcohol, or by dissolving terpeneless oil of lemon in diluted alcohol, and contains not less than 0.2 per cent by weight of citral derived from oil of lemon.

Nutmeg extract is the flavoring extract prepared from oil of nutmeg, and contains not less than 2 per cent by volume of oil of nutmeg.

Orange extract is the flavoring extract prepared from oil of orange, or from orange peel, or both, and contains not less than 5 per cent by volume of oil of orange.

Terpeneless extract of orange is the flavoring extract prepared by shaking oil of orange with diluted alcohol, or by dissolving terpeneless oil of orange in diluted alcohol, and corresponds in flavoring strength to orange extract.

Peppermint extract is the flavoring extract prepared from oil of peppermint, or from peppermint, or both, and contains not less than 3 per cent by volume of oil of peppermint.

Rose extract is the flavoring extract prepared from attar of rose, with or without red rose petals, and contains not less than 0.4 per cent by volume of attar of rose.

Savory extract is the flavoring extract prepared from oil of savory, or from savory, or both, and contains not less than 0.35 per cent by volume of oil of savory.

Spearmint extract is the flavoring extract prepared from oil of spearmint, or from spearmint, or both, and contains not less than 3 per cent by volume of oil of spearmint.

Star anise extract is the flavoring extract prepared from oil of star anise, and contains not less than 3 per cent by volume of oil of star anise.

Sweet basil extract is the flavoring extract prepared from oil of sweet basil, or from sweet basil, or both, and contains not less than 0.1 per cent by volume of oil of sweet basil.

Sweet marjoram extract, marjoram extract, is the flavoring extract prepared from oil of marjoram, or from marjoram, or both, and contains not less than 1 per cent by volume of oil of marjoram.

Thyme extract is the flavoring extract prepared from oil of thyme, or from thyme, or both, and contains not less than 0.2 per cent by volume of oil of thyme.

Tonka extract is the flavoring extract prepared from tonka beans, with or without one or more of the following: Sucrose, dextrose, glycerin. It contains not less than 0.1 per cent by weight of coumarin extracted from the tonka bean, together with a corresponding proportion of the other soluble matters thereof.

Vanilla extract is the flavoring extract prepared from vanilla bean, with or without one or more of the following: Sucrose, dextrose, glycerin. It contains in 100 cc. the soluble matter from not less than 10 Gm. of the vanilla bean.

Wintergreen extract is the flavoring extract prepared from oil of wintergreen, and contains not less than 3 per cent by volume of oil of wintergreen.

FLAVORING AGENTS

ALMOND EXTRACT

Benzaldehyde	20 cc.
Sherry Wine, a sufficient quantity,	
To make	1000 cc.

Mix.

CELERY SEED EXTRACT

Oil of Celery Seed	10 cc.
Alcohol	900 cc.
Distilled Water, a sufficient quantity,	
To make	1000 cc.

Dissolve the oil in the alcohol, add sufficient distilled water to make the product measure 1000 cc. and filter.

CINNAMON EXTRACT

Oil of Cinnamon . . . . 20 cc.
Alcohol . . . . 700 cc.
Distilled Water, a sufficient quantity,

To make . . . . 1000 cc.

Dissolve the oil in the alcohol, add sufficient distilled water to make the product measure 1000 cc. and filter.

CLOVE EXTRACT

Oil of Clove . . . . 20 cc.
Alcohol . . . . 600 cc.
Distilled Water, a sufficient quantity,

To make . . . . 1000 cc.

Dissolve the oil in the alcohol, add sufficient distilled water to make the product measure 1000 cc. and filter.

LEMON EXTRACT

Oil of Lemon . . . . 50 cc.
Lemon Peel, outer layer only . . . . 50 Gm.
Alcohol, a sufficient quantity,

To make . . . . 1000 cc.

Dissolve the oil in 900 cc. of alcohol, add the lemon peel, macerate for 48 hours, filter and pass sufficient alcohol through the filter to make the product measure 1000 cc.

TERPENELESS LEMON EXTRACT

Terpeneless Oil of Lemon . . . . 5 cc.
Turmeric . . . . 5 Gm.
Alcohol . . . . 500 cc.
Distilled Water, a sufficient quantity,

To make . . . . 1000 cc.

Dissolve the oil in the alcohol, add the turmeric, set aside for 24 hours, then add the distilled water and set aside again for 24 hours with occasional shaking, filter and pass sufficient distilled water through the filter to make the product measure 1000 cc.

NOTE—This must be labeled "Terpeneless Lemon Extract, Artificially Colored."

NUTMEG EXTRACT

Oil of Myristica	20 cc.
Alcohol	700 cc.
Distilled Water, a sufficient quantity,	
To make	1000 cc.

Dissolve the oil in the alcohol, add sufficient distilled water to make the product measure 1000 cc. and filter.

ORANGE EXTRACT

Oil of Orange	50 cc.
Orange Peel, outer layer only	50 Gm.
Alcohol, a sufficient quantity,	
To make	1000 cc.

Dissolve the oil in 900 cc. of alcohol, add the orange peel, macerate for 48 hours with occasional shaking, filter and pass sufficient alcohol through the filter to make the product measure 1000 cc.

TERPENELESS ORANGE EXTRACT

Terpeneless Oil of Orange	5 cc.
Solution of Cochineal.	1 cc.
Tincture of Caramel, R.B.	2 cc.
Alcohol	500 cc.
Distilled Water, a sufficient quantity,	
To make	1000 cc.

Dissolve the oil in the alcohol, add 400 cc. of distilled water gradually and then the colors. Filter and pass sufficient distilled water through the filter to make the product measure 1000 cc.

NOTE—This must be labeled "Terpeneless Orange Extract, Artificially Colored."

IMITATION PISTACHIO EXTRACT
I

Oil of Orange Flowers	0.4 cc.
Almond Extract, R.B..	350 cc.
Tincture of Vanilla, a sufficient quantity,	
To make	1000 cc.

Mix and filter.

II

Terpeneless Oil of Orange	1 cc.
Terpeneless Oil of Lemon	6 cc.
Oil of Myristica	6 cc.
Oil of Sassafras	4 cc.
Oil of Clove	1 cc.
Oil of Bitter Almond	4 cc.
Tincture of Vanilla, a sufficient quantity,	
To make	1000 cc.

Mix and filter.

IMITATION VANILLA EXTRACT
I

Vanillin	7.50 Gm.
Coumarin	0.08 Gm.
Alcohol	37.50 cc.
Glycerin	45 cc.
Tincture of Caramel, R.B.	100 cc.
Distilled Water, a sufficient quantity,	
To make	1000 cc.

Dissolve the vanillin and coumarin in the alcohol, add the glycerin and tincture of caramel and sufficient distilled water to make the product measure 1000 cc. and filter.

NOTE—This must be labeled "Imitation Vanilla Extract, Artificially Flavored and Colored."

II

Vanillin	6.5 Gm.
Coumarin	0.4 Gm.
Alcohol	200 cc.
Glycerin	125 cc.
Syrup	125 cc.
Compound Tincture of Cudbear	16 cc.
Distilled Water, a sufficient quantity,	
To make	1000 cc.

Dissolve the vanillin and coumarin in the alcohol, add the glycerin, syrup and compound tincture of cudbear, and lastly, sufficient distilled water to make the product measure 1000 cc.

NOTE—This formula was in the N.F. III as "Compound Tincture of Vanillin"; it must not be labeled with this title when sold for flavoring purposes; it must be labeled "Imitation Vanilla Extract, Artificially Flavored and Colored."

EXTRACT OF VANILLA AND TONKA

Vanilla Beans, cut fine	100 Gm.
Tonka Beans, in coarse powder	40 Gm.
Diluted Alcohol, a sufficient quantity,	
To make	1000 cc.

Prepare a tincture by Process P (see N. F. VII, page 439), using diluted alcohol as the menstruum.

SYRUPY CARAMEL
Caramel Syrup
Sugar Coloring

Sucrose.	1000 Gm.
Distilled Water	500 cc.

Melt the sucrose in an iron frying pan; by the time the sucrose is melted it is caramelized. Add the distilled water, previously heated to boiling, and boil to the consistency of a syrup.

FLAVORING POWDERS AND PASTES

These are used to avoid the alcohol in the extracts. They are more sensitive to exposure than the extracts and must be kept in tightly stoppered bottles.

The powders are made by triturating the volatile oils with sucrose; they correspond in strength to the flavoring extracts.

To make the pastes the powders are mixed with the required quantity of either glycerin or a mixture of equal volumes of glycerin and syrup.

COUMARIN SUGAR
Saccharum Coumarini
(D.M.)

Coumarin.	1 Gm.
Sucrose, in fine powder	999 Gm.
To make	1000 Gm.

Triturate well and keep in tightly stoppered bottles.

VANILLIN SUGAR
Saccharum Vanillini
(D.M.)

Vanillin.	30 Gm.
Sucrose, in fine powder.	970 Gm.
To make	1000 Gm.

Triturate well and keep in tightly stoppered bottles.

PART III

TABLE OF CERTIFIED (COLORS) COAL TAR DYES

COAL TAR COLORS (DYES) PERMITTED FOR FOODS, DRUGS AND COSMETICS

The following colors (dyes) are certified for use by the Food, Drug and Cosmetic Administration.

ABBREVIATIONS EMPLOYED

S   —soluble (1% or more)

I   —insoluble

M.S.—moderately soluble (usually less than 1%)

S.S. —sparingly soluble (usually less than 0.25%)

S.A. —soluble in alkaline solutions

Federal Name	Common Name	Water	Glycerin	Alcohol	Ether	Carbon Tetra-chloride	Special
FD & C Blue No. 1	Brilliant Blue	S	S	S	I	I	
FD & C Blue No. 2	Indigo Carmine	S	S	S.S.	I		
FD & C Green No. 1	Guinea Green	S	S	M.S.	I		
FD & C Green No. 2	Light Green SF Yellowish	S	S	M.S.	I		
FD & C Green No. 3	Fast Green FCF	S	S	M.S.	I		
FD & C Orange No. 1	Orange I	S	S	M.S.	I		
FD & C Orange No. 2	Orange SS	I	S.S.	M.S.	S	S	
FD & C Red No. 1	Ponceaux 3R	S	S	S.S.	I		
FD & C Red No. 2	Amaranth	S	S	S.S.	I		
FD & C Red No. 3	Erythrosine	S	S	S	I		
FD & C Red No. 4	Ponceaux SX	S	S	S.S.	I		
FD & C Red No. 32	Oil Red XO	I	S.S.	S.S.	S.S.	S	
FD & C Yellow No. 1	Naphthol Yellow S	S	S	S.S.	I		
FD & C Yellow No. 2	Naphthol Yellow S	S	S	S.S.	I		
FD & C Yellow No. 3	Oil Yellow AB	I	S.S.	S.S.	S	S	
FD & C Yellow No. 4	Oil Yellow OB	S	S.S.	S.S.	S		
FD & C Yellow No. 5	Tartrazine	S	S	S.S.	I		
FD & C Yellow No. 6	Sunset Yellow FCF	S	S	S.S.	I		

COAL TAR COLORS (DYES) PERMITTED ONLY FOR EXTERNALLY APPLIED DRUGS AND COSMETICS

The following colors (dyes) are certified by the Food, Drug and Cosmetic Administration *for use in externally applied drugs and cosmetics only.*

Federal Name	Common Name	Water	Glycerin	Alcohol	Ether	Carbon Tetra-chloride	Special
Ext. D & C Black No. 1	Fast Black BB	S	S	S.S.	I		
Ext. D & C Blue No. 1	Methylene Blue	S	S	S	I		
Ext. D & C Blue No. 2	Methylene Blue - Zinc Double Chloride	S	S	S.S.	I		
Ext. D & C Blue No. 3	Erioglaucine X	S	S	S	I		
Ext. D & C Blue No. 4	Alizarin Saphirol	S	S	S.S.	I		
Ext. D & C Blue No. 5	Hexyl Blue	I	I	S.S.	S.S.		Soluble in Toluene
Ext. D & C Green No. 1	Naphthol Green B	S	S	S.S.	I		
Ext. D & C Orange No. 1	Fanchon Orange	I	I	I	I		Soluble in Toluene
Ext. D & C Orange No. 2	Indelible Orange	I	I	M.S.	M.S.		Soluble in Alkalies
Ext. D & C Red No. 1	Amidonaphthol Red 6B	S	S	S.S.	I		
Ext. D & C Red No. 2	Pigment Scarlet NA	S	S	S.S.	I		
Ext. D & C Red No. 3	Violamine R	S	S	S	S.S.		
Ext. D & C Red No. 4	Dichloro-tetraiodofluorescein	I	I	S.S.	S.S.		Soluble in Alkalies
Ext. D & C Red No. 5	Rose Bengale TD	S	S	S	S.S.		
Ext. D & C Red No. 6	Rose Bengale TDK	S	S	S	S.S.		
Ext. D & C Red No. 7	Alizarine Carmine	S	S	S.S.	I		
Ext. D & C Red No. 8	Fast Red S, Fast Red A	S	S	S.S.	I		
Ext. D & C Red No. 9	Bordeaux Red	S	S.S.	I	I		
Ext. D & C Red No. 10	Azo Rubin Extra (A)	S	S	S.S.	I		
Ext. D & C Red No. 11	Fast Crimson GR	S	S	S.S.	I		
Ext. D & C Red No. 12	Royal Scarlet	S	S	S.S.	I		
Ext. D & C Red No. 13	Crocein Scarlet MOO	S	S	S.S.	I		
Ext. D & C Violet No. 1	Anthraquinone Violet	S	S	S.S.	I		
Ext. D & C Violet No. 2	Alizurol Purple	S	S	S.S.	I		
Ext. D & C Yellow No. 1	Metanil Yellow	S	S	S	I		
Ext. D & C Yellow No. 2	Metanil Yellow CA	S.S.	S.S.	S.S.	I		
Ext. D & C Yellow No. 3	Fast Light Yellow 3G	S	S	S	I		
Ext. D & C Yellow No. 4	Polar Yellow 5G	S	S	S.S.	I		
Ext. D & C Yellow No. 5	Fanchon Yellow (Hansa)	I	I	I	I		Soluble in Toluene

COAL TAR COLORS (DYES) PERMITTED ONLY FOR EXTERNALLY APPLIED DRUGS AND COSMETICS

The following colors (dyes) are certified by the Food, Drug and Cosmetic Administration *for use in externally applied drugs and cosmetics only.*

Federal Name	Common Name	Water	Glycerin	Alcohol	Ether	Carbon Tetrachloride	Special
D & C Black No. 1	Naphthol Blue Black	S	S	S.S.	I		
D & C Blue No. 4	Alphazurine FG	S	S	S	I		
D & C Blue No. 5	Alizarine Astrol B	S	S	S.S.	I		
D & C Blue No. 6	Indigotin	I	I	I	I		Soluble in Dichlorohydrin
D & C Blue No. 7	Patent Blue NA	S	S	S	I		
D & C Blue No. 8	Patent Blue CA	S	S	S	I		
D & C Blue No. 9	Carbanthrene Blue	I	I	I	I		
D & C Brown No. 1	Resorcin Brown	S	S	S.S.	S.S.		
D & C Green No. 4	Light Green CF Yellowish	S	S	M.S.			
D & C Green No. 5	Alizarine Cyanine Green F	S	S	S.S.	I		
D & C Green No. 6	Quinazarine Green SS	I	I	S.S.	S.S.	S	
D & C Green No. 7	Acid Fast Green	S	S	S.S.	I		
D & C Orange No. 3	Orange G	S	S	M.S.	I		
D & C Orange No. 4	Orange II	S	S	M.S.	I		
D & C Orange No. 5	Dibromofluorescein	I	S.S.	M.S.	M.S.		Soluble in Alkalies
D & C Orange No. 6	Dibromofluorescein NA	S	S	S	I		
D & C Orange No. 7	Dibromofluorescein K	S	S	S	I		
D & C Orange No. 8	Dichlorofluorescein	I	S.S.	M.S.	M.S.		Soluble in Alkalies
D & C Orange No. 9	Dichlorofluorescein NA	S	S	M.S.	I		
D & C Orange No. 10	Diiodofluorescein	I	S.S.	M.S.	M.S.		Soluble in Alkalies
D & C Orange No. 11	Erythrosine Yellowish NA	S	S	S	I		
D & C Orange No. 12	Erythrosine Yellowish K	S	S	S	I		
D & C Orange No. 13	Erythrosine Yellowish NH	S	S	S	I		
D & C Orange No. 14	Orange TR	I	S.S.	M.S.	M.S.		Soluble in Alkalies
D & C Orange No. 15	Alizarin	S.S.	I	S.S.	S		
D & C Orange No. 16	Dibromodiiodofluorescein	I	S.S.	M.S	M.S.		Soluble in Alkalies
D & C Orange No. 17	Permanent Orange	I	I	I	I		Soluble in Toluene
D & C Red No. 5	Ponceau 2R	S	S	S.S.	I		
D & C Red No. 6	Lithol Rubin B	S	S	I	I		
D & C Red No. 7	Lithol Rubin BCA	I	I	I	I		
D & C Red No. 8	Lake Red C	I	I	I	I		
D & C Red No. 9	Lake Red CBA	I	I	I	I		
D & C Red No. 10	Lithol Red	S.S.	S.S.	S.S.	I		
D & C Red No. 11	Lithol Red CA	I	I	I	I		
D & C Red No. 12	Lithol Red BA	I	I	I	I		
D & C Red No. 13	Lithol Red SR	I	I	I	I		
D & C Red No. 14	Lake Red D	S.S.	S.S.	M.S.	I		
D & C Red No. 15	Lake Red DBA	I	I	I	I		
D & C Red No. 16	Lake Red DCA	I	I	I	I		

Federal Name	Common Name	Water	Glycerin	Alcohol	Ether	Carbon Tetra-chloride	Special
D & C Red No. 17	Toney Red	I	S.S.	S.S.	S.S.		Soluble in Toluene
D & C Red No. 18	Oil Red OS	I	S.S.	S.S.	S.S.	S	
D & C Red No. 19	Rhodamine B	S	S	S	S		
D & C Red No. 20	Rhodamine B–Acetate	S	S	S	S		
D & C Red No. 21	Tetrabromofluorescein	I	I	S.S.	M.S.		Soluble in Alkalies
D & C Red No. 22	Eosin YS	S	S	S	I		
D & C Red No. 23	Eosine YSK	S	S	S	I		
D & C Red No. 24	Tetrachlorofluorescein	I	I	S.S.	I		Soluble in Alkalies
D & C Red No. 25	Tetrachlorofluorescein NA	S	S	M.S.	I		
D & C Red No. 26	Tetrachlorofluorescein K	S	S	M.S.	I		
D & C Red No. 27	Tetrachloro Tetrabromo-fluorescein	I	I	S.S.	I		Soluble in Alkalies
D & C Red No. 28	Phloxine B	S	S	S	I		
D & C Red No. 29	Bluish Orange TR	I	I	S.S.	I		Soluble in Alkalies
D & C Red No. 30	Helindon Pink CN	I	I	I	I		Soluble in Xylene
D & C Red No. 31	Brilliant Lake Red R	M.S.	S.S.	S.S.	I		
D & C Red No. 33	Acid Fuchsin D, Magenta B	S	S	S.S.	I		
D & C Red No. 34	Deep Maroon (Fanchon Maroon)	I	I	I	I		
D & C Red No. 35	Toluidine Red	I	I	I	I		Soluble in Toluene
D & C Red No. 36	Flaming Red, Permaton Red	I	I	I	I		Soluble in Toluene
D & C Red No. 37	Rhodamine B Stearate	I	S.S.	S	S		Soluble in Benzene
D & C Violet No. 1	Wool Violet 5BN, Acid Violet 6B	S	S	S	I		
D & C Violet No. 2	Alizurol Purple SS	I	I	S.S.	S.S.	S	
D & C Yellow No. 7	Fluorescein	I	S.S.	S.S.	S.S.		Soluble in Alkalies
D & C Yellow No. 8	Uranine	S	S	M.S.	I		
D & C Yellow No. 9	Uranine K	S	S	M.S.	I		
D & C Yellow No. 10	Quinoline Yellow WS	S	S	S.S.	I		
D & C Yellow No. 11	Quinoline Yellow SS	I	S.S.	S	S		

The following vegetable coloring agents may be used, see R.B. page 283.

Solution Cochineal	Bright red	For acid, alkaline and neutral solutions.
Tincture Cudbear		For acid, alkaline and neutral solutions.
Solution Carmine		For acid and alkaline solutions only.
Comp. Tr. Cudbear	Reddish brown	For acid, alkaline and neutral solutions.
Caramel	Brown	For acid, alkaline and neutral solutions.
Tincture Caramel R.B.		For acid, alkaline and neutral solutions.
Tincture Saffron R.B.	Golden-yellow	For acid, alkaline and neutral solutions.

PART IV

COSMETIC FORMULAS

The formulas given herein are intended to be used by pharmacists and others for small-scale manufacture. While many of the formulas can be adapted to large-scale production, most of them will require modification before this can be accomplished. All of the formulas, however, can be used as guides in developing satisfactory cosmetics, when correctly processed.

Variations in raw materials and in individual technic may result in unsatisfactory products. Due note must be taken to include antioxidants or preservatives where such are needed to keep a product from spoiling if it is to be packaged for any length of time before it is used. Strict observance of temperature control must be maintained.

Due to the excellence and complexity of modern perfumes, it is not possible to give definite formulas for them. The pharmacist is advised to purchase the finished perfume oil from a reputable essential oil supply company or perfume manufacturer. The type of perfume to be used for a cosmetic must be left largely to the best judgment of the compounder, or he may seek the advice of the perfume manufacturer. Perfume oils will be supplied by names, such as: "Lavender Bouquet," "Rose Type," "Lilac Type," "Violet Type," "Cream Bouquet," etc.

Antioxidants are substances that act against oxidation, preventing rancidity. When an antioxidant is added to an oil, and the mixture is exposed to the air, the antioxidant either prevents the oxygen from being absorbed or it takes up the oxygen itself.

Some fats and oils such as soy bean oil, wheat germ oil, etc., contain a natural antioxidant. These natural antioxidants have been called tocopherols and inhibitols.

Some of the more commonly used antioxidants are: thymol, isothymol, hydroquinone, pyrogallol and stannous salts.

Water-soluble antioxidants which have been suggested as having possibilities are: sorbitol, mannitol, glycerin, dextrose, aldehydes, alcohols, water-soluble soaps, ethanolamines, pyrophosphates, monoglycerides, methenamine and certain proprietory products.

In many of the cosmetic formulas in this section, there is a need for a preservative. Below is a tabulation of several preservatives which may be used to advantage by the compounder. A careful study should be made of the various preservatives listed and use made of the one which best meets the requirements of the cosmetic.

Chemical Name	Benzoic Acid	Sodium Benzoate	Salicylic Acid
Physical Form	White, odorless or slightly odorous crystals	White, odorless, granular or crystalline powder	White, odorless crystals or a white crystalline powder
Stability	Stable in air	Stable in air	Stable in air
Solubility Water Alcohol Other Solvents	1 Gm. in 275 cc. 1 Gm. in 2.3 cc.	1 Gm. in 1.8 cc. 1 Gm. in 47.5 cc.	1 Gm. in 460 cc. 1 Gm. in 2.7 cc.
Concentration as preservative	0.1–0.2%	0.1–0.2%	0.2%
Type of media in which effective	Acid	Acid and alkaline	Acid
Type of preparation for which usually used	Face lotions, wave set. Also elixirs, tonics, emulsions	Food products and fruit juices	Wave set, elixirs and tonics

Chemical Name	Tertiary Butyl p-Metacresol	Chlorthymol	Alcohol
Physical Form	Liquid, amber colored, characteristic odor	Crystalline, characteristic thymol-like odor	Liquid, sharp penetrating odor
Stability	Stable	Stable	Volatile
Solubility Water Alcohol Other Solvents	1:3000 30%:1:1000 Soluble in soaps, glycol, mineral and vegetable oils	1:7500 Soluble Soluble	All proportions
Concentration as preservative	1:5000	1:5000 1:7500	In acid and neutral media use 15%. In alkaline media use 17.5–20%
Type of media in which effective	Neutral, acid or alkaline	Acid and neutral	Acid, neutral and alkaline
Type of preparation for which usually used	Drugs and medicated soaps	Drugs and cosmetics	Drugs and cosmetics

Chemical Name	Methyl p-Hydroxy Benzoate	Propyl p-Hydroxy Benzoate	n-Butyl p-Hydroxy Benzoate
Physical Form	White crystalline powder	White crystalline powder	White, odorless powder
Stability	Stable	Stable	Stable in air
Solubility Water	Cold water: 1:400 Hot water: 1:100	Hot water: 1:1500	1:5000
Alcohol Other Solvents	1:25 Oils and fats: 1:50	1:5 Oils: 1:50	Readily soluble in alcohol
Concentration as preservative	1:750 or 0.15%	1:2000 to 1:1500	0.02%
Type of media in which effective	Acid, neutral or alkaline	Acid, neutral or alkaline	All types of liquid preparations, including face lotions, hand lotions, wave set, and cosmetic creams
Type of preparation for which usually used	Cosmetics in general	Oil containing cosmetics	

Chemical Name	Benzyl p-Hydroxy Benzoate	Formaldehyde	Oxyquinoline Benzoate
Physical Form	White crystalline powder	Usually sold as 40% solution	White to faint yellow colored powder, characteristic odor
Stability	Stable	Volatilizes	Stable
Solubility Water Alcohol Other Solvents	(1:10,000) Soluble Soluble	Miscible Miscible	Soluble Soluble Soluble
Concentration as preservative	1:10,000 to 1:5000	0.1% to 0.2%	1:2500
Type of media in which effective	Acid, neutral or alkaline	Neutral, acid or alkaline	Acid media, oils
Type of preparation for which usually used	Cosmetics containing a large % of oils or fats	Hair waving preparations	Oils such as baby oil

(Tables by courtesy of D. Van Nostrand Co., Inc., from "Chemistry and Manufacture of Cosmetics," by Maison G. de Navarre.)

BATH SALTS

While the literature indicates that bath salts may be prepared from sodium carbonate and sodium bicarbonate, sodium sesquicarbonate, borax, sodium chloride, sodium sulfate, buffered sodium hexametaphosphate, trisodium phosphate and tetrasodium pyrophosphates, the ingredients that have the most generally suitable properties are sodium sesquicarbonate and buffered sodium hexametaphosphate. Sodium sesquicarbonate is a fine needle-like crystalline mass which possesses an elegant appearance and is easily handled.

Sodium carbonate and trisodium phosphate are better water softeners than the sesquicarbonate, but do not produce so elegant a product. Even though water softening is the main reason for using a bath salt, appearance is probably a more important consideration. Perfume and coloring likewise play an important role and both should be checked for stability in alkali, because alkalies cause most dyestuffs and perfumes to deteriorate very quickly. All dyestuffs used must be certified and following are some that have been found stable to both light and alkali:

D & C Red No. 14	D & C Green No. 5
D & C Red No. 28	D & C Green No. 6
D & C Yellow No. 8	Ext. D & C Red No. 5
D & C Yellow No. 9	Ext. D & C Blue No. 4
Ext. D & C Violet No. 2	

By suitably blending these colors other tints are produced. The following formulas make satisfactory color spraying and perfuming solutions for bath salts.

For a representative list of certified colors permitted for cosmetics (see R.B., page 342).

COLOR SPRAYING LIQUID

Certified Color . . . .   2 Gm.
Acetone . . . .   80 cc.
Diluted Alcohol, a sufficient quantity,
                    To make . . . .   1000 cc.
    Dissolve.

PERFUMING SOLUTION

Perfume . . . .   100 cc.
Alcohol, a sufficient quantity,
                    To make . . . .   1000 cc.

Mix the materials and filter until brilliantly clear. Set aside in amber bottles for future use.

When coloring bath salts, it is best to spray the dyestuff on the salts, tumbling the mixture until the mass is uniformly colored. Now spray on a suitable amount of perfuming solution and mix by tumbling until the perfume has been dispersed throughout the mass. Spread on a tray to allow the alcohol and water to evaporate, then package.

BATH SALTS

Sodium Sesquicarbonate . . . .   1000 Gm.
Perfume and color, a sufficient quantity,
                    To make . . . .   1000 Gm.

BRILLIANTINES

Brilliantines are of two types—liquid and solid. The liquid type may be made from a mixture of vegetable and mineral oils, suitably perfumed and colored. Among the vegetable oils that may be used in brilliantines are oils of avocado, sweet almond, walnut, olive, cottonseed and peanut. Animal oils such as refined whale oil fractions may also be used. Usually a light mineral oil with a low pour point is the preferred ingredient. Some liquid brilliantines are alcoholic solutions of vegetable oils, colored and perfumed.

Solid brilliantines are the same as liquid brilliantines except that the oils are solidified with waxes, such as spermaceti, ceresin, ozokerite, microcrystalline wax or other suitable higher melting waxy substances. In the past, many brilliantines were solidified with spermaceti, resulting in a type of "crystallized" gel. While some of these are still popular, they have been for the most part replaced by special types of petrolatum of predetermined fiber length, melting point and consistency. The following formulas will indicate the types of products now in vogue.

LIQUID BRILLIANTINE
I

Castor Oil . . . .   35 cc.
Expressed Almond Oil . . . .   250 cc.
Glycerin . . . .   110 cc.
Perfume . . . .   12.5 cc.
Alcohol, a sufficient quantity,
                  To make . . . .   1000 cc.

Mix the oils, add the glycerin and perfume to 500 cc. of the alcohol and mix. Finally add sufficient alcohol to make the product measure 1000 cc.

NOTE—Attach a "shake well" label to the container.

II

Oil-soluble Chlorophyll . . . .   0.5 Gm.
Vegetable Oil . . . .   200 cc.
Perfume and color, as desired,
Light Liquid Petrolatum, a sufficient quantity,
                  To make . . . .   1000 cc.

Triturate the chlorophyll in a warmed mortar with the vegetable oil. Allow the insoluble matter to settle, pour off the clear liquid and add it to 700 cc. of the light liquid petrolatum. Finally stir in the perfumes, and add sufficient light liquid petrolatum to make the product measure 1000 cc.

III

Light Liquid Petrolatum	995 cc.
Perfume and color, as desired,	
To make about	1000 cc.

Mix.

IV

Castor Oil	200 cc.
Tincture of Benzoin	20 cc.
Benzyl Benzoate	25 cc.
Perfume and color, as desired,	
Alcohol, a sufficient quantity,	
To make	1000 cc.

Dissolve all ingredients in the alcohol.

SOLID BRILLIANTINE

Light Amber Petrolatum, Medium Fibre	1000 Gm.
Perfume, a sufficient quantity,	
To make about	1000 Gm.

Mix.

SEMI-SOLID BRILLIANTINE

Castor Oil	750 Gm.
Spermaceti	250 Gm.
Perfume, as desired,	
To make about	1000 Gm.

Melt the spermaceti, then add the castor oil, heating until a uniform mixture results. Add the perfume and stir until congealed.

CAMPHOR PREPARATIONS

CAMPHOR AND WAX BLOCK

Benzaldehyde	5 Gm.
Oil of Eucalyptus	5 cc.
White Beeswax	460 Gm.
Camphor	160 Gm.
Spermaceti	160 Gm.
Vegetable Oil, a sufficient quantity,	
To make	1000 Gm.

Melt the spermaceti and white wax, add the vegetable oil and camphor. Stir until the camphor is dissolved, then as the mass begins to solidify add the benzaldehyde and oil of eucalyptus.. Cool by circulating cold water and pour into molds at once just before the product chills. This avoids loss of camphor.

CAMPHOR ICE

I

Camphor	60 Gm.
Spermaceti	460 Gm.
Vegetable Oil	240 Gm.
White Beeswax, a sufficient quantity,	
To make	1000 Gm.

Melt the white beeswax and spermaceti, add the vegetable oil and camphor. Stir and continue the heating until the camphor is dissolved. Cool by circulating cold water and pour into molds at once just before the product chills. This avoids loss of camphor.

II

Heavy Liquid Petrolatum	110 Gm.
Paraffin	360 Gm.
White Petrolatum	480 Gm.
Camphor	50 Gm.
To make	1000 Gm.

Melt the paraffin, add the white petrolatum and heavy liquid petrolatum. When all are liquefied, add the camphor and stir until dissolved.

CLEANSING PREPARATIONS

ALMOND MEAL CLEANSER WITH BORAX

Almond Meal	650 Gm.
Kaolin, in fine powder	325 Gm.
Sodium Borate, in fine powder.	25 Gm.
Perfume and color, as desired,	
To make about	1000 Gm.

Triturate together the almond meal, kaolin and sodium borate until well mixed, then incorporate the perfume and color.

HAND CLEANER

Borax, powdered	600 Gm.
Pumice, in fine powder	25 Gm.
Hard Soap, in fine powder	375 Gm.
To make	1000 Gm.

Mix intimately by sifting.

ANTI-PERSPIRANTS

Anti-perspirants are applied in the forms of lotions and creams. The following formulas for lotions will give satisfactory anti-perspirants. The directions should include the following statement or its equivalent: "Apply and allow to dry, remove excess with damp wash cloth." Most powerful anti-perspirant solutions, such as the solution of aluminum chloride, mentioned below, should not be applied to broken skin or used immediately after shaving under the arms.

Used in anti-perspirant preparations are the following salts of aluminum: acetate, chloride, sulfate, phosphate, citrate and tartrate. Salts of zinc and magnesium may sometimes be used.

CAUTION—*Many anti-prespirants are destructive to textiles and in such cases, the label should bear a suitable warning.*

ALUMINUM CHLORIDE LOTION

Aluminum Chloride	225	Gm.
Hydrochloric Acid	0.5	cc.
Distilled Water, a sufficient quantity,		
To make	1000	cc.

Dissolve and filter if necessary. Color if desired.

NOTE—Most colors are unstable in this solution.

ALUMINUM SULFOCARBOLATE LOTION

Aluminum Sulfocarbolate . . . . 200 Gm.
Phenylethyl Alcohol . . . . 1 Gm.
Distilled Water, a sufficient quantity,

                 To make . . . . 1000 cc.

Dissolve and filter until brilliantly clear.

CAUTION—*Avoid traces of iron and other metals, as discolorations will result.*

DEODORANT CREAM

Zinc Oxide . . . . 200 Gm.
Benzoic Acid . . . . 20 Gm.
Perfume, as desired,
Petrolatum, a sufficient quantity,

                 To make . . . . 1000 Gm.

Mix below a temperature of 65° C. Triturate to a smooth paste.

DEPILATORIES

Depilatories are usually alkaline preparations containing barium, calcium, strontium or sodium sulfide. They act by causing the cellular structure of the hair to become soft and to disintegrate; they may irritate the skin if not used as directed.

Other forms known as epilating waxes have been used; they consist of a resinous wax material; they are melted, spread on the skin and subsequently removed by pulling quickly. This type simply pulls out the hairs.

Depilatories are sold as powders, pastes and creams. They generally contain sulfides or hydrosulfides as the active ingredient. When using powder depilatories, the powder is mixed into a stiff paste with water just before being applied; it is allowed to remain on the skin for 3 to 8 minutes and then scraped or washed off with as little water as possible. Neutral cream or a borated talc may be applied to the treated area.

NOTE—These products do not remove hair permanently.

EPILATING WAX

Yellow Wax. . . . . 200 Gm.
Rosin, in fine powder. . . . . 800 Gm.

                 To make . . . . 1000 Gm.

Heat the yellow wax until it is melted and add the powdered rosin, continuing the heat until the whole is melted. Mold into sticks or blocks. Color as desired.

FACE POWDERS

Face powders must have the following properties: (*a*) covering power, (*b*) absorbency, (*c*) adhesiveness, (*d*) slip, (*e*) pleasant odor, (*f*) color. Opacity may be obtained from titanium or zinc oxides. Absorbency may be had by using precipitated chalk, magnesium oxide, carbonate or kaolin. The stearates of zinc, magnesium and aluminum will give adhesiveness. Slip is best obtained with talc. The perfumes used in face powders should be used in concentrations of from 0.6 to 1% of the total and should contain deodorizing agents along with good fixatives to overcome the characteristic earthy odor of such powders.

The terms light, medium and heavy weight powders refer to powders having low, medium and high covering power, respectively. Dry skin usually requires powders with low covering power (light weight); oily skin usually takes a powder with high covering power (heavy weight).

All face powders should be made to pass through a No. 200 sieve or its equivalent. The colors must be uniformly dispersed and must be selected from the list of certified colors allowed by the Food, Drug and Cosmetic Act (see R.B., page 342). There should be no streaking or bleeding of color.

FACE POWDER—LIGHT WEIGHT
I

Zinc Oxide	100 Gm.
Light Magnesium Carbonate	50 Gm.
Purified Talc, in fine powder.	750 Gm.
Zinc Stearate	100 Gm.
Perfume and color, as desired,	
To make about	1000 Gm.

Mix thoroughly and pass the mixed powders through a No. 200 sieve or its equivalent.

II

Purified Talc, in fine powder.	530 Gm.
Kaolin	200 Gm.
Zinc Oxide	120 Gm.
Zinc Stearate	100 Gm.
Light Magnesium Carbonate	50 Gm.
Perfume and color, as desired,	
To make about	1000 Gm.

Mix thoroughly and pass through a No. 200 sieve or its equivalent.

FACE POWDER—HEAVY WEIGHT—MEXICAN TYPE POWDER

Zinc Stearate	75 Gm.
Zinc Oxide	300 Gm.
Precipitated Calcium Carbonate	125 Gm.
Rice Starch	50 Gm.
Perfume and color, as desired,	
Purified Talc, a sufficient quantity,	
To make about	1000 Gm.

Mix intimately and pass through a No. 200 sieve or equivalent.

LIQUID FACE POWDERS

It is essential in the manufacture of liquid face powders to use powdered material of the highest quality. Air-floated, impalpable powders are especially desired. Water-soluble resins or sodium caseinate are sometimes used to render the powder more permanent.

LIQUID FACE POWDER
Eau Cosmetique
I

Zinc Oxide	50 Gm.
Purified Talc	200 Gm.
Mannitol Borate	5 Gm.
Rose Water, a sufficient quantity,	
To make	1000 cc.

Triturate the dry ingredients together, add while stirring the mannitol borate dissolved in the rose water and gradually add sufficient rose water to make the product measure 1000 cc.

II

Bentonite, cosmetic grade	30 Gm.
Prepared Calamine	54 Gm.
Precipitated Calcium Carbonate	54 Gm.
Sorbitol Syrup	20 cc.
Perfume and color, as desired,	
Water, a sufficient quantity,	
To make	1000 cc.

Triturate the prepared calamine, bentonite and calcium carbonate until intimately mixed, then incorporate with the sorbitol syrup and enough water to make the product measure 1000 cc. Perfume and color as desired.

HAIR AND SCALP LOTIONS

Hair and scalp lotions are intended for application to the scalp with the aid of massage. Some are intended for dry hair, some for oily hair and some for normal scalps. Each lotion should be labeled accordingly.

Some of these lotions are hair dressings in addition to being scalp lotions and in such cases the words "hair lotion" will indicate the use. The lotions not so marked are intended for application directly to the scalp for whatever effect the medicinal agents may have.

All hair lotions should be allowed to set in a container after compounding for at least a week before bottling. This will cause any precipitation that would normally take place to develop, and so be removed before bottling. Scalp and hair lotions should be packaged in bottles with a shaker top.

ALKALINE SCALP LOTION

Oily Scalp Lotion

Quillaja, in powder	37.5 Gm.
Capsicum, in powder	5.6 Gm.
Ammonium Carbonate	7.5 Gm.
Distilled Water	15 cc.
Perfumed Spirit	75 cc.
Alcohol, a sufficient quantity,	
To make	1000 cc.

Macerate for 8 days and filter.

CANTHARIDIN SCALP LOTION

Dry Scalp Lotion

Cantharidin	0.2 Gm.
Acetone	50 cc.
Castor Oil	200 cc.
Alcohol, a sufficient quantity,	
To make	1000 cc.

Dissolve the cantharidin in the acetone, add the castor oil and sufficient alcohol to make the product measure 1000 cc.

COAL TAR AND RESORCINOL SCALP LOTION

Scalp Cleansing Lotion

Resorcinol.	32 Gm.
Solution of Coal Tar	32 cc.
Diluted Alcohol, a sufficient quantity,	
To make	1000 cc.

Dissolve the resorcinol in 500 cc. of diluted alcohol. Add the solution of coal tar and sufficient diluted alcohol to make the product measure 1000 cc., and filter.

CHLORAL AND TANNIN SCALP LOTION

Chloral Hydrate	20 Gm.
Tannic Acid.	10 Gm.
Tartaric Acid	10 Gm.
Castor Oil.	20 cc.
Alcohol	890 cc.
Distilled Water, a sufficient quantity,	
To make	1000 cc.

Dissolve the first four ingredients in the alcohol and add sufficient distilled water to make the product measure 1000 cc.

DETERGENT SCALP LOTION
Lotio Crinalis Detergens

Cleansing Lotion

Sodium Borate	25 Gm.
Tincture of Quillaja	75 cc.
Bay Rum, R.B.	150 cc.
Orange Flower Water, a sufficient quantity,	
To make	1000 cc.

Dissolve the sodium borate in the mixed liquids.

OLD TYPE SCALP LOTION

Tincture of Cantharides.	15	cc.
Tincture of Cinchona, R.B.	200	cc.
Glycerin	60	cc.
Potassium Carbonate.	4	Gm.
Diluted Alcohol, a sufficient quantity,		
To make	1000	cc.

Dissolve the potassium carbonate in 500 cc. of diluted alcohol, add the tinctures and glycerin. Finally add sufficient diluted alcohol to make the product measure 1000 cc.

SCALP LOTION WITH QUININE
I

Quinine Hydrochloride	5 Gm.
Chloroform	5 cc.
Alcohol	200 cc.
Glycerin	15 cc.
Bay Rum, R.B.	250 cc.
Tincture of Cudbear	30 cc.
Rose Water, a sufficient quantity,	
To make	1000 cc.

Dissolve the quinine hydrochloride in 400 cc. of rose water, add the other ingredients and then filter, using purified talc.   Finally add sufficient rose water through the filter to make the product measure 1000 cc.

II

Quinine Sulfate	5 Gm.
Cologne Water, R.B.	100 cc.
Alcohol	150 cc.
Glycerin	50 cc.
Rose Water, a sufficient quantity,	
To make	1000 cc.

Dissolve the quinine sulfate in the alcohol and add the other ingredients, and then sufficient rose water to make the product measure 1000 cc.

SCALP LOTION OF RESORCINOL AND BETANAPHTHOL WITH CANTHARIDES AND PILOCARPUS

Resorcinol	20 Gm.
Tincture of Cantharides	20 cc.
Fluidextract of Pilocarpus, R.B.	20 cc.
Betanaphthol	20 Gm.
Oil of Bergamot	2 cc.
Glycerin	120 cc.
Alcohol	400 cc.
Rose Water, a sufficient quantity,	
To make	1000 cc.

Dissolve the resorcinol and betanaphthol in the alcohol, add the other ingredients and 400 cc. of rose water.   Filter if necessary, passing sufficient rose water through the filter to make the product measure 1000 cc.

SCALP LOTION OF RESORCINOL, CANTHARIDES AND CAPSICUM

Tincture of Cantharides	30 cc.
Tincture of Capsicum.	15 cc.
Resorcinol.	8 Gm.
Alcohol	440 cc.
Perfume, as desired,	
Infusion of Sage,* a sufficient quantity,	
To make	1000 cc.

To 400 cc. of the infusion of sage add the tinctures and the resorcinol dissolved in the perfume and alcohol. Add sufficient infusion of sage to make the product measure 1000 cc.

SCALP LOTION OF RESORCINOL MONOACETATE

Resorcinol Monoacetate	40 cc.
Alcohol	500 cc.
Cologne Water, R.B.	50 cc.
Distilled Water, a sufficient quantity,	
To make	1000 cc.

Dissolve the resorcinol monoacetate in the alcohol, add the cologne water and sufficient distilled water to make the product measure 1000 cc.

SCALP LOTION OF RESORCINOL MONOACETATE AND SALICYLIC ACID

Resorcinol Monoacetate.	50 cc.
Castor Oil.	50 cc.
Salicylic Acid	1 Gm.
Spirit of Formic Acid	200 cc.
Oil of Bergamot	4 cc.
Alcohol, a sufficient quantity,	
To make	1000 cc.

Dissolve the salicylic acid in 500 cc. of alcohol, then add the other ingredients and sufficient alcohol to make the product measure 1000 cc.

* Prepared according to the general formula for Infusions (see U.S.P. XII, page 218).

SOLUTION OF RESORCINOL MONOACETATE, BETANAPHTHOL AND CASTOR OIL

Resorcinol Monoacetate.	**44 Gm.**
Betanaphthol	**22 Gm.**
Castor Oil.	**33 cc.**
Alcohol, a sufficient quantity,	
To make	**1000 cc.**

Dissolve the resorcinol monoacetate and betanaphthol in 400 cc. of alcohol, and the castor oil in another 400 cc. Mix these two solutions, then add sufficient alcohol to make the product measure 1000 cc.

SAGE LOTION

Scalp Wash

Oil of Sage	1.5	cc.
Liniment of Soft Soap	50	cc.
Tincture of Cantharides.	12	cc.
Glycerin	30	cc.
Menthol	15	Gm.
Bay Rum, R.B.	125	cc.
Oil of Bergamot	15	cc.
Alcohol	250	cc.
Distilled Water, a sufficient quantity,		
To make	1000	cc.

Dissolve the menthol and oils in the alcohol, add the other ingredients in the order given and then sufficient distilled water to make the product measure 1000 cc. Filter.

LOTION OF SALICYLIC AND BORIC ACIDS WITH RESORCINOL

Salicylic Acid	10 Gm.
Resorcinol.	20 Gm.
Boric Acid.	50 Gm.
Glycerin	60 cc.
Alcohol	500 cc.
Distilled Water, a sufficient quantity,	
To make	1000 cc.

Dissolve the resorcinol and boric acid in the glycerin, and the salicylic acid in the alcohol. Mix the solutions and add sufficient distilled water to make the product measure 1000 cc. Filter if necessary.

LOTION OF SALICYLIC ACID WITH CANTHARIDES AND CAPSICUM

Salicylic Acid	1 Gm.
Tincture of Cantharides	20 cc.
Tincture of Capsicum.	20 cc.
Castor Oil.	50 cc.
Alcohol, a sufficient quantity,	
To make	1000 cc.

Dissolve the salicylic acid in 500 cc. of alcohol, add the other ingredients and sufficient alcohol to make the product measure 1000 cc.

SCALP LOTION OF SALICYLIC ACID AND CAPSICUM

Salicylic Acid	10 Gm.
Tincture of Capsicum.	50 cc.
Castor Oil.	10 cc.
Alcohol, a sufficient quantity,	
To make	1000 cc.

Dissolve the salicylic acid in 500 cc. of alcohol, add the tincture of capsicum and castor oil. Finally add sufficient alcohol to make the product measure 1000 cc.

LOTION OF SALICYLIC ACID AND RESORCINOL WITH CHLORAL HYDRATE

Salicylic Acid	1 Gm.
Resorcinol.	25 Gm.
Castor Oil.	3 cc.
Chloral Hydrate	32 Gm.
Hamamelis Water	400 cc.
Bay Rum, R.B., a sufficient quantity,	
To make	1000 cc.

Dissolve the resorcinol and chloral hydrate in the hamamelis water, and the salicylic acid in 400 cc. of bay rum. Mix the solutions, add the castor oil and sufficient bay rum to make the product measure 1000 cc.

PERMANENT WAVE LOTIONS

Formulas for permanent waving lotions are difficult to give without knowledge of the method of permanent waving and the type of hair to which the solution is to be applied. Every texture of hair requires a different *strength* of lotion, and the various methods of waving hair such as preheat, chemical heating pad or electrical heating will all require a different type of solution because each has a different heating time.

The following formulas are intended for general use and are known to work with the electrical heating systems. For coarse hair the solutions may have to be diluted because coarse hair waves easier than fine hair. None of the solutions is recommended for use on bleached or otherwise damaged hair for the reason that such hair requires special handling and in many cases may not be waved at all.

LOTION FOR PERMANENT WAVING
I

Sodium Borate	40 Gm.
Sulfonated Castor Oil	20 cc.
Strong Solution of Ammonia	200 cc.
Water, a sufficient quantity,	
To make	1000 cc.

Dissolve the sodium borate in the water, add the strong solution of ammonia and the sulfonated oil, mix well, and add sufficient water to make the product measure 1000 cc.

II

Monoethanolamine sulfite (60% solution)	100 cc.
Sodium Sulfite, anhydrous	40 Gm
Sulfonated Castor Oil	150 cc.
Water, a sufficient quantity,	
To make	1000 cc.

Mix the sulfonated oil with the monoethanolamine sulfite solution and add the anhydrous sodium sulfite previously dissolved in the water.

POMADES
CASTOR OIL POMADE

Yellow Wax	100 Gm.
Petrolatum	200 Gm.
Castor Oil	700 Gm.
Perfume and color, as desired,	
To make about	1000 Gm.

Melt the yellow wax and petrolatum, add the castor oil and finally, as the product cools, the perfume and color.

WHITE POMADE

White Wax . . . . 300 Gm.
Heavy Liquid Petrolatum . . . . 700 Gm.
Perfume, as desired,
To make about . . . . 1000 Gm.

Melt the white wax, add the heavy liquid petrolatum and the perfume and stir until the pomade congeals.

WOOL FAT POMADE

Wool Fat . . . . 250 Gm.
Petrolatum . . . . 750 Gm.
Perfume and color, as desired,
To make about . . . . 1000 Gm.

Melt the wool fat, add the petrolatum and incorporate the perfume and color with the melted mixture as it is cooling.

EYEBROW AND EYELASH POMADE

Oil of Lavender . . . . 5 cc.
Petrolatum, short fibre, light amber . . . . 995 Gm.
To make about . . . . 1000 Gm.

Incorporate the oil in the petrolatum.

MUSTACHE WAX

Glycerin . . . . 122 Gm.
Triethanolamine . . . . 10 Gm.
Hard Soap, in fine powder . . . . 100 Gm.
Mucilage of Acacia . . . . 290 Gm.
White Wax . . . . 250 Gm.
Perfume and color, as desired,
Distilled Water, a sufficient quantity,
To make about . . . . 1000 Gm.

Melt the wax and heat to 70° C. Dissolve the triethanolamine in one-half the water and heat to 70° C. Add the solution to the wax and mix well. Dilute the mucilage with the remainder of the water and triturate with the hard soap. Heat to 70° C. and slowly work this mixture into the white wax emulsion, stirring constantly until the mass becomes homogeneous. Finally add the perfume and color and pour the mass into suitable moulds.

For a black color, add 10 per cent of finely powdered lampblack or 0.5 per cent of oil black. For brown, add 5 to 10 per cent of powdered sienna.

NAIL PREPARATIONS

Only certain types of nail preparations lend themselves to easy manufacture. Nail lacquer is best purchased from private label houses who have checked the product for the many physical properties it must possess.

CUTICLE SOFTENER

Potassium Hydroxide	20 Gm.
Glycerin	200 cc.
Oil of Bergamot	1 cc.
Distilled Water, a sufficient quantity,	
To make	1000 cc.

Dissolve the potassium hydroxide in 500 cc. of distilled water, add the glycerin and oil and finally sufficient distilled water to make the product measure 1000 cc. Allow to stand for 48 hours, strain or draw off the clear liquid and fill into frosted bottles.

NAIL BLEACH—NAIL STAIN REMOVER

Tartaric Acid	20 Gm.
Perfume, as desired,	
Distilled Water, a sufficient quantity,	
To make	1000 cc.

Dissolve and filter.

CUTICLE LUBRICATING CREAM

Petrolatum	580 Gm.
White Ceresin	125 Gm.
White Wax	75 Gm.
Wool Fat	85 Gm.
Oil of Orange Flowers	1 cc.
Distilled Water	134 cc.
To make about	1000 Gm.

Melt the fats and waxes together and while warm, incorporate the distilled water and lastly the oil of orange flowers. Pass through an ointment mill or otherwise triturate until smooth and creamy.

NAIL POLISH CREAM

Tin Oxide	250 Gm
Kaolin	250 Gm
Hydrogenated Cottonseed Oil	50 Gm
Paraffin	25 Gm
Carnauba Wax	50 Gm
Benzyl Alcohol	375 Gm
To make	1000 Gm.

Dissolve the oil, paraffin and wax in the benzyl alcohol with the aid of heat. While still hot, incorporate the mixed tin oxide and kaolin. Dispense in air-tight containers.

NAIL POLISHING POWDER

Tin Oxide, in fine powder.	600 Gm.
Purified Talc, in fine powder.	240 Gm.
Rice Starch	150 Gm.
Carmine, in fine powder.	10 Gm.
To make	1000 Gm.

Mix thoroughly by trituration.

The intensity of the carmine coloring in the three powders above may be increased by the addition of a small quantity of powdered ammonium carbonate.

NAIL POLISH REMOVER
(Oily Type)
I

Butyl Stearate	50 cc.
Diethylene Glycol Mono-Ethyl Ether	150 cc.
Acetone	250 cc.
Perfume, as desired,	
Alcohol, a sufficient quantity,	
To make	1000 cc.

Mix.

II

Perfume Oil	4 cc.
Olive Oil	125 cc.
Acetone, a sufficient quantity,	
To make	1000 cc.

Dissolve the oils in the acetone.

LIP PREPARATIONS

LIP STICK

A lipstick is a mixture of liquid, soft and solid fats, containing from 8 to 10% of insoluble color lake and up to 2% of bromo acid. A lipstick should not sweat, it should not be brittle, and the color must be uniformly dispersed. It should have a melting point of from 50° to 60° C.

The perfume used in lipstick is chosen for its taste as well as its odor. For this reason, fruity perfume compounds, such as raspberry, have been popular.

LIP STICK
I

Wool Fat	50 Gm.
Light Liquid Petrolatum	390 Gm.
White Wax	275 Gm.
Spermaceti	225 Gm.
Perfume and color, as desired,	
To make about	1000 Gm.

Rub the color to a smooth paste with the liquid petrolatum added gradually; melt the wool fat, wax and spermaceti and add the color lake mixture. Mill or otherwise triturate until smooth and uniform while warm and fluid. Remove from the mill, stirring constantly, and pour into molds.

II

White Wax	240 Gm.
Spermaceti	100 Gm.
Cetyl Alcohol	40 Gm.
Hydrogenated Cotton Seed Oil	80 Gm.
White Petrolatum	165 Gm.
Absorption Base	200 Gm.
Castor Oil, tasteless	55 Gm.
Bromo Acid	10 Gm.
Certified Color	100 Gm.
Perfume and Preservative, as desired,	
To make about	1000 Gm.

Mix the coloring matter with the petrolatum and absorption base very thoroughly using an ointment mill, then warm the mixture until it is quite fluid. Now stir in the solution of the bromo acid in the castor oil and mix well. Next heat the white wax, spermaceti, cetyl alcohol and hydrogenated oil, and when just liquid, stir in the color mass. Add the preservative and the perfume last. Careful control of the temperature, also that of the chilled mold is essential.

COLORLESS LIP STICK BASE

White Wax . . . . 300 Gm.
Spermaceti . . . . 300 Gm.
Light Liquid Petrolatum . . . . 400 Gm.

To make . . . . 1000 Gm.

Melt the wax and spermaceti, then add the liquid petrolatum, heating until the mixture is uniform. Remove from the source of heat and stir until it congeals.

ROUGES

LIQUID ROUGE

I

Castor Oil . . . . 2 cc.
Tincture of Benzoin . . . . 100 cc.
Alcohol Soluble Certified Color, as desired,
Alcohol, a sufficient quantity,

To make . . . . 1000 cc.

Mix and dissolve. Filter clear and bottle.

II

Erythrosine . . . . 1 Gm.
Glycerin . . . . 500 cc.
Alcohol . . . . 100 cc.
Rose Water, a sufficient quantity,

To make . . . . 1000 cc.

Dissolve the erythrosine in 300 cc. of rose water, add the glycerin and alcohol and sufficient rose water to make the product measure 1000 cc.

The amount of erythrosine in this formula may be increased by any quantity up to 5 Gm., if desired.

PASTE ROUGE

Base

White Ceresin . . . . 500 Gm.
Heavy Liquid Petrolatum . . . . 500 Gm.
Perfume and color, as desired,

To make about . . . . 1000 Gm.

Fuse the white ceresin on a water bath, add the heavy liquid petrolatum and continue the heat until the mixture is liquefied. Triturate to smoothness with the color and digest on a water bath for 20 minutes. Allow to cool almost to the congealing point, add the perfume and triturate to a smooth consistency.

ROUGE POWDER

Certified Color	40 Gm.
Purified Talc, in fine powder.	890 Gm.
Acacia, in fine powder	70 Gm.
To make	1000 Gm.

Mix the ingredients by prolonged trituration, and add gradually sufficient water to form a doughy mass. Transfer this to a shallow porcelain dish, dry on a water bath and triturate the product to a very fine powder.

SHAMPOOS

In the formulation of any soap shampoo made by saponification, it is impossible to give an exact formula because the concentration of alkali varies slightly from batch to batch and the saponification value of the fats varies likewise. Accordingly, in the manufacture of shampoos, it is best to analyze the product for alkalinity or excess fat after the saponification is considered complete. If there is a slight excess of fat, a little more alkali may be added. If there is an excess of alkali, the addition of coconut fatty acids or oleic acid may be used to make the product neutral.

It is most important that soap shampoo be allowed to settle for at least a week, or longer if possible, before bottling. This allows the colloidal unsaponifiables and other extraneous matter to settle out and be filtered off.

DRY SHAMPOO

Starch	500 Gm.
Sodium Bicarbonate	500 Gm.
Perfume, as desired,	
To make about	1000 Gm.

Mix intimately.

Keep in tightly sealed containers.

LIQUID SHAMPOO SOAP
I

Coconut Oil	66 Gm.
Cottonseed Oil	78 cc.
Oleic Acid	36 Gm.
Potassium Hydroxide	42 Gm.
Potassium Carbonate	9 Gm.
Alcohol	42 cc.
Purified Talc	10 Gm.
Perfume, as desired,	
Distilled Water, a sufficient quantity,	
To make	1000 cc.

Heat the oleic acid with the oils to about 82° C. Add the alkalis dissolved in 100 cc. of distilled water, then the alcohol and heat until saponified. Check for complete saponification. When cool, add the perfume and sufficient distilled water to make the product measure 1000 cc. Set aside for at least a week. Add the purified talc and filter.

II

Coconut Oil Fatty Acids	150 Gm.
Castor Oil Fatty Acids	50 Gm.
Potassium Hydroxide	35 Gm.
Triethanolamine	60 Gm.
Purified Talc	30 Gm.
Water, a sufficient quantity,	
To make	1000 cc.

Dissolve the potassium hydroxide and triethanolamine in 400 cc. of water and warm to a temperature of 60° C., add the fatty acids previously melted. Continue heating until the mixture becomes clear. Add the remainder of the water and check for the presence of excess alkali or fat. Allow to stand for one week or longer, add the purified talc and filter until brilliantly clear.

LIQUID SHAMPOO WITH TAR

I

Rectified Oil of Tar	10 cc.
Liquid Shampoo Soap, R.B., a sufficient quantity,	
To make	1000 cc.

II

Coconut Oil Soap*	60 Gm.
Potassium Tetrapyrophosphate	20 Gm.
Rectified Oil of Tar	2 cc.
Alcohol	500 cc.
Distilled Water, a sufficient quantity,	
To make	1000 cc.

Dissolve the soap in 400 cc. of distilled water by the aid of heat, add the potassium tetrapyrophosphate and stir until dissolved. Cool. Dissolve the rectified oil of tar in the alcohol and add to the soap solution, lastly adding sufficient distilled water to make the product measure 1000 cc. Set aside for one week and filter.

* Coconut oil soap may be made in the same way as U.S.P. Soft Soap, using coconut oil instead of the oil directed and the needed quantity of alkali.

LIQUID SHAMPOO WITH HENNA

Henna Leaves, in moderately coarse powder. . . . .   10 Gm.
Medicinal Soft Soap . . . .   300 Gm.
Alcohol . . . .   250 cc.
Oil of Lavender . . . .   20 cc.
Distilled Water, a sufficient quantity,
                    To make . . . .   1000 cc.

Infuse the henna leaves in 100 cc. of boiling distilled water and filter. Dissolve the soft soap in the alcohol and add the oil, the henna infusion and sufficient distilled water to make the product measure 1000 cc. Set aside for 7 days and filter.

SHAMPOO WITH CHAMOMILE

Peanut Oil . . . .   190 cc.
Solution of Potassium Hydroxide, 40% . . . .   70 cc.
Alcohol . . . .   100 cc.
Glycerin . . . .   40 cc.
Tincture of Chamomile, 20% . . . .   120 cc.
Distilled Water, a sufficient quantity,
                    To make . . . .   1000 cc.

Heat the peanut oil to about 90° C. Add the potassium hydroxide-alcohol mixture heated to 80° C. Stir. When the saponification is complete, add the water. The chamomile tincture and a suitable perfume are added last. Check for excess fat or alkali, adjust, set aside for one week and filter until brilliantly clear.

SOAPLESS SHAMPOO

Soapless shampoos are of two types, foaming and non-foaming. The foaming type is made from materials generally called wetting agents or soap substitutes. Wetting agents are compounds which lower the surface tension, and as a rule do not form insoluble calcium and magnesium compounds. consequently will rinse out thoroughly, leaving the hair soft and very glossy.

The non-foaming shampoos are prepared from sulfonated oils such as sulfonated castor oil or sulfonated olive oil, to which is added a small amount of liquid petrolatum in order to leave a gloss on the hair.

SOAPLESS SHAMPOO
I

Sodium Alkyl Aryl Sulfonate . . . .   200 Gm.
Glycerin . . . .   80 cc.
Perfume and color, as desired,
Water, a sufficient quantity,
                    To make . . . .   1000 cc.

Dissolve and set aside for one week and filter until brilliantly clear.

II

Sodium Dihexylsulfosuccinate*	100 Gm.
Sulfonated Castor Oil, 75%	200 Gm.
Oleic Acid	50 Gm.
Perfume and color, as desired,	
Water, a sufficient quantity,	
To make	1000 cc.

Dissolve and set aside for one week and filter until brilliantly clear.

III

Non-Lathering Oil Shampoo

Sulfonated Castor Oil, 75%	650 cc.
Sulfonated Olive Oil, 75%	310 cc.
Light Liquid Petrolatum	40 cc.
Perfume and color, as desired,	
Preservative, a sufficient quantity,	
Water, a sufficient quantity,	
To make	1000 cc.

Dissolve the light liquid petrolatum in the mixed sulfonated oils, perfume, color and preservative. Set aside for at least two weeks and draw off the clear portion.

This product may be diluted with water, thus reducing the cost of manufacture.

Satisfactory preservatives are benzoic acid 1:1000 (in acid media) or butyl *p*-hydroxybenzoic acid 1:5000.

SHAVING PREPARATIONS

There are two types of shaving preparations: (*a*) the brushless (non-lathering) and (*b*) the lathering type. In the compounding of a brushless shaving product, it is essential that a beard softener be used in conjunction with a lubricant and such bodying agents as will produce a cream of desired consistency. The cream should rinse off the razor readily with cold water. The formulas which follow will indicate the types of products that are in demand today.

In compounding a lathering shaving cream, it is essential that the product lather easily, and that such lather as is produced, remain fairly permanent. To obtain this effect, coconut oil is used for its ability to produce quick lather when saponified and stearic acid for its lasting properties. Glycerin may or may not be added and usually a small amount of mucilage is added to prevent the cream from getting hard and gummy in hot weather or in a heated bathroom. The cream should be so made as to contain 1.5% or more of free fatty acids. The comments made under shampoos will apply here as well, namely, that after the saponification has been completed, the product should be checked for excess fat or excess alkali and then properly adjusted so that there is a slight excess of fatty acids.

* Aerosol M.A.

BRUSHLESS SHAVING CREAM
I

Stearic Acid	150 Gm.
Spermaceti	20 Gm.
Petrolatum	30 Gm.
Triethanolamine	25 Gm.
Glycerin	50 cc.
Perfume, as desired,	
Water, a sufficient quantity,	
To make	1000 Gm.

Melt the waxes and fats and heat to 70° C. and add the triethanolamine previously dissolved in the water and heated to 70° C. Stir the mixture until cooled to 40° C., and then add the glycerin and perfume.

II

Sodium Borate	10 Gm.
Stearic Acid	150 Gm.
White Petrolatum	50 Gm.
Spermaceti	20 Gm.
Strong Solution of Ammonia	20 cc.
Sorbitol, syrupy	60 Gm.
Distilled Water	690 cc.
Perfume, as desired,	
To make about	1000 Gm.

Melt the waxes and fats. Boil the distilled water and dissolve the sodium borate; add the strong solution of ammonia, and pour into the melted fat with constant agitation. When completely saponified add the syrupy sorbitol, stir slowly until quite cold, then add the perfume.

LATHERING SHAVING CREAM
I

Stearic Acid	336 Gm.
Coconut Oil	64 Gm.
Glycerin	40 Gm.
Sodium Alginate, 2% mucilage	30 cc.
Boric Acid	14 Gm.
Potassium Hydroxide, 40% solution	184 cc.
Sodium Hydroxide, 36% solution	28 cc.
Water	299 cc.
Perfume, as desired,	
To make about	1000 Gm.

Melt half of the stearic acid and all of the coconut oil and warm to 75° C. In another container, mix the two alkaline solutions and heat to 75° C. Slowly add the alkaline mixture to the liquid stearic acid-coconut oil mixture. Heat and stir until saponification is complete. Add slowly the remainder of the stearic acid warmed to 70° C. and continue stirring. Dissolve the boric acid in the water, heat to 65° C. and add slowly until the cream is quite uniform and smooth. Mix the glycerin with the sodium alginate mucilage and work into the cream. Perfume. Allow the cream to set for at least two weeks then work until soft. Pack into tubes or jars.

II

Stearic Acid	300 Gm.
Coconut Fatty Acids	100 Gm.
Glycerin	50 Gm.
Sodium Alginate Mucilage, 2%	50 Gm.
Boric Acid	10 Gm.
Potassium Hydroxide, 40% Solution	150 Gm.
Sodium Hydroxide, 36% Solution	25 Gm.
Perfume, as desired,	
Water, a sufficient quantity,	
To make about	1000 Gm.

Melt the fatty acids and heat to 65° C. Heat the alkaline solution to the same temperature and add with stirring to the fatty mixture, maintaining the same temperature. Dissolve the boric acid in water, warm to 60° C. and add to the mixture of fatty acids and alkalies. Mix the sodium alginate mucilage with glycerin and add slowly. Allow to cool and add the perfume. Set the cream aside for two weeks, work up again and pack into jars or tubes.

SHAVING POWDER

Coumarin	0.2 Gm.
Oil of Bergamot	1 cc.
Methyl Salicylate	0.2 cc.
Spermaceti, in fine powder	18 Gm.
Coconut Oil Soap, in powder, a sufficient quantity,	
To make about	1000 Gm.

Mix intimately.

SKIN CREAMS

There are two types of skin creams in common use today, "day" and "night" creams, respectively. Day creams are usually of a greaseless or vanishing type, whereas night creams are greasy.

The day creams may be based on stearic acid, suitably saponified so that from 20 to 30% of the stearic acid has formed a soap and the remainder is emulsified within the mass. Within recent times, self-emulsifying glyceryl monostearates and other similarly behaving polyhydroxy stearates have been used. In this group of new stearates are sorbitol monostearate, mannitol monostearate, propylene glycol stearate, diethylene glycol stearate and mixtures of these, all containing a sufficient amount of soap to render them self-emulsifying.

Night creams have formerly been sold under such names as cleansing creams, skin food, eye cream, massage cream and so forth. They may be made along the lines of ointment of rose water, suitably modified to obtain the desired texture, or may be made from absorption bases, or with such new emulsifiers as sorbitol and mannitol oleates that give emulsions of water-in-oil type.

ALMOND OIL COLD CREAM

Borax	6 Gm.
Spermaceti	80 Gm.
White Wax	80 Gm.
Expressed Oil of Almond or Persic Oil	640 cc.
Distilled Water	196 cc.
Perfume, as desired,	
Preservative, a sufficient quantity,	
To make about	1000 Gm.

Melt the spermaceti and white wax with the aid of gentle heat and add the preservative. Add the expressed oil of almond to the melted waxes and warm the mixture to 70° C. Dissolve the borax in the water, bring to the same temperature as the melted oily mixture and add gradually. Allow to cool and stir in the perfume. When the cream cools to 42° C. pour into jars.

CLEANSING CREAM

Stearic Acid	145 Gm.
Wool Fat	40 Gm.
Triethanolamine	18 Gm.
Light Liquid Petrolatum	250 cc.
Distilled Water	550 cc.
Perfume, as desired,	
To make about	1000 Gm.

Heat the stearic acid, wool fat and liquid petrolatum to 70° C., in a separate vessel heat to 70° C. the distilled water and triethanolamine. Add the melted mixture to the aqueous solution, stirring vigorously to obtain a uniform emulsion. Stir until the mixture cools to 45° C., add the perfume, triturate thoroughly, then stir occasionally until cold.

EMOLLIENT CREAM

Wool Fat	200 Gm.
White Petrolatum	450 Gm.
Rose Water	350 Gm.
Antioxidant, a sufficient quantity,	
Perfume, as desired,	
To make about	1000 Gm.

Melt the wool fat, antioxidant and petrolatum; incorporate the rose water slowly, triturate thoroughly after each addition. Perfume and pack into jars.

GALEN'S CERATE
Ceratum Galeni
Cold Cream, Paragon Cold Cream

Sodium Borate	8 Gm.
White Petrolatum	120 Gm.
White Wax	120 Gm.
Expressed Oil of Almond or Persic Oil	500 Gm.
Rose Water	249 cc.
Perfume, as desired,	
Antioxidant, a sufficient quantity,	
To make about	1000 Gm.

Melt the wax, petrolatum and antioxidant in the oil and dissolve the sodium borate in the rose water by the aid of gentle heat. When both solutions are at approximately the same temperature, add the aqueous liquid gradually to the wax and oil, and stir until the mixture stiffens. Pour into a slightly warmed mortar containing the petrolatum, stirring until mixed. Add the perfume and stir until cold.

LIQUID ALMOND CREAM

Tragacanth	17.5	Gm.
Mucilage of Quince Seed, 2%	220	cc.
Boric Acid	15	Gm.
Glycerin	60	cc.
Alcohol	200	cc.
Benzaldehyde	1	cc.
Oil of Rose Geranium	1	cc.
Stearic Acid	15	Gm.
Expressed Oil of Almond or Persic Oil	17.5	Gm.
Triethanolamine Solution, 20%	100	cc.
Preservative, a sufficient quantity,		
Distilled Water, a sufficient quantity,		
To make about	1000	cc.

Macerate the tragacanth in 650 cc. of distilled water, in which the boric acid has been dissolved, for 4 days and strain. Dissolve the benzaldehyde and oil of rose geranium in the alcohol. Mix these two solutions, add the glycerin and add this mixture to the mucilage of tragacanth; mix well and warm to 60° C. Melt the stearic acid, add the expressed oil of almond and warm to 70° C. Heat the triethanolamine solution to 70° C. and add with stirring to the mixture of stearic acid and almond oil. Now add the tragacanth mixture a little at a time and finally add the quince seed mucilage and strain.

The preservative may be dissolved in the water used to prepare the mucilage of tragacanth.

MINERAL OIL COLD CREAM
I

Spermaceti	83 Gm.
White Wax	110 Gm.
Light Liquid Petrolatum	500 Gm.
Sodium Borate	7 Gm.
Distilled Water	300 cc.
Perfume, as desired,	
To make about	1000 Gm.

Melt the spermaceti and white wax at the lowest possible temperature and add the liquid petrolatum. Dissolve the sodium borate in the distilled water, bringing it to the same temperature as the melted mixture. Add it all at once with constant stirring. Avoid very rapid stirring as it will beat in too much air and make the cream too fluffy. When nearly cold, add the perfume.

II

White Wax	126 Gm.
White Ceresin	35 Gm.
Light Liquid Petrolatum	550 cc.
Sodium Borate	8 Gm.
Distilled Water	281 cc.
Perfume, as desired,	
To make about	1000 Gm.

Melt the white wax and ceresin, and add the liquid petrolatum. Warm to 70° C. Dissolve the sodium borate in the distilled water and warm to 70° C. Add this solution to the mixture of fats and waxes and beat rapidly until the cream cools to 50° C., add the perfume and mix until cold.

PETROLATUM PROTECTIVE CREAM
I—With Zinc Oxide and Stearate

White Petrolatum	780 Gm.
Wool Fat	100 Gm.
White Wax	40 Gm.
Zinc Stearate	40 Gm.
Zinc Oxide	40 Gm.
Perfume, as desired,	
To make about	1000 Gm.

Melt the first three ingredients together in order of their melting points and strain into a steam-jacketed mixer. Start the agitator and sift in gradually the powders, previously mixed and sifted. Continue mixing until a smooth white cream is formed, add the perfume and pour into jars.

II—With Zinc Oxide and Stearate

White Petrolatum	438.5 Gm.
Wool Fat	438.5 Gm.
White Wax	17.5 Gm.
Spermaceti	53 Gm.
Zinc Stearate	17.5 Gm.
Zinc Oxide	35 Gm.
Perfume, as desired,	
To make about	1000 Gm.

Melt the first four ingredients in order of their melting points. Mix the powders, sift, then add to the melted mixture, stirring until cold. Pack into jars.

III

Zinc Stearate	80 Gm.
White Wax	40 Gm.
Spermaceti	120 Gm.
Wool Fat	80 Gm.
White Petrolatum	480 Gm.
Rose Water	200 cc.
To make about	1000 Gm.

Heat the first five ingredients together until melted, cool to 45° C. When cold, add the rose water gradually, triturating thoroughly after each addition.

IV

Glyceryl Monostearate (self emulsifying)	120 Gm.
Light Liquid Petrolatum	65 Gm.
Petrolatum	50 Gm.
Glycerin	35 cc.
Titanium Dioxide	50 Gm.
Distilled Water	630 cc.
Perfume, as desired,	
To make about	1000 Gm.

Place all the ingredients (except perfume) in a porcelain vessel and heat with constant agitation until the glyceryl monostearate has melted and the cream has become white and homogeneous. Strain and continue agitating slowly until cool; add the perfume.

THEATRICAL COLD CREAM

I

Glycerin	10 cc.
Sodium Borate	9 Gm.
White Wax	141 Gm.
Heavy Liquid Petrolatum	620 Gm.
Perfume, as desired,	
Distilled Water, a sufficient quantity,	
To make	1000 Gm.

Melt the white wax with the liquid petrolatum on a water bath. Dissolve the sodium borate and glycerin in the distilled water, warm it to the same temperature as the melted mixture and add it to this with constant stirring. Then add the perfume and pour the cream immediately into ointment jars or tubes.

II

Glycerin	10 cc.
Sodium Borate	10 Gm.
White Wax	130 Gm.
White Petrolatum	120 Gm.
Heavy Liquid Petrolatum	530 Gm.
Distilled Water	200 cc.
Perfume, as desired,	
To make	1000 Gm.

Melt the white wax and white petrolatum with the heavy liquid petrolatum on a water bath. Dissolve the sodium borate and glycerin in the distilled water, warm it to the same temperature as the melted mixture and add it to this with constant stirring, continued until the cream congeals.

III

Glycerin	10 cc.
Sodium Borate	8 Gm.
Spermaceti	125 Gm.
White Wax	120 Gm.
Heavy Liquid Petrolatum	560 Gm.
Distilled Water, a sufficient quantity,	
To make	1000 Gm.

Melt the spermaceti and white wax on a water bath, add the heavy liquid petrolatum and continue the heat until a uniform mixture is obtained. Dissolve the sodium borate and glycerin in the distilled water and heat to bring this solution to the same temperature as that of the oily solution. Pour the aqueous solution all at once into the oily solution and stir until congealed.

LUBRICATING CREAM

White Wax	114	Gm.
Spermaceti	85	Gm.
Hydrous Wool Fat	156	Gm.
Expressed Oil of Almond or Persic Oil	463.5	Gm.
Rose Water	175	cc.
Sodium Borate	2.5	Gm.
Antioxidant, a sufficient quantity,		
Perfume, as desired,		
To make about	1000	Gm.

Melt the white wax and spermaceti with the antioxidant on a water bath, add the expressed oil of almond and warm to 70° C. Dissolve the sodium borate in the rose water and bring to the same temperature as the melted mixture, to which it should be added gradually, with constant stirring. Pour into a slightly warmed mortar containing the wool fat and stir. Add the perfume and stir until cold.

The hydrous wool fat may be replaced by theobroma oil, if desired.

ZINC OXIDE AND BORIC ACID CREAM

Boric Acid	40 Gm.
Zinc Oxide	80 Gm.
Expressed Oil of Almond or Persic Oil	140 Gm.
Glycerin	100 Gm.
Wool Fat	480 Gm.
Rose Water	160 cc.
To make	1000 Gm.

Triturate the wool fat with the expressed oil of almond or persic oil in a warm mortar. Add the zinc oxide and boric acid and rub until a smooth mixture results. Finally incorporate the glycerin and rose water.

SKIN CLEANSING AND LUBRICATING CREAM

Mannitol Mono-oleate	40	Gm.
Petrolatum	310	Gm.
Wool Fat	30	Gm.
White Wax	70	Gm.
Light Liquid Petrolatum	200	cc.
Methyl Parahydroxybenzoic Acid	1.5	Gm.
Water	350	cc.
Perfume, as desired,		
To make	1000	Gm.

Melt the white wax, wool fat and petrolatum, add the light liquid petrolatum and the mannitol mono-oleate, and heat to 65° C. Dissolve the methyl parahydroxy-benzoic acid in the water heated to 65° C. Add the water solution to the oily solution with constant stirring and add the perfume when it begins to congeal. Continue stirring until cool.

VANISHING OR NON-GREASY CREAMS, POWDER BASE CREAMS

Creams of this type are primarily stearate soaps of ammonium, potassium, sodium, triethanolamine or other alkaline substances capable of neutralizing stearic acid. Vanishing creams acquired their name because of their ability to disappear into the skin upon rubbing. Their high water content aids in producing this illusion Because of the dry film left on the skin by vanishing creams, they are used a great deal as powder bases and hand creams. Vanishing creams are also the base for brushless shaving creams and many other cosmetics.

The most important ingredient in vanishing creams is the stearic acid, which should be the triple pressed variety if the finest white cosmetic is to be produced. Depending upon the purpose for which the cream is intended, it will contain varying quantities of moistening agent, such as glycerin or commercial sorbitol syrup.

VANISHING CREAM
I

Stearic Acid	190 Gm.
Glycerin	75 cc.
Potassium Hydroxide	10 Gm.
Perfume, as desired,	
Distilled Water, a sufficient quantity,	
To make	1000 Gm.

Melt the stearic acid on a water bath, heated to a temperature of 80° C. Dissolve the potassium hydroxide and glycerin in the distilled water, warm to 85° C. and pour gradually into the melted acid, stirring briskly. Keep at the same temperature and continue stirring for 10 minutes to insure complete saponification and absence of free alkali. Then remove the heat and stir until cold, at the same time incorporating the perfume. Beat for a time, preferably by mechanical means, and then place in jars or tubes.

II

Stearic Acid.	142	Gm.
Glycerin	100	cc.
Sodium Borate.	2.5	Gm.
Triethanolamine	10	Gm.
Perfume, as desired,		
Distilled Water, a sufficient quantity,		
To make about	1000	Gm.

Prepare as directed under I, mixing the glycerin and distilled water together with the sodium borate and triethanolamine.

III

Stearic Acid	150 Gm.
Triethanolamine	20 Gm.
Sorbitol, syrupy	20 cc.
Perfume, as desired,	
Water, a sufficient quantity,	
To make	1000 Gm.

Heat the stearic acid to 80° C.; in a separate vessel, heat the water and triethanolamine to 85° C. Add the melted stearic acid to the aqueous solution, stirring constantly until a smooth cream is obtained. Add the syrupy sorbitol and cool to 45° C., perfume, triturate and stir occasionally until cold.

WITCH HAZEL CREAM OR "SNOW"
Cremor Hamamelidis
Hamamelis Cream

Stearic Acid.	100	Gm.
Monohydrated Sodium Carbonate	7.5	Gm.
Glycerin	15	Gm.
Hamamelis Water	500	Gm.
Distilled Water, a sufficient quantity,		
To make	1000	Gm.

NOTE—Use a kettle much larger than the batch requires or the effervescence may cause the cream to go over the top.

Melt the stearic acid on a water bath heated to 70° C. Add the sodium carbonate dissolved in the glycerin and 10 cc. of hot water. Continue heating for an hour, make up the weight to 500 Gm. with water heated to 75° C. and then add 500 Gm. of hamamelis water heated to 70° C. Stir until smooth.

Keep in well-closed containers or the cream will become dry.

ROLLING OR MASSAGE CREAMS

These are generally made of freshly precipitated milk casein, though some are said to be largely composed of starch or to have been made from dried casein. Their preparation is difficult. Casein is prone to decompose when in a moist state so it is necessary to add a preservative, such as formaldehyde.

When rubbed on the skin these creams apparently disappear, but upon continued friction they "roll out" in small particles carrying with them the dirt and dust.

ROLLING OR MASSAGE CREAM
I

Skimmed Milk 1280   cc.
Solution of Formaldehyde . . . .   1.25 cc.
Sodium Borate, in fine powder.   20   Gm.
Alum, in fine powder   40   Gm.
Sodium Benzoate.   20   Gm.
Boric Acid, in fine powder.   45   Gm.
Distilled Water 260   cc.
Perfume and color, as desired.

Add the solution of formaldehyde to the skimmed milk, warm gently to 50° C. on a water bath and stir in quickly a solution of the sodium borate in 100 cc. of warm distilled water. Warm to 55° C. and strain through unbleached muslin, previously wetted. Prepare a solution of the alum in 160 cc. of boiling distilled water, strain through cotton and add immediately to the milk, stirring it in slowly and keeping the temperature at 55° C. When cool, and the supernatant liquid is colorless, collect the precipitate on a strainer. Allow to drain, wash thoroughly with distilled water, drain again, and then press until the product is of proper consistence. Finally incorporate the sodium benzoate and boric acid, and the perfume and color.

Skim milk will not produce as smooth a cream as does whole milk, but it is much cheaper to use than the whole milk and does not become rancid so easily.

II

Skimmed Milk . . . .   920 cc.
Sodium Borate, in fine powder . . . .   21 Gm.
Boric Acid, in fine powder . . . .   21 Gm.
Sodium Benzoate, in fine powder . . . .   4 Gm.
Tartaric Acid, in fine powder . . . .   50 Gm.
Glycerin . . . .   15 cc.
Perfume and color, as desired.

Mix the sodium borate, boric acid and sodium benzoate with the milk and heat the mixture to the boiling point. Remove from the source of heat, add the tartaric acid and allow to stand for 24 hours. Strain and mix the glycerin with the residue. Add the perfume and color.

STARCH MASSAGE CREAM

Starch	100 Gm.
Cold Water	500 cc.
Theobroma Oil	20 Gm.
Vanishing Cream, R.B.	50 Gm.
Perfume and Color, as desired.	

Heat the starch with the water on a water bath until a uniform paste has formed. Then add the liquefied theobroma oil and, lastly, the vanishing cream. Color and perfume when cold.

LIQUID MASSAGE CREAM

Paraffin	160 Gm.
Stearic Acid	20 Gm.
Triethanolamine	3.2 Gm.
Perfume, as desired,	
Water, a sufficient quantity,	
To make	1000 Gm.

Melt the fats and heat to 90° C. Dissolve the triethanolamine in water and heat to the same temperature. Add the water solution to the melted fats with rapid stirring, mixing until cold. Perfume at about 55° C. Stir again the next day.

SMELLING SALTS

Ammonia in some form is the medicinal agent in most types of smelling salts, dry or liquid type.

Dry Type

These generally consist of granular ammonium carbonate in a combination of granular ammonium chloride and potassium carbonate. They are usually perfumed and occasionally colored.

GRANULAR SMELLING SALT

Potassium Carbonate, granular	470 Gm.
Ammonium Carbonate, granular	100 Gm.
Ammonium Chloride, granular.	380 Gm.
Camphor, in powder	45 Gm.
Oil of Bergamot	5 cc.
Oil of Clove	5 cc.
To make about	1000 Gm.

Mix by gentle trituration.

Keep in glass or rubber stoppered bottles.

Liquid Type

I

Suitable containers are filled with small cubes of ammonium carbonate or large crystals of potassium sulfate.   The following solution is then poured over them:

Strong Solution of Ammonia.	40 cc.
Oil of Lemon	10 cc.
Oil of Lavender	20 cc.
Oil of Clove.	10 cc.
Alcohol, a sufficient quantity,	
To make	1000 cc.

Mix.

II

Ammonium Carbonate, powder	800 Gm
Strong Solution of Ammonia	125 cc.
Cologne Water, R.B., a sufficient quantity,	
To make	1000 cc.

Dissolve the ammonium carbonate in the strong solution of ammonia and add the cologne water.

ENGLISH SMELLING SALT

Ammonium Carbonate, in small cubes	700 Gm.
Ammonium Chloride, in fine powder	200 Gm.
Oil of Lavender	30 cc.
Oil of Lemon	20 cc.
Oil of Bergamot	10 cc.
Alcohol	35 cc.
Glycerin, a sufficient quantity,	
To make	1000 cc.

Place the ammonium carbonate in a wide-mouthed glass-stoppered bottle.   Add the ammonium chloride and the oils dissolved in the alcohol.   Finally add sufficient glycerin to make the product measure 1000 cc.

Solidified Type

This form consists of a dilute spirit of ammonia, solidified with sodium stearate:

Sodium Hydroxide.	13.5 Gm.
Strong Solution of Ammonia.	20 cc.
Oil of Lavender	10 cc.
Stearic Acid.	85 Gm.
Color,* as desired,	
Alcohol.	900 cc.
To make about	1000 Gm.

Dissolve the sodium hydroxide in 400 cc. of alcohol, warm, add the strong solution of ammonia, oil and color. Dissolve the stearic acid in 500 cc. of alcohol by the aid of heat, add this to the alkaline solution and warm until clear. Pour while hot into suitable containers.

TALCUM POWDERS

BORATED TALC
I

Boric Acid, in fine powder.	100 Gm.
Purified Talc, in very fine powder	900 Gm.
Perfume, as desired,	
To make about	1000 Gm.

Mix intimately and pass through a No. 150 sieve.

II—With Zinc Stearate

Boric Acid, in fine powder.	50 Gm.
Zinc Stearate	50 Gm.
Purified Talc, in very fine powder	900 Gm.
Perfume, as desired,	
To make about	1000 Gm.

Mix intimately, after having first incorporated the perfume with the boric acid, and pass through a No. 150 sieve.

COMPOUND TALCUM POWDER
I

Magnesium Carbonate,
Alum, in fine powder,
Purified Talc, in very fine powder, of each, an equal weight.

Mix intimately and pass through a No. 150 sieve.

* The color used must be an alcohol-soluble, alkali-fast certified aniline dye.

II

Purified Talc, in very fine powder	885 Gm.
Boric Acid, in fine powder	40 Gm.
Zinc Stearate	15 Gm.
Magnesium Carbonate	60 Gm.
Perfume, as desired,	
To make	1000 Gm.

Mix thoroughly and pass through a No. 150 sieve. Perfume should be added at the beginning of the mixing.

TOILET LOTIONS

AFTER-SHAVING LOTION

Menthol	0.5	Gm.
Alum	2	Gm.
Glycerin	110	cc.
Hamamelis Water	160	cc.
Perfumed Spirit	500	cc.
Alcohol, a sufficient quantity,		
To make	1000	cc.

Dissolve the alum in the hamamelis water, add the glycerin and perfumed spirit and sufficient alcohol in which the menthol is dissolved to make the product measure 1000 cc.

BENZOIN LOTION
Lotio Benzoini
Lait Virginal
(B.P.C. 1934)

Tincture of Benzoin	25 cc.
Rose Water, a sufficient quantity,	
To make	1000 cc.

Place the rose water in a bottle and add the tincture of benzoin in a thin stream, with continuous agitation.

NOTE—Dispense with a "shake well" label.

COMPOUND BENZOIN LOTION

I

Tincture of Benzoin . . . . 62.5 cc.
Sodium Lauryl Sulfate (salt free)* . . . . 1 Gm.
Cologne Water, R.B. . . . . 62.5 cc.
Distilled Water, a sufficient quantity,

To make . . . . 1000 cc.

Mix the first three ingredients and add gradually sufficient distilled water to make the product measure 1000 cc.

Note—Dispense with a "shake well" label.

II

Karaya Gum Powder . . . . 10 Gm.
Tragacanth, in powder . . . . 30 Gm.
Tincture of Benzoin . . . . 20 cc.
Glycerin . . . . 80 cc.
Alcohol . . . . 150 cc.
Benzoic Acid . . . . 1 Gm.
Distilled Water, a sufficient quantity,

To make . . . . 1000 cc.

Mix the tragacanth, karaya gum and benzoic acid with 60 cc. of the alcohol, add 700 cc. of distilled water and make a mucilage. Add the glycerin and the remainder of the alcohol, then the tincture of benzoin in small portions, mixing well after each addition. Lastly add sufficient distilled water to make the product measure 1000 cc. Pass through a hand homogenizer.

Note—Dispense with a "shake well" label.

BENZOIN AND GLYCERIN LOTION

Benzoin, Glycerin and Rose Water

Sodium Lauryl Sulfate (salt free)* . . . . 0.5 Gm.
Tincture of Benzoin . . . . 30 cc.
Glycerin . . . . 250 cc.
Rose Water, a sufficient quantity,

To make . . . . 1000 cc.

To 350 cc. of rose water, previously mixed with the glycerin, add gradually the tincture of benzoin in which the sodium lauryl sulfate is dissolved, and sufficient rose water to make the product measure 1000 cc.

Note—Dispense with a "shake well" label.

* Dupanol.

GLYCERIN LOTION
Lotio Glycerini
Glycerin and Rose Water

Rose Water,
Glycerin, of each, an equal volume.
  Mix.

GLYCERIN AND BENZOIN LOTION WITH ALMOND OIL

Tragacanth, in fine powder	27	Gm.
Glycerin	100	cc.
Expressed Oil of Almond or Persic Oil	20	cc.
Alcohol	120	cc.
Tincture of Benzoin	30	cc.
Sodium Alkyl Aryl Sulfonate	0.5	Gm.
Perfume, as desired,		
Distilled Water, a sufficient quantity,		
To make	1000	cc.

Form an emulsion with the tragacanth, expressed oil of almond and 50 cc. of distilled water, diluting with distilled water until the product measures approximately 500 cc., then add the glycerin. Dissolve the tincture of benzoin, the sodium alkyl aryl sulfonate and perfume in the alcohol. Add this solution to the emulsion in small portions, agitating thoroughly after each addition, then add sufficient distilled water to make the product measure 1000 cc.

GLYCERIN AND BORIC ACID LOTION
Lac Glycerini, Glycerin Milk

Hard Soap, in powder	10 Gm.
Alcohol	20 cc.
Boric Acid	25 Gm.
Glycerin	150 cc.
Perfume, as desired,	
Mucilage of Quince Seed, R.B., a sufficient quantity,	
To make	1000 cc.

Dissolve the soap in the alcohol and mix with 700 cc. of the mucilage. Heat the boric acid with the glycerin until dissolved; mix with the mucilage and soap and add the perfume. Add sufficient mucilage, if necessary, to make the product measure 1000 cc., and mix thoroughly.

COMPOUND HONEY AND ALMOND LOTION

Sodium Borate, in fine powder.	3.75	Gm.
Hard Soap, in fine powder	33.75	Gm.
White Wax	7.50	Gm.
Spermaceti	41.25	Gm.
Expressed Oil of Almond or Persic Oil	30	cc.
Honey	12.50	cc.
Hamamelis Water	15	cc.
Glycerin	20	cc.
Alcohol	15	cc.
Quince Seed, bruised.	5	Gm.
Perfume, as desired,		
Distilled Water, a sufficient quantity,		
To make	1000	cc.

Macerate the quince seed in 500 cc. of water for 24 hours, stirring frequently and strain through muslin. Warm to 60° C. and set aside. Melt the wax, spermaceti and almond oil, bring to 70° C. add the glycerin, add the mucilage quickly and mix thoroughly. Dissolve the soap and borax in 300 cc. of boiling water, add the hamamelis water and honey which have been mixed; add this to the first mixture and mix. When luke warm add the perfume; set aside for 4 days, stirring frequently and strain, adding sufficient distilled water to make the product measure 1000 cc.

LANOLIN LOTION

Wool Fat	275	Gm.
Stearic Acid	50	Gm.
Triethanolamine	16	Gm.
Rose Water, a sufficient quantity,		
To make	1000	cc.

Melt the wool fat and stearic acid on a water bath and warm to 70° C. Add the triethanolamine to the rose water and heat to 72° C. Add the rose water, gradually, stirring after each addition to make the product measure 1000 cc.

MENTHOL LOTION
Lotio Mentholis
Shaving Lotion

Menthol	7.5	Gm.
Tragacanth	25	Gm.
Benzoic Acid	1	Gm.
Glycerin	36	cc.
Alcohol	45	cc.
Distilled Water, a sufficient quantity,		
To make	1000	cc.

Macerate the tragacanth in 900 cc. of distilled water to form a homogeneous mucilage. Add the glycerin, benzoic acid, perfume and the menthol dissolved in the alcohol, and sufficient distilled water to make the product measure 1000 cc.

PASCHKIS' LOTION

Potassium Carbonate	60 Gm.
Potassium Chlorate	20 Gm.
Sodium Borate	15 Gm.
Sorbitol, syrupy	60 Gm.
Glycerin	120 cc.
Rose Water	330 cc.
Orange Flower Water, a sufficient quantity,	
To make	1000 cc.

Dissolve the salts in the rose water, add the glycerin, syrupy sorbitol and finally sufficient orange flower water to make the product measure 1000 cc. and filter.

QUINCE SEED LOTION
I

Quince Seed	16 Gm.
Sodium Borate	6 Gm.
Benzoic Acid	1 Gm.
Boric Acid	6 Gm.
Glycerin	120 cc.
Alcohol	120 cc.
Perfume and color, as desired,	
Distilled Water, a sufficient quantity,	
To make	1000 cc.

Wash the quince seed quickly with cold water and strain, then macerate it with 500 cc. of distilled water overnight, and strain. Dissolve the sodium borate and boric acid in 250 cc. of distilled water, add to the mucilage and incorporate the benzoic acid dissolved in the alcohol, glycerin, perfume and color. Add sufficient distilled water to make the product measure 1000 cc.

II

Quince Seed	30 Gm.
Sodium Borate	5 Gm.
Benzoic Acid	1 Gm.
Alcohol	120 cc.
Distilled Water, a sufficient quantity,	
To make	1000 cc.

Wash the quince seed quickly with cold water and strain, then macerate it with 500 cc. of distilled water overnight and strain. Dissolve the sodium borate in 250 cc. of distilled water and add this solution to the mucilage; incorporate the alcohol which contains the benzoic acid and add sufficient distilled water to make the product measure 1000 cc.

ROSE FRAGRANCE LOTION

Hard Soap, in fine powder	7 Gm.
White Wax	7 Gm.
Expressed Oil of Almond or Persic Oil	6 cc.
Alcohol	150 cc.
Quince Seed Mucilage, 2%	350 cc.
Perfume, as desired,	
Rose Water, a sufficient quantity,	
To make	1000 cc.

Melt together the first three ingredients and warm to 70° C. Heat 250 cc. of rose water to the same temperature. Add rose water to the melted fats and when emulsified by stirring, add the quince seed mucilage and finally the perfume dissolved in the alcohol, and the remainder of the water to make the product measure 1000 cc.

VIRGINAL ROSE FRAGRANCE LOTION

Sodium Alkyl Aryl Sulfonate	0.5 Gm.
Tincture of Tolu Balsam	15 cc.
Rose Water, a sufficient quantity,	
To make	1000 cc.

Place the rose water in a container and gradually add with stirring the tincture of tolu balsam containing the dissolved sodium alkyl aryl sulfonate. Strain if necessary.

SUN TAN PREPARATIONS

Lotions intended to protect the skin from the burning rays of the sun usually contain a screening agent capable of filtering out the wave length 2900–3200 Å. Chemical screens capable of filtering out this wave length are butyl benzal acetone oxalate $\frac{1}{2}\%$, isobutyl para-aminobenzoate $1\frac{1}{2}\%$, menthyl salicylate 10%, and menthyl anthranilate $3\frac{1}{2}\%$ among many other chemicals that could be used for this purpose. The salts of quinine are well known for their effectiveness as sun screens but they have a tendency to irritate certain skins. Phenol salicylate has likewise been recommended as a sun screen in quantities of 7% but it likewise irritates certain skins. Aesculin is useless as a sun screen because its effectiveness is short lived.

Sun tan preparations usually take the form of oils, alcoholic lotions, emulsions or creams. The most popular products on the market are the alcoholic lotions and oils, although recently a few emulsified products have begun to appear.

The oils are usually a mixture of ⅓ vegetable oil and ⅔ mineral oil, in as much as sun screens are not always soluble in mineral oil alone. In the case of alcoholic lotions, a film-forming agent must be added to the composition or the screen may be rendered useless. For this purpose, castor oil, propylene glycol laurate and other glycol fatty acid esters may be used.

SUNBURN LOTION

Heat Lotion

I

Liquefied Phenol	10 cc.
Glycerin	25 cc.
Witch Hazel Water	360 cc.
Solution of Calcium Hydroxide, a sufficient quantity,	
To make	1000 cc.

Mix the liquefied phenol with the glycerin and add the witch hazel water and sufficient solution of calcium hydroxide to make the product measure 1000 cc.

II

Menthol	0.5 Gm.
Zinc Oxide	50 Gm.
Sodium Borate	25 Gm.
Glycerin	100 cc.
Bay Rum, R.B.	150 cc.
Distilled Water, or Aromatic Water, a sufficient quantity,	
To make	1000 cc.

Dissolve the menthol in a small amount of alcohol. Triturate the other solids with the glycerin and add the other liquids gradually so as to obtain a smooth mixture.

III

Calamine	100 Gm.
Glycerin	30 cc.
Sambucus Water*	30 cc.
Solution of Cochineal	1 cc.
Rose Water, a sufficient quantity,	
To make	1000 cc.

Triturate the calamine with the glycerin, added gradually, to a smooth cream, add the sambucus water and solution of cochineal and finally sufficient rose water to make the product measure 1000 cc.

* Prepared as directed in either of the general processes for Aromatic Waters (see U.S.P. XII, page 62).

PROTECTIVE SUN TAN LOTION

Menthyl Salicylate . . . . 60 cc.
Expressed Oil of Almond or Persic Oil . . . . 400 cc.
Light Liquid Petrolatum . . . . 540 cc.
Perfume, a sufficient quantity,

To make about . . . . 1000 cc.

Mix.

NOTE—Peanut oil, olive oil or other vegetable oils may be used in place of the expressed oil of almond. It is advisable to add an antioxidant if the product is not to be used shortly after its preparation.

SUN TAN LOTION

Menthyl Anthranilate . . . . 35 Gm.
Propylene Glycol Laurate . . . . 100 Gm.
Perfume and color, as desired,
Alcohol, a sufficient quantity,

To make . . . . 1000 cc.

Dissolve the ingredients in the alcohol and filter until clear.

SUN TAN OIL

Isobutyl Paraaminobenzoate . . . . 15 Gm.
Sesame Oil . . . . 350 Gm.
Perfume and color, as desired,
Light Liquid Petrolatum, a sufficient quantity,

To make . . . . 1000 cc.

Mix.

ZINC PHENOLSULFONATE LOTION

Zinc Phenolsulfonate. . . . . 10 Gm.
Glycerin . . . . 20 cc.
Alcohol . . . . 10 cc.
Spirit of Camphor . . . . 1 cc.
Rose Water, a sufficient quantity,

To make . . . . 1000 cc.

Dissolve the zinc phenolsulfonate in 500 cc. of rose water, then add the other ingredients and sufficient rose water to make the product measure 1000 cc.

COSMETIC LOTION, LILIONESE

Purified Talc	100 Gm.
Sodium Borate	15 Gm.
Potassium Carbonate	5 Gm.
Glycerin	50 cc.
Cologne Water, R.B.	25 cc.
Rose Water, a sufficient quantity,	
To make	1000 cc.

Dissolve the salts in 800 cc. of rose water and add the cologne water. Triturate the purified talc with the glycerin, then add gradually the solution of salts and sufficient rose water to make the product measure 1000 cc.

HAND LOTION

Hamamelis Water	65 cc.
Glycerin	60 cc.
Alcohol	65 cc.
Tincture of Benzoin	4 cc.
Quince Seed	16 Gm.
Preservative, a sufficient quantity,	
Perfume, as desired,	
Distilled Water, a sufficient quantity,	
To make about	1000 cc.

Macerate the quince seed overnight in 500 cc. of distilled water in which the preservative has been dissolved, and strain. Add to the alcohol the tincture of benzoin, perfume and glycerin. Incorporate the strained mucilage in the alcohol mixture and add with constant shaking, sufficient distilled water to make the product measure 1000 cc.

If color is desired, a water-soluble certified color should be used. (See R.B., page 341, for a representative list of certified colors.)

CITRIC ACID HAND LOTION

Citric Acid	4.8 Gm.
Compound Tincture of Lavender	96 cc.
Alcohol	240 cc.
Distilled Water	240 cc.
Glycerin, a sufficient quantity,	
To make	1000 cc.

Dissolve the citric acid in the distilled water, add the alcohol, compound tincture of lavender and sufficient glycerin to make the product measure 1000 cc.

TRAGACANTH HAND LOTION

Tragacanth, in ribbons . . . .   18 Gm.
Boric Acid . . . .   16 Gm.
Glycerin . . . .   120 cc.
Alcohol . . . .   120 cc.
Preservative, a sufficient quantity,
Perfume and color, as desired,
Distilled Water, a sufficient quantity,
To make . . . .   1000 cc.

Dissolve the boric acid in 750 cc. of distilled water, add the tragacanth and macerate with frequent stirring until dissolved and strain through muslin or cheese-cloth, and add the glycerin. Dissolve the preservative and perfume in the alcohol and add color as desired. Dilute with sufficient water to make the product measure 1000 cc. Pass through a hand homogenizer to obtain proper viscosity.

WITCH HAZEL AND BENZOIN HAND LOTION

Tragacanth, in ribbons . . . .   18 Gm.
Hamamelis Water . . . .   65 cc.
Glycerin . . . .   60 cc.
Alcohol . . . .   65 cc.
Tincture of Benzoin . . . .   4 cc.
Preservative, a sufficient quantity,
Perfume, as desired,
Distilled Water, a sufficient quantity,
To make . . . .   1000 cc.

Macerate the tragacanth in 750 cc. of distilled water containing the preservative, then heat gently until a uniform mixture is obtained. Cool and add the hamamelis water and glycerin. Then add the alcohol in which the tincture of benzoin and perfume have been dissolved. Add sufficient distilled water to make the product measure 1000 cc. Pass through a hand homogenizer to obtain proper viscosity.

LOHSE'S LILY MILK

Lohse's Lilienmilch

Zinc Oxide, in fine powder . . . .   10 Gm.
Purified Talc . . . .   10 Gm.
Glycerin . . . .   20 cc.
Preservative, a sufficient quantity,
Rose Water, a sufficient quantity,
To make . . . .   1000 cc.

Triturate the zinc oxide and purified talc with the glycerin, perfume and rose water, adding sufficient rose water to make the product measure 1000 cc.

TOILET AND COSMETIC WATERS

COLOGNE WATER

Oil of Bergamot	12 cc.
Oil of Lemon	6 cc.
Oil of Orange Flowers	4 cc.
Oil of Orange	2 cc.
Oil of Rosemary	2 cc.
Tincture of Benzoin	8 cc.
Orange Flower Water	100 cc.
Alcohol, a sufficient quantity,	
To make	1000 cc.

Dissolve the oils and the tincture in 800 cc. of alcohol, add the orange flower water and sufficient alcohol to make the product measure 1000 cc. Allow to blend for 7 days or more and filter.

AMMONIATED COLOGNE

Ethyl Acetate	100 cc.
Strong Solution of Ammonia	14 cc.
Oil of Peppermint	7 cc.
Perfume, as desired,	
Alcohol, a sufficient quantity,	
To make	1000 cc.

Mix.

MENTHOLATED COLOGNE

Menthol	40 Gm.
Perfumed Spirit, a sufficient quantity,	
To make	1000 cc.

Dissolve.

FLORIDA WATER

I

Oil of Bergamot	7 cc.
Oil of Lemon	4 cc.
Oil of Orange	3 cc.
Oil of Lavender	5 cc.
Oil of Clove	0.7 cc.
Oil of Cinnamon	0.7 cc.
Oil of Orange Flowers	0.7 cc.
Distilled Water	200 cc.
Alcohol, a sufficient quantity,	
To make	1000 cc.

Dissolve the oils in 700 cc. of alcohol, add the distilled water and sufficient alcohol to make the product measure 1000 cc. and filter, using purified talc, if necessary.

II

Oil of Orange Flowers	5 cc.
Oil of Lavender	5 cc.
Oil of Bergamot	30 cc.
Oil of Clove	2 cc.
Oil of Cinnamon	3 cc.
Oil of Rose	5 cc.
Orange Flower Water.	100 cc.
Alcohol, a sufficient quantity,	
To make	1000 cc.

Dissolve the oils in 800 cc. of alcohol and add the orange flower water and sufficient alcohol to make the product measure 1000 cc. Allow to blend for a week or more and filter, using purified talc.

HONEY WATER
Aqua Mellis
I

Oil of Bergamot	7.8	cc.
Oil of Lavender	2.6	cc.
Oil of Clove	2.6	cc.
Oil of Santal.	0.5	cc.
Tincture of Musk, 2%	30	cc.
Stronger Rose Water.	150	cc.
Orange Flower Water	150	cc.
Honey	5	cc.
Color, as desired,		
Alcohol, a sufficient quantity,		
To make	1000	cc.

Dissolve the oils in 650 cc. of alcohol, add the tincture of musk and color, the honey mixed with the rose and orange flower waters, and sufficient alcohol to make the product measure 1000 cc. Set aside for 7 days and filter, using purified talc if necessary.

II

Lavender Water, R.B.	60	cc.
Honey	74	cc.
Distilled Water	250	cc.
Oil of Orange	6	cc.
Oil of Clove	1.5	cc.
Tincture of Saffron, R.B.	5.8	cc.
Rose Water, a sufficient quantity,		
To make	1000	cc.

Mix the honey with the distilled water, add the oils, lavender water, tincture of saffron and sufficient rose water to make the product measure 1000 cc. and filter.

LAVENDER WATER

I

Oil of Lavender	25	cc.
Oil of Bergamot	5	cc.
Oil of Orange	1	cc.
Oil of Orange Flowers	0.5	cc.
Coumarin	0.5	Gm
Tincture of Benzoin	7	cc.
Distilled Water	110	cc.
Alcohol, a sufficient quantity,		
To make	1000	cc.

Add the oils, coumarin and tincture of benzoin to 800 cc. of alcohol. Now add the distilled water and sufficient alcohol to make the product measure 1000 cc.

II

Tincture of Musk, 2%	12	cc.
Ambergris	0.1	Gm.
Oil of Bergamot	15	cc.
Oil of Lavender	15	cc.
Oil of Myristica	2	cc.
Alcohol, a sufficient quantity,		
To make	1000	cc.

Add the tincture of musk and ambergris to the solution of the oils in 900 cc. of alcohol. Blend for 7 or more days, then filter, passing sufficient alcohol through the filter to make the product measure 1000 cc.

III

Oil of Lavender, English	15 cc.
Oil of Lavender, French	5 cc.
Oil of Bergamot	10 cc.
Oil of Clary Sage	1 cc.
Civet Extract, 10 per cent	4 cc.
Oleoresin of Orris, Concrete	2 Gm.
Oil of Myristica	1 cc.
Alcohol, a sufficient quantity,	
To make	1000 cc.

Dissolve the oils, civet extract and oleoresin of orris in 900 cc. of alcohol. Allow to blend for 7 or more days and filter, passing sufficient alcohol through the filter to make the product measure 1000 cc.

HUFELAND'S COSMETIC WATER
Aqua Cosmetica Hufelandi
Hufeland's Schönheitswasser

Bitter Almond, blanched	32.5 Gm.
Rose Water	450 cc.
Sodium Borate	39 Gm.
Tincture of Benzoin	90 cc.
Orange Flower Water, a sufficient quantity,	
To make	1000 cc.

Prepare an emulsion with the bitter almond and the rose water and 400 cc. of orange flower water in which the sodium borate has been dissolved. Add the tincture of benzoin and sufficient orange flower water to make the product measure 1000 cc.; mix well.

Note—Dispense with a "shake well" label.

VIENNA TYPE COSMETIC WATER

Sweet Almonds, blanched	120 Gm.
Rose Water	480 cc.
Sodium Borate	8 Gm.
Tincture of Benzoin	16 cc.
Orange Flower Water, a sufficient quantity,	
To make	1000 cc.

Prepare an emulsion with the almond and rose water and add 400 cc. of orange flower water in which the sodium borate has been dissolved. Add the tincture of benzoin and sufficient orange flower water to make the product measure 1000 cc., mix well.

Note—Dispense with a "shake well" label.

BAY RUM

Citric Acid	5	Gm.
Oil of Myrcia	2	cc.
Oil of Myristica	0.1	cc.
Oil of Orange	1	cc.
Alcohol	500	cc.
Glycerin	30	cc.
Purified Talc	20	Gm.
Distilled Water, a sufficient quantity,		
To make	1000	cc.

Dissolve the oils in the alcohol, add the glycerin and citric acid, then add sufficient distilled water to make the product measure 1000 cc. Add the purified talc. Filter, returning the first portions until the liquid filters clear.

TOILET AMMONIA

Medicinal Soft Soap	120 Gm.
Strong Solution of Ammonia	250 cc.
Oleic Acid	10 cc.
Oil of Myrcia	1 cc.
Oil of Rosemary	1 cc.
Oil of Verbena	5 cc.
Distilled Water, a sufficient quantity,	
To make	1000 cc.

Dissolve the medicinal soft soap in 500 cc. of boiling distilled water, cool and add the strong solution of ammonia and oleic acid. Add the perfume oils after the mixture cools, and sufficient distilled water to make the product measure 1000 cc.

TOILET VINEGAR
Acetum Odoratum
I

Oil of Lemon	7 cc.
Oil of Bergamot	7 cc.
Oil of Clove	1 cc.
Oil of Rose	1 cc.
Acetic Ether	12 cc.
Alcohol	300 cc.
Diluted Acetic Acid, a sufficient quantity,	
To make	1000 cc.

Mix the oils and acetic ether with the alcohol. Then add the diluted acetic acid, shake well and filter until clear, using purified talc if necessary.

MISCELLANEOUS PREPARATIONS

BANDOLINE

Tragacanth, in ribbons	56 Gm.
Benzaldehyde	1.5 cc.
Anisic Aldehyde	1.5 cc.
Benzoic Acid	1 Gm.
Rose Water, a sufficient quantity,	
To make	1000 cc.

Reduce the tragacanth to small pieces and allow it to soak in the rose water in a warm place, add the benzoic acid, occasionally stirring until it has swollen. Press the mass through a cloth and incorporate the aromatics; color as desired.

ODOROUS OIL

I

Mistura Odorifera, Oleum Milleflorum, Perfume Oil

Coumarin.	5 Gm.
Oil of Lemon . . . , ...	300 cc.
Oil of Lavender	200 cc.
Oil of Cinnamon.	20 cc.
Oil of Clove	20 cc.
Methyl Salicylate	10 cc.
Oil of Bergamot, a sufficient quantity,	
To make	1000 cc.

Dissolve the coumarin in the mixed oils.

II

Oil of Bergamot	430 cc.
Oil of Lemon	350 cc.
Oil of Clove.	150 cc.
Oil of Cinnamon.	50 cc.
Oil of Orange Flowers	20 cc.
To make	1000 cc.

Mix the oils.

HAIR WAVING FLUID

Karaya Gum, powdered	20 Gm.
Sodium Borate	5 Gm.
Glycerin	5 Gm.
Benzoic Acid	1 Gm.
Alcohol	50 cc.
Perfume and color, as desired,	
Water, a sufficient quantity,	
To make	1000 cc.

Place the gum, perfume, alcohol and benzoic acid in a large container. Add with stirring the water containing sodium borate and glycerin. Color to suit and strain.

NOTE—This fluid should be prepared fresh as it changes its viscosity on standing.

HAIR WAVING CONCENTRATE LOTION

Karaya Gum, powdered	375 Gm.
Sodium Borate	75 Gm.
Perfume, as desired,	
Color, as desired,	
Alcohol, a sufficient quantity,	
To make	1000 Gm.

Mix the gum and borax with the alcohol; perfume and color as desired.

POWDER BASE

Glycerol Mono-Stearate (self-emulsifying)	120 Gm.
Glycerin	50 Gm.
Light Liquid Petrolatum	25 cc.
Spermaceti	30 Gm.
Titanium Dioxide	20 Gm.
Preservative, a sufficient quantity,	
Perfume, as desired,	
Water, a sufficient quantity,	
To make	1000 Gm.

Place all the ingredients in a container and heat to boiling. Triturate the mixture and allow to cool. Add the perfume when the temperature drops to 55° C. and mix well.

SKIN FRESHENER

Benzoic Acid	1.5 Gm.
Boric Acid	5 Gm.
Alcohol	150 cc.
Orange Flower Water, a sufficient quantity,	
To make	1000 cc.

Mix the ingredients, allow to set a few days and filter until clear.

PART V

TECHNICAL AND MISCELLANEOUS FORMULAS

CEMENTS

CEMENT FOR ATTACHING GLASS LABELS TO BOTTLES
I

Rosin	34 Gm.
Yellow Wax	66 Gm.
To make	100 Gm.

Melt the rosin and wax by the aid of gentle heat and stir until congealed.

II

Paraffin	25 Gm.
Rosin	75 Gm.
To make	100 Gm.

Melt together with the aid of gentle heat and stir until of the consistency of syrup.

Apply warm to the moisture-free glass surface and gently press the glass label into place.

CHINA CEMENT

Isinglass, finely cut	24 Gm.
Hide Glue, in fine powder	3 Gm.
Salicylic Acid	1 Gm.
Acetic Acid	24 cc.
Water	48 cc.
To make	100 Gm.

Soak the isinglass in 25 cc. of water, then add the glue, salicylic acid and remainder of the water and heat on a boiling water bath, while stirring, until the isinglass and glue are dissolved. Then add the acetic acid and mix well.

403

CEMENT FOR BROKEN MORTARS
I

Gutta Percha,
Shellac, of each, an equal weight.

Fuse together in an iron dish.

To mend broken mortars or similar utensils, heat the fractured surfaces, apply a little of the cement and bring the pieces together under pressure.

II

Litharge,
Glycerin, a sufficient quantity.

Triturate the litharge with sufficient glycerin to make a soft paste.

CLEANING ACCESSORIES

DETERGENT SOLUTION OF AMMONIA
Liquor Ammoniæ Detergens

Strong Solution of Ammonia . . . .   300 cc.
Oleic Acid . . . .   60 cc.
Alcohol . . . .   60 cc.
Distilled Water, a sufficient quantity,
            To make . . . .   1000 cc.

Mix.

About 50 Gm. of sodium borate may be added if desired, together with a little oil of lavender or other suitable perfume. If a cloudy preparation is desired, about half of the distilled water should be replaced by hard tap water, the exact proportion depending on the amount of total solids in the hard water.

GLASS CLEANING FORMULA

Sodium Perborate,
Sodium Borate,
Trisodium Phosphate, of each, an equal weight.

Mix.

For use, dissolve 2 teaspoonfuls in a quart of water.

LABORATORY GLASSWARE CLEANING SOLUTIONS

These solutions are to be used when the usual methods of water and soap are not effective.

SULFURIC ACID-DICHROMATE CLEANING SOLUTION

I

Sulfuric Acid (sp. gr. 1.84)	200 cc.
Cold Water	150 cc.
Potassium or Sodium Dichromate, technical, powdered, a sufficient quantity,	

To make a saturated solution.

With stirring, cautiously pour the concentrated sulfuric acid into the cold water. Saturate the resulting hot solution, without further heating, with the powdered dichromate salt. This solution may be used cold or hot, but used with caution.

II

Potassium Dichromate	100 Gm.
Sulfuric Acid (sp. gr. 1.84)	100 cc.
Distilled Water, a sufficient quantity,	
To make	1000 cc.

Dissolve the potassium dichromate in 800 cc. of distilled water. Add the sulfuric acid, mix and add sufficient distilled water to make the product measure 1000 cc.

III

NITRIC-SULFURIC ACID CLEANING SOLUTION

Nitric Acid, concentrated	30 cc.
Sulfuric Acid, concentrated	70 cc.

Mix the acids carefully. This solution, when heated carefully, will usually remove stains and debris from glassware that are unaffected by the sulfuric acid-dichromate cleaning solution.

JEWELERS' CLEANSING SOLUTION

I

For Gold

Oleic Acid	30 cc.
Acetone.	60 cc.
Strong Solution of Ammonia	120 cc.
Water, a sufficient quantity,	
To make	1000 cc.

Dissolve the oleic acid in the strong solution of ammonia, add 500 cc. of water, then the acetone and, lastly, sufficient water to make the product measure 1000 cc.

II

For Silver

Ammonium Chloride . . . .   150 Gm.
    Dissolve in solution I.

The articles to be cleaned are first dipped in the cleansing solution, then in benzene or naphtha, afterwards they are dried, preferably in boxwood sawdust.

MOTORISTS' HAND SOAP

Medicinal Soft Soap . . . .   700 Gm.
Diluted Solution of Ammonia . . . .   40 Gm.
Gasoline . . . .   50 Gm.
Pumice, in fine powder . . . .   210 Gm.
                    To make . . . .   1000 Gm.

Mix the diluted solution of ammonia thoroughly with the medicinal soft soap, then incorporate the gasoline and finally the pumice.

SOAP POWDER FOR WASHING

Dried Soap, in powder . . . .   460 Gm.
Exsiccated Sodium Carbonate . . . .   270 Gm.
Sodium Metasilicate . . . .   180 Gm.
Sodium Borate, in powder . . . .   90 Gm.
                    To make . . . .   1000 Gm.

Mix and sift.

BENZIN SOAP

Oleic Acid . . . .   370 Gm.
Stearic Acid . . . .   80 Gm.
Potassium Carbonate . . . .   80 Gm.
Water . . . .   70 Gm.
Benzin* . . . .   395 Gm.
Strong Solution of Ammonia . . . .   5 Gm.
                    To make . . . .   1000 Gm.

Melt the stearic acid and incorporate with it the warmed oleic acid. To this mixture add the warm benzin and mix thoroughly. Dissolve the potassium carbonate in the water and briskly stir this solution into the benzin mixture. Finally add the strong solution of ammonia and beat into a homogeneous paste.

* The benzin used for this purpose is of the type of Stoddard Solvent, a high flash point fraction. It is not so dangerous to handle as the low flash point, high test naphthas and is more efficient as a dirt remover.

DRY CLEANERS' BENZIN-SOLUBLE SOAP

Benzin Soap, R.B.	925 Gm.
Ethylene Dichloride	75 Gm.
To make	1000 Gm.

Incorporate the ethylene dichloride in the benzin soap.

DRY CLEANERS' WATER-SOLUBLE SOAP

Soft Soap	650 Gm.
Ethylene Dichloride	325 Gm.
Oleic Acid	25 Gm.
To make	1000 Gm.

Incorporate the liquids with the soap.

COLORS FOR SHOW GLOBES

ANILINE COLORS

These are convenient for use in liquids for show globes and although more or less fugitive are still desirable. With a little attention in the way of adding more color from time to time, the liquids may be kept in good condition. (For a representative list of colors, see R.B., page 341.)

SHOW GLOBE SOLUTIONS

BLUE

Cupric Sulfate	30 Gm.
Sulfuric Acid	11 cc.
Distilled Water, a sufficient quantity,	
To make	1000 cc.

Dissolve the cupric sulfate in the distilled water and add the sulfuric acid. Mix.

DARK BLUE

Cupric Sulfate	10 Gm.
Diluted Solution of Ammonia*	40 cc.
Distilled Water, a sufficient quantity,	
To make	1000 cc.

Dissolve the cupric sulfate in the distilled water and add the diluted solution of ammonia and mix well.

* It may be necessary to replenish the ammonia from time to time to avoid turbidity.

GREEN
I

Cupric Sulfate	35 Gm.
Ammonium Chloride	35 Gm.
Distilled Water, a sufficient quantity,	
To make	1000 cc.

Dissolve the cupric sulfate in the distilled water. Add the ammonium chloride and shake until dissolved.

II

Nickel Nitrate	100 Gm.
Distilled Water, a sufficient quantity,	
To make	1000 cc.

Dissolve.

SEA GREEN

Cupric Acetate	4 Gm.
Acetic Acid	34 cc.
Distilled Water, a sufficient quantity,	
To make	1000 cc.

Triturate the cupric acetate with the acetic acid and dissolve in the distilled water.

GREEN, VARIOUS SHADES

Cupric Sulfate	90 Gm.
Hydrochloric Acid	69 cc.
Distilled Water, a sufficient quantity,	
To make	1000 cc.

Dissolve the cupric sulfate in the distilled water, add the hydrochloric acid and mix.

Various shades of green (permanent) may be produced by adding Solution of Ferric Chloride in varying quantities to the above.

ORANGE

Potassium Dichromate	32 Gm.
Nitric Acid	6 cc.
Distilled Water, a sufficient quantity,	
To make	1000 cc.

Dissolve the potassium dichromate in the distilled water and add the nitric acid. Mix.

PINK

Cobalt Nitrate. . . . .   40 Gm.
Nitric Acid . . . .   10 cc.
Distilled Water, a sufficient quantity,

To make . . . .   1000 cc.

Dissolve the cobalt nitrate in the distilled water and add the nitric acid. Mix.

PURPLE

Salicylic Acid . . . .   0.1 Gm.
Alcohol.   11   cc.
Diluted Solution of Ferric Chloride (1 in 5) . . . .   0.4 cc.
Distilled Water, a sufficient quantity,

To make 1000   cc.

Dissolve the salicylic acid in the alcohol, add the diluted solution of ferric chloride and sufficient distilled water to make the product measure 1000 cc.

RED

Iodine . . . .   2 Gm.
Potassium Iodide . . . .   2 Gm.
Hydrochloric Acid . . . .   31 cc.
Distilled Water, a sufficient quantity,

To make . . . .   1000 cc.

Dissolve the iodine and potassium iodide in the distilled water and add the hydrochloric acid. Mix.

YELLOW

Potassium Chromate . . . .   50 Gm.
Distilled Water, a sufficient quantity,

To make . . . .   1000 cc.

Dissolve.

FUMIGATORS

CHLORINE FUMIGATOR

Sodium Chloride, in powder. . . . .   125 Gm.
Manganese Dioxide, in powder . . . .   125 Gm.
Sulfuric Acid . . . .   150 cc.

Mix the sodium chloride and manganese dioxide and spread on a saucer, then add the sulfuric acid.

This quantity is sufficient to disinfect a room of 1000 cubic feet content. It should be tightly closed during, and for 24 hours after, the fumigation.

CAUTION—*Chlorine in the presence of moisture, is a powerful bleaching agent.*

FORMALDEHYDE FUMIGATOR

Solution of Formaldehyde. . . . .   430 cc.
Sulfuric Acid . . . .   45 cc.
Sodium Dichromate, in powder . . . .   300 Gm.

Add the acid slowly to the formaldehyde solution in small portions. Pour the mixture into a vessel containing the sodium dichromate. Because of the heat generated it is well to float this vessel in a larger one containing water.

This quantity generates sufficient gas to disinfect a room of 1000 cubic feet content. It should be tightly closed during, and for 24 hours after, the fumigation.

INCENSES

INCENSE PASTILLES

Benzoin, in moderately coarse powder . . . .   60 Gm.
Cascarilla, in moderately coarse powder. . . . .   60 Gm.
Myrrh, in moderately coarse powder . . . .   300 Gm.
Charcoal, in moderately coarse powder . . . .   360 Gm.
Oil of Myristica . . . .   15 cc.
Oil of Clove . . . .   15 cc.
Potassium Nitrate . . . .   100 Gm.
Mucilage of Tragacanth, a sufficient quantity.

Mix the first four ingredients, pass through a No. 20 sieve and incorporate the oils and potassium nitrate. Mix with just sufficient mucilage to make a stiff paste and heat on a water bath. When uniformly warmed, make into pastilles and dry.

INCENSE POWDER

I

Olibanum, in coarse powder. . . . .   700 Gm.
Benzoin, in coarse powder. . . . .   200 Gm.
Cascarilla, in coarse powder . . . .   100 Gm.
                              To make . . . .   1000 Gm.
Mix.

II

Olibanum, in coarse powder . . . .   525 Gm.
Benzoin, in coarse powder. . . . .   285 Gm.
Cascarilla, in coarse powder . . . .   142 Gm.
Potassium Nitrate, in coarse powder . . . .   48 Gm.
                              To make . . . .   1000 Gm.
Mix together on a flat surface, using a wooden spatula.

ARABIAN INCENSE POWDER

Clove, in coarse powder.	50 Gm.
Cassia Bark, in coarse powder	50 Gm.
Cascarilla, in coarse powder.	100 Gm.
Benzoin, in coarse powder.	100 Gm.
Olibanum, in coarse powder.	700 Gm.
To make	1000 Gm.

Mix.

INKS

BLACK INK

Pyrogallol.	20 Gm.
Ferrous Sulfate	16 Gm.
Sodium Sulfite.	8 Gm.
Mucilage of Acacia.	24 cc.
Water, a sufficient quantity,	
To make	1000 cc.

Dissolve the first two ingredients in 500 cc. of water, add the mucilage of acacia and mix this solution with 400 cc. of water in which the sodium sulfite has been dissolved. Add sufficient water to make the product measure 1000 cc. and mix thoroughly.

BLACK GALL INK

Nutgall, bruised	90 Gm.
Ferrous Sulfate	60 Gm.
Acacia	120 Gm.
Water, a sufficient quantity,	
To make	1000 cc.

Boil the nutgall in 600 cc. of water for 3 hours, using a copper boiler, and replacing the evaporated water from time to time. Filter, and add the acacia, dissolved in 250 cc. of water, to the filtrate. Add the ferrous sulfate, dissolved in 100 cc. of water, and sufficient water to make the product measure 1000 cc.

BLACK STENCIL INK

Amber Shellac.	166 Gm.
Sodium Borate	125 Gm.
Lampblack	83 Gm.
Acacia, in fine powder	83 Gm.
Water, a sufficient quantity,	
To make	1000 Gm.

Boil the shellac and sodium borate in the water until the resulting solution weighs 834 Gm. Incorporate gradually, the lampblack and acacia and mix thoroughly.

BLUE BLACK INK
(U. S. Public Document Ink, Permanent)
I

Tannic Acid.	23.7 Gm.
Gallic Acid	7.7 Gm.
Ferrous Sulfate	30 Gm.
Liquefied Phenol	1 cc.
Acacia, in fine powder	10 Gm.
Methylene Blue	5 Gm.
Glycerin	30 cc.
Hydrochloric Acid	12 cc.
Water, a sufficient quantity,	
To make	1000 cc.

Mix the acacia with 200 cc. of water, added gradually to make a smooth mucilage. Dissolve the tannic acid and ferrous sulfate separately in water and the gallic acid in hot water, and add these solutions to the mucilage. Shake well, add the hydrochloric acid and then the liquefied phenol dissolved in the glycerin. Add the methylene blue dissolved in water, and lastly, sufficient water to make the product measure 1000 cc.

II

Tannic Acid	11.7 Gm.
Gallic Acid	3.8 Gm.
Ferrous Sulfate, granular	15 Gm.
Hydrochloric Acid, diluted	12.5 cc.
Phenol	1 Gm.
Soluble Blue (Schultz No. 539)	3.5 Gm.
Water, a sufficient quantity,	
To make	1000 cc.

Dissolve the two acids in 400 cc. of water and the ferrous sulfate in 200 cc. of warm water. Dissolve the phenol and the dye in 200 cc. of warm water. Mix the solutions and allow to cool, make to volume and allow to stand for several days before using. Use the decanted liquid.

INDELIBLE MARKING INK

Silver Nitrate	310 Gm.
Acacia, in fine powder	186 Gm.
Lampblack	23 Gm.
Strong Solution of Ammonia, a sufficient quantity,	
To make	1000 cc.

Dissolve the acacia in 475 cc. of strong ammonia water by frequent agitation. Add this to the solution of silver nitrate in 250 cc. of strong solution of ammonia. Triturate the lampblack with this mixture, added gradually, and add sufficient strong solution of ammonia to make the product measure 1000 cc.

This ink should be used with a quill pen, and a hot iron should be drawn over the dried characters.

RED INDELIBLE MARKING INK

Silver Nitrate	66.7 Gm.
Tartaric Acid	66.7 Gm.
Diluted Solution of Ammonia	250 cc.
Acacia	100 Gm.
Sucrose	66.7 Gm.
Carmine	2.5 Gm.
Water, a sufficient quantity,	
To make	1000 cc.

Dissolve the silver nitrate and tartaric acid, each separately, in 200 cc. of water, mix the solutions and add the diluted solution of ammonia. Dissolve the acacia and sucrose in 200 cc. of water, incorporate the carmine, add the silver solution and sufficient water to make the product measure 1000 cc.

WATERPROOF INDIA INK

Lampblack	30 Gm.
Gelatin	7.5 Gm.
Potassium Dichromate	1 Gm.
Water, a sufficient quantity.	

Dissolve the gelatin in a small amount of water, warm the solution and stir in the lampblack until a smooth paste is formed. Add water in sufficient amount to make the ink of the desired fluidity. Dissolve the potassium dichromate in a small amount of water and add to the gelatin solution and mix well. Add a small amount of oil of clove or phenol to preserve the solution.

SHOW CARD INK BASE

Mucilage of Acacia	135 cc.
Alcohol	90 cc.
Oil of Clove	0.3 cc.
Mercury Bichloride	1.5 Gm.
Water, a sufficient quantity,	
To make	1000 cc.

Dissolve the mercury bichloride in 500 cc. of water, add the alcohol with which the oil of clove has been mixed, then sufficient water to make 865 cc. Add the mucilage and shake well.

Any water-soluble dye may be used with this vehicle.

STERILIZER INK

Carmine	1.5 Gm.
Silver Nitrate, in fine powder	14.5 Gm.
Potassium Bitartrate	14.5 Gm.
Strong Solution of Ammonia	58 cc.
Syrup.	7 cc.
Mucilage of Acacia, a sufficient quantity,	
To make	100 cc.

Add to the silver nitrate the carmine, previously triturated with the strong solution of ammonia until dissolved. Mix, add the potassium bitartrate and stir briskly. Add the syrup and then sufficient mucilage of acacia to make the product measure 100 cc., transfer to a bottle and shake well until thoroughly mixed.

This ink is deep purplish-red and prints light red letters.

Method of Using—Before the dressings are placed in the sterilizer, a piece of paper, upon which the date of sterilization is written with this ink, is attached and the sterilizing is conducted in the usual way. If sterilizing temperature (approximately 127° C.—20 pounds pressure) is attained, when the dressings are withdrawn, the ink, originally red, will have changed to black, indicating the completion of proper sterilizing procedure.

SYMPATHETIC OR INVISIBLE INK

Cobalt Chloride	120 Gm.
Glycerin	24 cc.
Water, a sufficient quantity,	
To make	1000 cc.

Dissolve the cobalt chloride in 500 cc. of water, add the glycerin and sufficient water to make the product measure 1000 cc.

The characters traced with this ink become blue when heated gently.

FUNGICIDES, INSECTICIDES AND RODENTICIDES

ARSENIC FLY KILLER

Molasses	100 Gm.
Sodium or Potassium Arsenite.	20 Gm.
Water, a sufficient quantity,	
To make	1000 cc.

Dissolve the arsenite in 500 cc. of hot water, add the molasses and sufficient water to make the product measure 1000 cc.

FORMALDEHYDE FLY KILLER

Solution of Formaldehyde. . . . . 35 cc.
Sucrose. . . . . 60 Gm.
Water, a sufficient quantity,

To make . . . . 1000 cc.

Dissolve.

Place in shallow dishes.

FLY REPELLENT

I

Eucalyptol . . . . 100 cc.
Oil of Bergamot . . . . 30 cc.
Ethyl Acetate . . . . 100 cc.
Cologne Water, R.B. . . . . 50 cc.
Denatured Alcohol, a sufficient quantity,

To make . . . . 1000 cc.

Mix.

II

Pyrethrum Flowers, in coarse powder. . . . . 200 Gm.
Camphor . . . . 25 Gm.
Oil of Cedar Wood. . . . . 75 cc.
Oil of Citronella . . . . 12.5 cc.
Oil of Lavender . . . . 12.5 cc.
Denatured Alcohol, a sufficient quantity,

To make . . . . 1000 cc.

Macerate the pyrethrum flowers with the alcohol for 3 or 4 days and dissolve the camphor and oils in the product; filter and add sufficient alcohol to make the product measure 1000 cc.

FLUID INSECTICIDE

Pyrethrum Flowers, in coarse powder. . . . . 100 Gm.
Kerosene . . . . 1000 cc.

To make about . . . . 1000 cc.

Macerate for 3 or 4 days, shaking occasionally. Filter.
NOTE—This liquid is inflammable.

JAPANESE BEETLE SPRAY

Sulfurated Potash . . . . 50 Gm.
Solution of Calcium Hydroxide, a sufficient quantity,

To make . . . . 1000 cc.

Dissolve.

LOUSE REPELLENT
Crude Oil Emulsion

Crude Petroleum . . . .   610 Gm.
Medicinal Soft Soap . . . .   325 Gm.
Water . . . .   65 cc.
                    To make . . . .   1000 Gm.

Triturate the soap and water to a smooth paste, and add the crude petroleum gradually.

This should be rubbed into the hair and applied to all clothing that touches the skin. As it contains a large proportion of soft soap it may be used as a detergent for washing vermin-infested clothes.

SMALL INSECT REPELLENT

Oil of Clove . . . .   125 cc.
Oil of Cinnamon . . . .   125 cc.
Oil of Cedar Wood . . . .   375 cc.
Oil of Eucalyptus, a sufficient quantity,
                    To make . . . .   1000 cc.

Mix the oils.

Use with an electrical deodorizer, or spray.

MOSQUITO REPELLENT

Oil of Citronella . . . .   32 cc.
Oil of Pennyroyal . . . .   32 cc.
Oil of Eucalyptus . . . .   64 cc.
Denatured Alcohol, a sufficient quantity,
                    To make . . . .   1000 cc.

Dissolve.

BORDEAUX MIXTURE

Cupric Sulfate . . . .   15 Gm.
Lime . . . .   10 Gm.
Water, a sufficient quantity,
                    To make . . . .   1000 cc.

Dissolve the cupric sulfate in 500 cc. of water. Slake the lime and mix it thoroughly with the remainder of the water, then add the cupric sulfate solution. Molasses or soft soap is sometimes added to increase its adhesiveness.

This mixture is used as a fungicide, as a spray for potato blight and for combating mildew on plants resistant to copper injury.

MOTH PREPARATIONS

CAPSICUM, NAPHTHALENE AND PYRETHRUM POWDER

Capsicum, in powder	100 Gm.
Naphthalene, in powder	400 Gm.
Pyrethrum Flowers, in powder	500 Gm.
To make	1000 Gm.

Mix.

CEDAR AND NAPHTHALENE POWDER

Cedar Wood, ground,
Naphthalene, in powder, of each, an equal weight.
Mix.

LAVENDER AND NAPHTHALENE POWDER

Lavender Flowers, ground	100 Gm.
Naphthalene, in powder	900 Gm.
To make	1000 Gm.

Mix.

PARADICHLOROBENZENE AND NAPHTHALENE POWDER

Paradichlorobenzene	700 Gm.
Naphthalene, in powder	300 Gm.
To make	1000 Gm.

Mix.

CEDARTINE MOTH KILLER

Oil of Cedar Wood or Oil of Cedar Leaf	50 cc.
Oil of Turpentine, a sufficient quantity,	
To make	1000 cc.

Mix.

MOTH REPELLENT
I

Camphor	10 Gm.
Naphthalene	40 Gm.
Capsicum	100 Gm.
Oil of Clove	10 cc.
Oil of Turpentine	100 cc.
Denatured Alcohol, a sufficient quantity,	
To make	1000 cc.

Macerate the solids in the mixed liquids for 48 hours, and strain.

II

Phenol	50 Gm.
Naphthalene	200 Gm.
Ethyl Acetate	50 cc.
Denatured Alcohol, a sufficient quantity,	
To make	1000 cc.

Dissolve the solids in the mixed liquids.

III

Phenol	60 Gm.
Camphor	60 Gm.
Purified Benzin, a sufficient quantity,	
To make	1000 cc.

Dissolve.

NOTE—This preparation is inflammable.

IV

Camphor	25 Gm.
Naphthalene	50 Gm.
Nitrobenzene	10 cc.
Denatured Alcohol	815 cc.
Oil of Turpentine, a sufficient quantity,	
To make	1000 cc.

Dissolve the camphor and naphthalene in the mixed liquids.

V

Phenol	10 Gm.
Camphor	30 Gm.
Carbon Tetrachloride	500 cc.
Purified Benzin, a sufficient quantity,	
To make	1000 cc.

Dissolve the camphor and phenol in the mixed liquids.

NOTE—This preparation is inflammable.

MOTH POWDER

White Pepper, in powder	100 Gm.
Camphor, in fine powder	200 Gm.
Pyrethrum Flowers, in powder	350 Gm.
Naphthalene, in fine powder	350 Gm.
To make	1000 Gm.

Mix.

ROACH POWDER

Sodium Fluoride	40 Gm.
Sodium Borate	40 Gm.
Starch	10 Gm.
Cocoa	10 Gm.
To make	100 Gm.

Powder the ingredients finely and mix well.

CAUTION—*This preparation must be used with care due to its poisonous nature.*

ROACH SPRAY
I

Paradichlorobenzene	50 Gm.
Cresylic Acid	250 cc.
Kerosene, a sufficient quantity,	
To make	1000 cc.

Dissolve.

NOTE—This liquid is inflammable.

II

Cresylic Acid	200 cc.
Kerosene, a sufficient quantity,	
To make	1000 cc.

Mix.

NOTE—This liquid is inflammable.

III

Paradichlorobenzene	100 Gm.
Methyl Salicylate	20 cc.
Kerosene, a sufficient quantity,	
To make	1000 cc.

Dissolve the paradichlorobenzene in the mixed liquids.

NOTE—This liquid is inflammable.

RAT POISONS

(Fish and Wildlife Service)

CAUTION—*In distributing any of these poisons, great care must be exercised to prevent possible injury to other animals or to small children.*

PLAIN BAIT

Bread Crumbs	80 Gm.
Peanut Butter	10 Gm.
Creamed Cheese or Black Strap Molasses, a sufficient quantity,	
To make	100 Gm.

Mix the bread crumbs with the peanut butter and add the creamed cheese or black strap molasses.

POISONED BAIT NO. 1

Red Squill, powdered	10 Gm.
Plain Bait, R.B., a sufficient quantity,	
To make	100 Gm.

Mix.

POISONED BAIT NO. 2

Thallium Sulfate	2 Gm.
Plain Bait, R.B., a sufficient quantity,	
To make	100 Gm.

Mix.

POISONED BAIT NO. 3

Barium Carbonate	20 Gm.
Plain Bait, R.B., a sufficient quantity,	
To make	100 Gm.

Mix.

POISONED BAIT NO. 4

Arsenous Oxide	2.5 Gm.
Plain Bait, R.B., a sufficient quantity,	
To make	100 Gm.

Mix.

CAUTION—*All poisoned baits must be thoroughly mixed and adequately labeled.*

LAUNDRY ACCESSORIES

CLEANING FLUIDS

CAUTION—*The use of these preparations without proper ventilation must be avoided.*

BIJOU CLEANING FLUID

Methyl Salicylate	8 cc.
Chloroform	160 cc.
Ethyl Oxide	80 cc.
Purified Benzin, a sufficient quantity,	
To make	1000 cc.

Mix.

NOTE—This mixture is inflammable.

CLEAN-ALL

Ethyl Oxide	250 cc.
Strong Solution of Ammonia	250 cc.
Oil of Turpentine	250 cc.
Denatured Alcohol	250 cc.
To make	1000 cc.

Mix the ethyl oxide, oil of turpentine and denatured alcohol, then add the strong solution of ammonia.

NOTE—This liquid is inflammable.

TETRAZINE CLEANER

Purified Benzin,	
Carbon Tetrachloride, of each	500 cc.

Mix the liquids.

HATTER'S CLEANING FLUID

Benzol,
Acetone,
Ethylene Dichloride, of each, an equal volume.

Mix.

NOTE—This liquid is inflammable.

IRON-RUST STAIN REMOVER

Cream of Tartar	350 Gm.
Potassium Binoxalate, powdered	350 Gm.
Oil of Lemon	1 cc.

Mix the powders well and incorporate the oil of lemon.

Rub the moistened spot with the powder.

WATER-SOFTENERS

Certain waters fail to produce a lather with soap because they contain dissolved salts which react with the soap and render it insoluble. Such waters are said to be "hard." This hardness may be only "temporary," in which case it can be corrected by boiling, or it may be "permanent" and requires the addition of certain chemicals, like washing soda, borax, ammonia and sodium phosphate for its correction. Such chemicals are called "water-softeners" since they precipitate the dissolved salts which cause the hardness and enable the water to lather well with soap. One of the best water-softeners for general use is tribasic sodium phosphate. The following mixture has also been used as a water-softener.

Calcium Hydroxide. . . . . 100 Gm.
Anhydrous Sodium Carbonate . . . . 200 Gm.

Reduce the two ingredients to a fine powder and mix them.

Earthy materials specially treated, and known as Zeolites, have the property of removing hardness from water by a process of base exchange, generally substituting sodium for the calcium or magnesium. Elaborate installations such as the Permutit use this method and the process is cyclic, since the Zeolite can be continuously revivified with brine.

Many of the modern and most effective water-softeners contain sodium hexametaphosphate or tetra-sodium pyrophosphate as sequesterers for alkali earth metals.

FIREPROOFING SOLUTION FOR FABRICS

Sodium Borate . . . . 160 Gm.
Magnesium Sulfate. . . . . 120 Gm.
Water, a sufficient quantity,

To make . . . . 1000 cc.

Dissolve.

Immerse the fabric in this solution and wring it out.

SCHWEITZER'S REAGENT (TEST FOR WOOL)

Copper Sulfate . . . . 10 Gm.
Sodium Hydroxide . . . . 4 Gm.
Solution of Ammonia, 20 per cent . . . . 20 cc.
Water, a sufficient quantity.

Dissolve the copper sulfate in 100 cc. of water; add the sodium hydroxide dissolved in 50 cc. of water. Collect the precipitate and wash it with water. Allow to drain and dissolve the precipitate in the ammonia water, 20%, by shaking occasionally during a period of 24 hours.

NOTE—This solution dissolves silk, cotton and linen but will *not dissolve wool*.

ODORIZERS

ODORIZER FOR SICK ROOM

Coumarin.	5 Gm.
Oil of Lavender	6 cc.
Oil of Bitter Almond	12 cc.
Oil of Clove	35 cc.
Oil of Patchouli	2 cc.
Oil of Eucalyptus, a sufficient quantity,	
To make	1000 cc.

Dissolve the coumarin in the mixed oils.

Use as a spray.

PINE OIL ODORIZER

Oil of Dwarf Pine Needles	666 Gm.
Rosin.	266 Gm.
Sodium Hydroxide.	34 Gm.
Water	34 cc.
To make about	1000 Gm.

Melt the rosin and add to it the oil, adjusting the temperature to about 80° C. Then pour in the solution of sodium hydroxide in the water, heated to about 80° C., stirring briskly until the mixture is uniform.

PAINTS AND LACQUERS

BRONZING LIQUID

Fuchsin.	100 Gm.
Crystal Violet.	50 Gm.
Benzoic Acid	50 Gm.
Denatured Alcohol, a sufficient quantity,	
To make	1000 cc.

Dissolve the fuchsin and crystal violet in the alcohol, then add the benzoic acid and boil the mixture for a few minutes, or until the color changes to bronze-brown.

GOLD LACQUER

Shellac.	125 Gm.
Dragon's Blood	15 Gm.
Turmeric.	8 Gm.
Denatured Alcohol, a sufficient quantity,	
To make	1000 cc.

Mix, digest the mixture for a week at about 38° C. and filter.

LUMINOUS PAINT POWDER
Lennard's Compound

Strontium Carbonate	496.5 Gm.
Sublimed Sulfur	496.5 Gm.
Sodium Chloride	2.5 Gm.
Potassium Chloride	2.5 Gm.
Manganese Chloride	2 Gm.
To make	1000 Gm.

Mix, and heat the mixture to whiteness for half an hour.

This emits a golden-yellow light.

PAINT SOLUTION FOR LABELING BOTTLES

Gentian Violet	0.3 Gm.
White Shellac	25 Gm.
Alcohol, a sufficient quantity,	
To make	100 cc.

Shake thoroughly until dissolved.

For use, apply with either a very fine brush or a toothpick.

PAINT REMOVER
I

Potassium Hydroxide	165 Gm.
Denatured Alcohol	165 cc.
Oil of Turpentine	165 cc.
Gasoline	165 cc.
Castor Oil	85 cc.
Acetone, a sufficient quantity,	
To make	1000 cc.

Dissolve the potassium hydroxide in 300 cc. of acetone, add the other liquids and then sufficient acetone to make the product measure 1000 cc. Mix by shaking.

Make two applications of this liquid to the painted surface, a few minutes apart, then remove the paint with a blunt spatula.

II

Castor Oil	5 cc.
Benzene	500 cc.
Acetone	300 cc.
Denatured Alcohol, a sufficient quantity,	
To make	1000 cc.

Mix.

POLISHES

FURNITURE POLISH

I

Linseed Oil, boiled	300 cc.
Glacial Acetic Acid	100 cc.
Oil of Turpentine	600 cc.
To make	1000 cc.

Add the glacial acetic acid to the boiled linseed oil and shake well, add the oil of turpentine and shake again.

II

Linseed Oil, boiled	550 cc.
Denatured Alcohol	138 cc.
Oil of Turpentine	138 cc.
Saturated Solution of Antimony Chloride	36 cc.
Diluted Acetic Acid	138 cc.
To make	1000 cc.

Mix, adding the solution of antimony chloride last.

LINOLEUM POLISH

I

Light

White Ceresin	140 Gm.
Paraffin	280 Gm.
Oil of Turpentine	480 cc.
Purified Benzin	100 cc.
To make about	1000 Gm.

Melt the ceresin and paraffin with the aid of gentle heat. After extinguishing all open flames, incorporate the oil of turpentine and purified benzin in the mixture while still warm.

II

Dark

Yellow Ceresin	185 Gm.
Paraffin	115 Gm.
Linseed Oil, boiled	65 cc.
Oil of Turpentine	625 cc.
Nitrobenzene	10 cc.
To make about	1000 Gm.

Melt the ceresin and paraffin with the aid of gentle heat; while still warm incorporate the oils and nitrobenzene.

DRESSING FOR LEATHER BOOKS

Yellow Wax	29 Gm.
Oil of Lavender	14 cc.
Oil of Cedar Wood	60 cc.
Wool Fat	350 Gm.
Neatsfoot Oil, a sufficient quantity,	
To make	1000 Gm.

Melt the yellow wax with the wool fat, allow to cool and add the oils and mix well.

METAL POLISH
I

Red Iron Oxide, in very fine powder	312 Gm.
Pumice, in very fine powder	412 Gm.
Oleic Acid	82 Gm.
Benzin Soap, R.B.	182 Gm.
Nitrobenzene	12 cc.
To make about	1000 Gm.

Triturate the solids with the oleic acid, and incorporate the nitrobenzene and benzin soap.

II

Prepared Chalk	310 Gm.
Linseed Oil, boiled	180 cc.
Diluted Solution of Ammonia	120 cc.
Denatured Alcohol	130 cc.
Carbon Tetrachloride	260 cc.
To make about	1000 Gm.

Saponify the linseed oil with the diluted solution of ammonia and mix with the prepared chalk to make a smooth paste. Add gradually the denatured alcohol and carbon tetrachloride, previously mixed, and triturate to make a cream.

POLISHING POWDER FOR METALS
I

Siliceous Earth	265 Gm.
Red Iron Oxide	265 Gm.
Precipitated Calcium Carbonate	132 Gm.
Citric Acid	132 Gm.
Alum	132 Gm.
Purified Talc	74 Gm.
To make	1000 Gm.

Mix and triturate to a fine powder.

II

Prepared Chalk, in impalpable powder . . . .   475 Gm.
Kaolin, in impalpable powder . . . .   190 Gm.
Lead Carbonate, in impalpable powder . . . .   235 Gm.
Magnesium Carbonate, in impalpable powder . . . .   50 Gm.
Red Iron Oxide, in impalpable powder . . . .   50 Gm.
                              To make . . . .   1000 Gm.
  Mix intimately.

III

Ferric Oxide, in fine powder. . . . .   5 Gm.
Sodium Thiosulfate, in fine powder. . . . .   7 Gm.
Pipe Clay. . . . .   23 Gm.
Siliceous Earth . . . .   65 Gm.
                              To make . . . .   100 Gm.
  Mix the sodium thiosulfate with the ferric oxide.   Add the pipe clay and siliceous earth and mix well.

STAINS

EBONY STAIN FOR WOOD

A

Sodium Dichromate . . . .   100 Gm.
Water, a sufficient quantity,
                              To make . . . .   1000 cc.
  Dissolve.

B

Gallic Acid . . . .   11.5 Gm.
Water, a sufficient quantity,
                              To make . . . .   1000 cc.
  Dissolve.

  Smooth the wood with sandpaper and brush over it the hot solution A sparingly, so as not to leave any salt on the surface.   When dry apply the hot solution B in the same manner.   Repeat these two operations until the desired degree of blackness is obtained.   A dull ebony finish is obtained by rubbing with a rag and a trace of linseed oil; a bright surface may be produced by varnish.

LABORATORY DESK STAIN, BLACK

A

Cupric Sulfate.	125 Gm.
Potassium Chlorate.	125 Gm.
Water, a sufficient quantity,	
To make	1000 cc.

Dissolve the salts in boiling water.

A (Alternative)

Ferrous Sulfate	40 Gm.
Cupric Sulfate.	40 Gm.
Potassium Permanganate	80 Gm.
Water, a sufficient quantity,	
To make	1000 cc.

Dissolve the salts in boiling water.

B

Aniline	120 cc.
Hydrochloric Acid	180 cc.
Water, a sufficient quantity,	
To make	1000 cc.

Dissolve.

C

Linseed Oil, boiled.

Apply solution A boiling hot, and a second coat 24 hours later. When the boards have dried apply solution B and allow the stain to dry thoroughly. Sandpaper lightly and brush clean. The surface will now have a green tinge which upon vigorous rubbing with C will turn jet black.

The above quantities are sufficient for a surface of 75 square feet.

DESK STAIN RESISTANT TO CHEMICALS

Furfuryl Alcohol, a sufficient quantity,
Hydrochloric Acid, 15%, a sufficient quantity,
Linseed or China Wood Oil, a sufficient quantity.

Paint or spray a liberal amount of the furfuryl alcohol on the smooth clean wooden surface. After this application dries, apply the hydrochloric acid with a brush. The surface will gradually darken and become black. Apply as many coats as are desired and then buff and polish after several applications of the oil have been applied.

STAIN REMOVERS

IODINE STAIN REMOVER

Sodium Thiosulfate. . . . . 10 Gm.
Distilled Water, a sufficient quantity,
To make . . . . 100 cc.

Dissolve.

This may be applied to linen, etc., to remove an iodine stain completely.

FOR REMOVING MERCUROCHROME STAINS FROM COLORLESS COTTON OR LINEN CLOTH

A

Solution of Sodium Hypochlorite . . . . 10 cc.
Water . . . . 90 cc.
To make . . . . 100 cc.

Mix.

B

Diluted Acetic Acid . . . . 20 cc.

Soak the material in solution A for 2 minutes. Without taking out the fabric add solution B and mix thoroughly, agitating the cloth to hasten removal of the stain, which should take about 1 minute. Wash the material thoroughly in hot water.

MISCELLANEOUS FORMULAS

BLACK DYE FOR SILKWORM GUT SUTURE

Extract of Hematoxylon, R.B.. . . . . 20 Gm.
Cupric Sulfate. . . . . 8 Gm.
Water, a sufficient quantity,
To make . . . . 1000 cc.

Dissolve the extract of hematoxylon in 500 cc. of water and the cupric sulfate in 400 cc. of water. Mix the liquids and add sufficient water to make the product measure 1000 cc.

For use, first boil the white silkworm gut in sterile water for 30 minutes, and after bringing the dye to the boiling point, add the gut and boil for 5 minutes.

EXTINGUISHER FOR GASOLINE AND OIL FIRES

Sodium Bicarbonate	800 Gm.
Purified Talc	150 Gm.
Sodium Chloride	50 Gm.
To make	1000 Gm.

Mix.

A handful should be thrown with some force against the fire.

FERTILIZERS FOR POTTED PLANTS
I

Sodium Chloride	435 Gm.
Potassium Nitrate	218 Gm.
Magnesium Sulfate	218 Gm.
Magnesium Oxide	43 Gm.
Sodium Phosphate	86 Gm.
To make	1000 Gm.

Mix.

A teaspoonful in a quart of water makes a nutrient wash for ferns and other plants. It should be sprayed on the leaves by a sprinkler.

II

Ammonium Nitrate	220 Gm.
Potassium Phosphate	280 Gm.
Sodium Nitrate	500 Gm.
To make	1000 Gm.

Mix.

A teaspoonful is dissolved in a quart of water for watering the plants.

III

Ammonium Nitrate	335 Gm.
Ammonium Phosphate	165 Gm.
Potassium Nitrate	210 Gm.
Ammonium Chloride	40 Gm.
Calcium Sulfate	50 Gm.
Ferrous Sulfate	200 Gm.
To make	1000 Gm.

Mix.

For use, add about half a teaspoonful to a quart of water and spray with a sprinkler.

IV

Potassium Nitrate	220 Gm.
Potassium Phosphate.	280 Gm.
Ammonium Sulfate.	110 Gm.
Ammonium Nitrate	390 Gm.
To make	1000 Gm.

Mix.

For use, add a teaspoonful to a quart of water.

This mixture is to be used when leaf growth is deficient; if flowers are specially desired, do not add the last ingredient.

ROOTING MIXTURE FOR CONIFERS, RHODODENDRONS AND HOLLY

Indole-Butyric Acid	0.12 Gm.
Purified Talc, a sufficient quantity,	
To make	10 Gm.

Mix well by trituration.

For use, moisten the ends of the cuttings and dip into the rooting mixture prior to planting.

SOLUTION OF THIAMIN HYDROCHLORIDE AS A PLANT STIMULANT
(Boyce Thompson Institute)

Thiamin Hydrochloride	0.1 Gm.
Water, a sufficient quantity,	
To make	100 cc.

Dissolve.

For watering plants, use 1 drop of the solution per gallon of water.

For root shock in transplanting, use 15 drops of solution per quart of water and allow the plants to stand in this solution for 15 minutes before planting.

LABEL VARNISH
I

White Shellac	300 Gm.
Copaiba.	30 Gm.
Venice Turpentine	6 Gm.
Denatured Alcohol, a sufficient quantity,	
To make	1000 cc.

Dissolve the first three ingredients in the denatured alcohol by stirring continuously, then strain the solution.

II

Collodion	50	cc.
Camphor	0.8	Gm.
Ethyl Oxide	21.5	cc.
Denatured Alcohol, a sufficient quantity,		
To make	100	cc.

Dissolve the camphor in 10 cc. of alcohol and the collodion in a mixture of the ethyl oxide and 35 cc. of alcohol. Mix the solutions and add sufficient alcohol to make the product measure 100 cc.

III

Copal	24 Gm.
Ethyl Oxide	35 cc.
Acetone	35 cc.
Alcohol, a sufficient quantity,	
To make	100 cc.

Dissolve the copal in the mixed liquids.

QUICK DRYING LABEL VARNISH

Vinyl Resin	18 Gm.
Methylisobutyl Ketone	41 Gm.
Toluene	41 Gm.

Mix the solvents thoroughly and then pour on the resin in a suitable vessel and stir until dissolved, avoiding excessive evaporation. The varnish may be thinned or thickened by increasing or decreasing the amount of the mixed solvents.

LIQUID CELLULOID FOR CAPPINGS

Boric Acid	1 Gm.
Rosin	25 Gm.
Ethyl Oxide	10 cc.
Aniline Dye for Color (red, green, etc.), as desired,	
Collodion, a sufficient quantity,	
To make	100 cc.

Mix and allow to stand with occasional agitation to complete solution.

SEALING WAX

Amber Shellac	500 Gm.
Venice Turpentine	125 Gm.
Red Mercury Sulfide	375 Gm.
To make	1000 Gm.

Melt the shellac and add the Venice turpentine slowly. Incorporate the red mercury sulfide while stirring vigorously. Pour the molten mass into suitable molds and allow to solidify.

STOPCOCK GREASE—For General Use

Crepe Rubber . . . . 51.5 Gm.
Petrolatum . . . . 40 Gm.
Paraffin . . . . 8.5 Gm.

Melt the petrolatum and paraffin together and to the warm mixture add the rubber. It may be necessary to apply additional heat in order to make a uniform mixture.

STOPCOCK GREASE—For High Vacuum

Crepe Rubber . . . . 43 Gm.
Petrolatum . . . . 50 Gm.
Paraffin . . . . 7 Gm.

Melt the petrolatum and paraffin together and add the rubber to the warm mixture. It may be necessary to apply additional heat in order to make a uniform mixture.

SOLUTION FOR REMOVING GLASS STOPPERS

Chloral Hydrate . . . . 55 Gm.
Glycerin . . . . 22 cc.
Hydrochloric Acid . . . . 27 cc.
Water, a sufficient quantity,

To make . . . . 100 cc.

Dissolve the chloral hydrate in 20 cc. of water, add the glycerin and hydrochloric acid and sufficient water to make the product measure 100 cc.

Apply a few drops of the solution around the neck of the glass stopper. Allow it to spread and remain until the stopper can be removed by gentle rotation, or tapping, if necessary, with a light wooden mallet.

SPONGE BLEACH

A

Potassium Permanganate . . . . 1 Gm.
Hydrochloric Acid . . . . 8 cc.
Water, a sufficient quantity,

To make . . . . 1000 cc.

Dissolve the potassium permanganate in the water, add the hydrochloric acid and mix.

B

Potassium Carbonate. . . . . 62 Gm.
Water, a sufficient quantity,

　　　　　　To make . . . . 1000 cc.

Dissolve.

Immerse the sponges in solution A for a few minutes, then remove, press and wash them with cold water.　Finally soak the sponges in solution B, and rinse again several times in cold water.

ANTI-FREEZING SOLUTIONS FOR AUTOMOBILE RADIATORS

Many liquids have been suggested for this purpose, among the most satisfactory being the alcohols—denatured alcohol, wood alcohol, glycerin and ethylene glycol. All of these are miscible with water in all proportions and the addition of one of them to water considerably lowers its freezing point.　Solutions of inorganic salts should never be used for this purpose under any circumstances.

The following table has been compiled from information obtained from the United States Bureau of Standards.　It shows the quantities of alcohols required for protection at various temperatures, and also the specific gravities of the solutions so that it may be determined whether any alcohol, water, etc., has boiled off and needs to be replaced.

If the capacity of the radiator is known it can easily be calculated from the table how much of any alcohol is needed for protection at any given temperature.

Alcohol	For Protection at ° F.	Percentage by Volume	Pints to 1 Gallon of Water	Specific Gravity 60° F./60° F.
Denatured Alcohol (94% by volume)	+10°	29	3.3	0.968
	0°	37	4.7	0.959
	−10°	43	6.0	0.950
	−20°	49	7.7	0.942
	−30°	59	11.5	0.921
Wood Alcohol (97% by volume)	+10°	20	2.0	0.975
	0°	28	3.1	0.966
	−10°	35	4.3	0.958
	−20°	40	5.3	0.952
	−30°	45	6.5	0.945
Glycerin (95% by weight)	+10°	32	3.8	1.090
	0°	40	5.3	1.112
	−10°	47	7.1	1.131
	−20°	53	9.0	1.147
	−30°	57	10.6	1.158
Ethylene Glycol (95% by weight)	+10°	25	2.7	1.038
	0°	33	4.0	1.048
	−10°	39	5.1	1.056
	−20°	45	6.5	1.064
	−30°	50	8.0	1.069

FACTORY FIRST-AID OUTFITS

In a large number of states equipment of factories, workshops, etc., with First Aid Outfits is required by law. For example, the Industrial Code of the Department of Labor of the State of New York requires that in every factory employing more than 10 persons, in which power machinery is used, there shall be provided a First Aid Cabinet accessible at all times. The contents of the cabinet under these regulations are as follows:

Instruments

1 pair of scissors.
Thumb forceps.
Tourniquet.
Graduated medicine glass.

Drugs

2 oz. aromatic spirit of ammonia.
2 oz. 4 per cent boric acid solution.
2 oz. mild tincture of iodine.
2 (3 oz.) collapsible tubes of bicarbonate of soda (3 per cent), mixed with petrolatum (for burns).
2 oz. castor oil (for eye injuries).

Dressings

1 doz. assorted sizes, sterile gauze bandages.
1 spool of zinc oxide adhesive plaster, 1 inch by 5 yards.
3 (½ oz.) packages of absorbent cotton.
3 (1 yard) packages of sterile gauze.
Splints of assorted sizes for fractures.
Wooden applicators wound with cotton.
Wooden tongue depressors.

The Liability Insurance Acts of many states likewise require the installation of a First Aid Kit or Outfit; one containing the following articles has been stated to be suitable for factories employing 50 to 100 persons:

Instruments

1 pair of scissors.
3 pairs of splinter forceps.
Tourniquet.
Graduated medicine glass.
Medicine dropper.

Drugs

2 oz. (or a minimum of 10 ampuls) aromatic spirit of ammonia.

2 oz. 4 per cent boric acid solution.

2 oz. (or a minimum of 18 ampuls) iodine solution, $3\frac{1}{2}\%$ (for external use).

2 collapsible tubes (3 oz. each) petrolatum with 3 per cent sodium bicarbonate.

2 oz. castor oil (for eye injuries).

2 collapsible tubes (2 oz. each) tannic acid jelly.

Dressings

1 doz. assorted sizes, sterile gauze bandages.

3 assorted sizes, sterile muslin bandages.

2 triangular bandages.

3 (1 yard) packages of sterile gauze.

6 finger cots, assorted sizes.

1 spool zinc oxide adhesive plaster, 1 inch by 5 yards.

4 packages ($\frac{1}{2}$ oz.) absorbent cotton.

1 package ($\frac{1}{4}$ lb.) absorbent cotton.

4 wooden splints, assorted sizes, for fractures.

1 wire splint.

1 doz. wooden applicators wound with cotton.

1 doz. tongue depressors.

1 doz. assorted sizes, safety pins.

1 cake germicidal soap.

PART VI

AVERAGE DOSES OF UNOFFICIAL DRUGS†

	Metric		Apothecaries
Absinthium	2	Gm.	30 grains
Acid Acetyltannic	0.6	Gm.	10 grains
Acid Bromauric	0.006	Gm.	⅒ grain
Acid Cacodylic	0.06	Gm.	1 grain
Acid Camphoric	0.5	Gm.	8 grains
Acid Cinnamic	0.15	Gm.	2½ grains
Acid Nucleic	0.125	Gm.	2 grains
Acid Oxalic	0.03	Gm.	½ grain
Acid Sulfuric Aromatic	0.5	cc.	8 minims
Acid Sulphanilic	0.6	Gm.	10 grains
Acid Iso-Valeric	0.2	cc.	3 minims
Aconitine, Crystalline	0.00015	Gm.	¼₀₀ grain
Agaric	0.6	Gm.	10 grains
Albumin Tannate	2	Gm.	30 grains
Althea Leaves	2	Gm.	30 grains
Amiodoxyl Benzoate* (Ammonium orthoiodoxy-benzoate)	0.75	Gm.	12 grains
Ammoniac	1	Gm.	15 grains
Ammonium Benzoate	1	Gm.	15 grains
Ammonium Camphorate	0.06	Gm.	1 grain
Ammonium Phosphate	0 3	Gm.	5 grains
Amphotropin (Hexamethylenetetramine camphorate)	0.5	Gm.	8 grains
Iso-Amyl Salicylate	0.2	cc.	3 minims
Iso-Amyl Iso-Valerate	0.2	cc.	3 minims
Angelica Fruit	1	Gm.	15 grains
Angelica Root	2	Gm.	30 grains
Aniline Sulfate	0.06	Gm.	1 grain
Anthemis	2	Gm.	30 grains
Antimony Arsenate	0.00125	Gm.	¹⁄₅₀ grain
Antimony Iodide	0.015	Gm.	¼ grain
Antimony Oxide	0.06	Gm.	1 grain
Antimony Sodium Thioglycollate	0.06	Gm.	1 grain
Antimony, Sulfurated	0.06	Gm.	1 grain
Antimony Thioglycollamide**	0.08	Gm.	1⅓ grains

†NOTE—The doses given are average doses. The Association does not assume legal responsibility for them. Doses marked * are intravenous doses; those marked ** are intramuscular doses; those marked *** are subcutaneous doses. Doses not marked are doses for administration by mouth.

		Metric		Apothecaries
Arbutin		0.2	Gm.	3 grains
Arsenous Bromide		0.002	Gm.	1/30 grain
Asclepias		2	Gm.	30 grains
Aspidosperma		4	Gm.	60 grains
Baptisia		1	Gm.	15 grains
Barium Chloride		0.03	Gm.	1/2 grain
Barium Iodide		0.008	Gm.	1/8 grain
Bayberry Bark		0.5	Gm.	8 grains
Benzanilid		0.6	Gm.	10 grains
Benzene, Medicinal		0.5	cc.	8 minims
Benzosalin (Methylbenzoylsalicylate)		0.5	Gm.	8 grains
Benzyl Benzoate		0.3	cc.	5 minims
Benzyl Fumarate		0.3	Gm.	5 grains
Benzyl Succinate		0.6	Gm.	10 grains
Berberine Salts	Tonic	0.03	Gm.	1/2 grain
	Antiperiodic	0.6	Gm.	10 grains
Betaine Hydrochloride (Trimethylglycine hydrochloride)		0.5	Gm.	8 grains
Betanaphthol Benzoate		0.25	Gm.	4 grains
Betanaphthol Salicylate		0.3	Gm.	5 grains
Bismuth Benzoate		0.5	Gm.	8 grains
Bismuth Betanaphthol		0.5	Gm.	8 grains
Bismuth Citrate		0.125	Gm.	2 grains
Bismuth Ditannate		0.5	Gm.	8 grains
Bismuth Dithiosalicylate		0.3	Gm.	5 grains
Bismuth Oxide		0.3	Gm.	5 grains
Bismuth Phosphate, Soluble		0.3	Gm.	5 grains
Bismuth, Resorcinated		0.3	Gm.	5 grains
Bismuth Sodium Tartrate**		0.03	Gm.	1/2 grain
Bismuth Tribromphenate (1-3 Gm. per day)		0.5	Gm.	8 grains
Bismuth Valerate		0.03	Gm.	1/2 grain
Bismuth and Ammonium Citrate		0.125	Gm.	2 grains
Boldo		0.5	Gm.	8 grains
Brayera		15	Gm.	4 drachms
Bromoform		0.2	cc.	3 minims
Butylchloral Hydrate		0.3	Gm.	5 grains
Caffeine Hydrobromide		0.125	Gm.	2 grains
Caffeine Hydrochloride		0.125	Gm.	2 grains
Caffeine Salicylate		0.125	Gm.	2 grains
Caffeine Sulfate		0.125	Gm.	2 grains
Caffeine Triiodide		0.125	Gm.	2 grains
Calcium Acetylsalicylate		0.6	Gm.	10 grains
Calcium Bromide		1	Gm.	15 grains
Calcium Cacodylate**		0.045	Gm.	3/4 grain
Calcium Formate		0.3	Gm.	5 grains
Calcium Hydrochlorophosphate		0.06	Gm.	1 grain

	Metric		Apothecaries
Calcium Iodate	0.2	Gm.	3 grains
Calcium Lactophosphate	0.5	Gm.	8 grains
Calcium Permanganate	0.03	Gm.	$\frac{1}{2}$ grain
Calcium Peroxide	0.2	Gm.	3 grains
Calcium Phenolsulfonate	0.5	Gm.	8 grains
Calcium Saccharate	1	Gm.	15 grains
Calcium Santoninate	0.06	Gm.	1 grain
Calcium Sulfide	0.06	Gm.	1 grain
Canella	2	Gm.	30 grains
Cantharidin	0.0003	Gm.	$\frac{1}{200}$ grain
Cascara Amarga	1	Gm.	15 grains
Cascarilla	2	Gm.	30 grains
Cassia Fistula	4	Gm.	60 grains
Castor	0.6	Gm.	10 grains
Centaury	2	Gm.	30 grains
Cerebrin (Dried brain substance)	0.75	Gm.	12 grains
Cesium and Ammonium Bromide	1	Gm.	15 grains
Cevadilla	0.3	Gm.	5 grains
Chelidonium	2	Gm.	30 grains
Chenopodium	2	Gm.	30 grains
Chinoidin (Quinoidin)	0.5	Gm.	8 grains
Chirata	1	Gm.	15 grains
Cinchonidine Salicylate	0.2	Gm.	3 grains
Cinnamaldehyde	0.05	cc.	$\frac{3}{4}$ minim
Coca	2	Gm.	30 grains
Cocillana	1	Gm.	15 grains
Coffee	2	Gm.	30 grains
Coniine Hydrobromide	0.001	Gm.	$\frac{1}{60}$ grain
Conium	0.2	Gm.	3 grains
Copper Acetate	0.008	Gm.	$\frac{1}{8}$ grain
Copper Arsenite	0.0006	Gm.	$\frac{1}{100}$ grain
Copper Oxide, Black	0.06	Gm.	1 grain
Coptis	2	Gm.	30 grains
Cornus	2	Gm.	30 grains
Creosote Phosphate (6–8 Gm. per day)	2	cc.	30 minims
Creosote Valerate	0.3	cc.	5 minims
Cumin	1	Gm.	15 grains
Cusparia	1	Gm.	15 grains
Cypripedium	1	Gm.	15 grains
Diacetylmorphine Hydrochloride	0.003	Gm.	$\frac{1}{20}$ grain
Diastase	0.5	Gm.	8 grains
Digipoten	0.1	Gm.	$1\frac{1}{2}$ grains
Digitalein, Crude	0.001	Gm.	$\frac{1}{60}$ grain
Digitalin, French	0.00025	Gm.	$\frac{1}{240}$ grain
Digitalin, German	0.006	Gm.	$\frac{1}{10}$ grain
Drosera	4	Gm.	60 grains

		Metric	Apothecaries
Dulcamara	4	Gm.	60 grains
Elaterin	0.003	Gm.	$\frac{1}{20}$ grain
Emetine Bismuth Iodide	0.2	Gm.	3 grains
Ergotin	0.2	Gm.	3 grains
Ergotinine Citrate	0.0004	Gm.	$\frac{1}{150}$ grain
Ethylene Bromide	0.12	cc.	2 minims
Ethyl Iodide (Inhalation)	1.0	cc.	16 minims
Ethyl Salicylate	0.5	cc.	8 minims
Ethyl Valerate	0.06	cc.	1 minim
Eucalyptus	2	Gm.	30 grains
Eucalyptus Gum	0.6	Gm.	10 grains
Farfara	4	Gm.	60 grains
Fraxinus	2	Gm.	30 grains
Fucus	0.6	Gm.	10 grains
Galangal	1	Gm.	15 grains
Galbanum	0.6	Gm.	10 grains
Galega	4	Gm.	60 grains
Garlic	2	Gm.	30 grains
Gelseminine salts	0.0006	Gm.	$\frac{1}{100}$ grain
Geranium	1	Gm.	15 grains
Glycosal	0.5	Gm.	8 grains
Glycyrrhizin, Ammoniated	0.25	Gm.	4 grains
Gold Tribromide	0.008	Gm.	$\frac{1}{8}$ grain
Gold Trichloride	0.006	Gm.	$\frac{1}{10}$ grain
Gold and Potassium Cyanide	0.03	Gm.	$\frac{1}{2}$ grain
Gold Iodide	0.006	Gm.	$\frac{1}{10}$ grain
Gold Oxide	0.01	Gm.	$\frac{1}{6}$ grain
Gold Sodium Chloride	0.005	Gm.	$\frac{1}{12}$ grain
Guaiacol Phosphate	0.2	Gm.	3 grains
Guaiacol Salicylate	1	Gm.	15 grains
Guaiacol Valerate	0.3	cc.	5 minims
Hedeoma	8	Gm.	120 grains
Helianthemum	4	Gm.	60 grains
Helmitol	0.6	Gm.	10 grains
Hematoxylon	2	Gm.	30 grains
Hydrastinine Hydrochloride	0.03	Gm.	$\frac{1}{2}$ grain
Hydroquinone	0.3	Gm.	5 grains
Hyoscyamine Hydrobromide	0.0006	Gm.	$\frac{1}{100}$ grain
Hyssop	2	Gm.	30 grains
Ignatia	0.1	Gm.	$1\frac{1}{2}$ grains
Inula	2	Gm.	30 grains
Iodized Starch	4	Gm.	60 grains
Iodo-casein	0.6	Gm.	10 grains

	Metric		Apothecaries
Iron Acetate, Basic, Ferric	0.125	Gm.	2 grains
Iron, Albuminized	0.5	Gm.	8 grains
Iron Arsenate, Ferrous	0.006	Gm.	$\frac{1}{10}$ grain
Iron Arsenite and Ammonium Citrate,** Ferric	0.03	Gm.	$\frac{1}{2}$ grain
Iron Benzoate, Ferric	0.125	Gm.	2 grains
Iron Bromide, Ferrous	0.125	Gm.	2 grains
Iron Cacodylate, Ferric	0.03	Gm.	$\frac{1}{2}$ grain
Iron Chloride, Ferric	0.06	Gm.	1 grain
Iron Lactate, Ferrous	0.3	Gm.	5 grains
Iron Nucleinate	0.3	Gm.	5 grains
Iron Peptonate	0.3	Gm.	5 grains
Iron Salicylate, Ferric	0.3	Gm.	5 grains
Iron Succinate, Ferric	0.6	Gm.	10 grains
Iron Sulfate, Exsiccated, Ferrous	0.2	Gm.	3 grains
Iron Tannate, Ferric	0.5	Gm.	8 grains
Iron Valerate, Ferric	0.125	Gm.	2 grains
Iron and Ammonium Sulfate, Ferric	0.5	Gm.	8 grains
Iron and Ammonium Tartrate, Ferric	0.3	Gm.	5 grains
Iron and Magnesium Citrate, Ferric	0.3	Gm.	5 grains
Iron and Potassium Tartrate, Ferric	0.3	Gm.	5 grains
Iron and Quinine Citrate, Ferric	0.25	Gm.	4 grains
Iron and Strychnine Citrate, Ferric	0.125	Gm.	2 grains
Jamaica Dogwood	4	Gm.	60 grains
Jambul	0.6	Gm.	10 grains
Juglans	4	Gm.	60 grains
Kava	1	Gm.	15 grains
Kidney Substance, Dried	0.3	Gm.	5 grains
Lactucarium	1	Gm.	15 grains
Lecithin	0.25	Gm.	4 grains
Lithium Acetylsalicylate	0.5	Gm.	8 grains
Lithium Iodide	0.2	Gm.	3 grains
Lithium Metavanadate	0.002	Gm.	$\frac{1}{30}$ grain
Lovage Root	1	Gm.	15 grains
Mace	0.5	Gm.	8 grains
Magnesium Benzoate	0.3	Gm.	5 grains
Magnesium Borate	0.3	Gm.	5 grains
Magnesium Bromide	0.6	Gm.	10 grains
Magnesium Chloride	15	Gm.	4 drachms
Magnesium Glycerophosphate	0.3	Gm.	5 grains
Magnesium Hypophosphite	0.3	Gm.	5 grains
Magnesium Iodide	0.3	Gm.	5 grains
Magnesium Lactate	1	Gm.	15 grains
Magnesium Peroxide	1	Gm.	15 grains
Magnesium Salicylate	1	Gm.	15 grains

	Metric		Apothecaries
Magnesium Sulfite	1	Gm.	15 grains
Mammary Gland, Dried	0.3	Gm.	5 grains
Manaca	1	Gm.	15 grains
Manganese Carbonate	0.3	Gm.	5 grains
Manganese Dioxide	0.25	Gm.	4 grains
Manganese Iodide	0.125	Gm.	2 grains
Manganese Lactate	0.125	Gm.	2 grains
Manganese Phosphate	0.125	Gm.	2 grains
Manganese Sulfate	0.2	Gm.	3 grains
Marrubium	2	Gm.	30 grains
Matico	4	Gm.	60 grains
Melissa Leaves	2	Gm.	30 grains
Menyanthes	1	Gm.	15 grains
Merbaphen	0.15	Gm.	2½ grains
Mercury Acetate, Mercuric	0.01	Gm.	⅙ grain
Mercury Acetate, Mercurous	0.0125	Gm.	⅕ grain
Mercury Benzoate,** Mercuric	0.015	Gm.	¼ grain
Mercury Bromide, Mercuric	0.004	Gm.	¹⁄₁₅ grain
Mercury Cacodylate,** Mercuric	0.03	Gm.	½ grain
Mercury Cyanide, Mercuric	0.006	Gm.	¹⁄₁₀ grain
Mercury Oxycyanide, Mercuric	0.01	Gm.	⅙ grain
Mercury Tannate, Mercurous	0.06	Gm.	1 grain
Muira Puama	1	Gm.	15 grains
Mullein Flowers	8	Gm.	2 drachms
Mullein Leaves	4	Gm.	60 grains
Musk	0.25	Gm.	4 grains
Naphthalene	0.125	Gm.	2 grains
Nickel Bromide	0.3	Gm.	5 grains
Nicotine Tartrate***	0.001	Gm.	¹⁄₆₀ grain
Nutgall	0.5	Gm.	8 grains
Oil of Cajeput	0.5	cc.	8 minims
Oil of Cubeb	0.5	cc.	8 minims
Oil of Erigeron	1	cc.	15 minims
Oil of Gurjun	0.6	cc.	10 minims
Oil of Mace	0.12	cc.	2 minims
Oil of Rue	0.2	cc.	3 minims
Oil of Savin	0.06	cc.	1 minim
Olibanum	1	Gm.	15 grains
Ovarian Substance, Dried	0.125	Gm.	2 grains
Ovogal (Albumin cholate)	1	Gm.	15 grains
Oxyl-iodide (Cinchophen hydriodide)	0.4	Gm.	6 grains
Papain	0.2	Gm.	3 grains
Paracoto	0.3	Gm.	5 grains
Parathyroid, Dried	0.006	Gm.	¹⁄₁₀ grain

	Metric		Apothecaries
Pareira	2	Gm.	30 grains
Parsley Fruit	2	Gm.	30 grains
Parsley Root	2	Gm.	30 grains
Passion Flower	0.2	Gm.	3 grains
Pepo	30	Gm.	1 ounce
Pepper	0.5	Gm.	8 grains
Periplocin	0.001	Gm.	$\frac{1}{60}$ grain
Petroleum	2	cc.	30 minims
Physostigma	0.1	Gm.	1½ grains
Pichi	4	Gm.	60 grains
Pilocarpus	2	Gm.	30 grains
Pimenta	1	Gm.	15 grains
Pimpinella	1	Gm.	15 grains
Pineal Gland, Dried	0.006	Gm.	$\frac{1}{10}$ grain
Piperine	0.3	Gm.	5 grains
Pituitary, Dried Anterior Lobe	0.3	Gm.	5 grains
Platinum Sodium Chloride	0.03	Gm.	½ grain
Pomegranate	2	Gm.	30 grains
Poppy Capsules	1.25	Gm.	20 grains
Potassium Bisulfate	4	Gm.	60 grains
Potassium Cyanide	0.01	Gm.	⅙ grain
Potassium Dichromate	0.008	Gm.	⅛ grain
Potassium Ferrocyanide	0.5	Gm.	8 grains
Potassium Glycerophosphate	0.25	Gm.	4 grains
Potassium Iodate	0.3	Gm.	5 grains
Potassium Nitrite	0.06	Gm.	1 grain
Potassium Phosphate	1	Gm.	15 grains
Potassium Sulfite	1	Gm.	15 grains
Proferrin (Iron nucleo-proteid)	0.2	Gm.	3 grains
Proposote (Creosote phenylpropionate)	0.3	cc.	5 minims
Protan (Tannin nucleo-proteid)	0.3	Gm.	5 grains
Pyramidon Camphorate	0.5	Gm.	8 grains
Pyramidon Salicylate	0.5	Gm.	8 grains
Pyrethrum Root	2	Gm.	30 grains
Pyridine	0.125	cc.	2 minims
Quercus	1	Gm.	15 grains
Quinidine	0.1	Gm.	1½ grains
Quinine Acetylsalicylate	0.2	Gm.	3 grains
Quinine Arsenate	0.008	Gm.	⅛ grain
Quinine Arsenite	0.04	Gm.	⅔ grain
Quinine Glycerophosphate	0.1	Gm.	1½ grains
Quinine Tannate	0.2	Gm.	3 grains
Quinine Valerate	0.125	Gm.	2 grains
Rhus Glabra	1	Gm.	15 grains
Rhus Toxicodendron	0.6	Gm.	10 grains

	Metric		Apothecaries
Rubidium Bromide	0.6	Gm.	10 grains
Rubidium Iodide	0.2	Gm.	3 grains
Rubidium and Ammonium Bromide	1.5	Gm.	25 grains
Rubus	1	Gm.	15 grains
Rue	1	Gm.	15 grains
Rumex	4	Gm.	60 grains
Sabromin (Calcium dibrombehenate)	0.5	Gm.	8 grains
Safflower	4	Gm.	60 grains
Safrol	0.2	cc.	3 minims
Saligenin	0.5	Gm.	8 grains
Sanguinarine Nitrate	0.006	Gm.	$\frac{1}{10}$ grains
Santonica	1	Gm.	15 grains
Scammony Root	0.25	Gm.	4 grain
Scillaren	0.0015	Gm.	$\frac{1}{40}$ grains
Scillaren-B*	0.0005	Gm.	$\frac{1}{120}$ grains
Scoparius	1	Gm.	15 grain
Scopola	0.06	Gm.	1 grain
Senecio	4	Gm.	60 grains
Silver Arsphenamine*	0.1	Gm.	1$\frac{1}{2}$ grain
Silver Chloride	0.06	Gm.	1 grain
Silver Iodate	0.008	Gm.	$\frac{1}{8}$ grain
Silver Iodide	0.06	Gm.	1 grain
Silver Lactate	0.01	Gm.	$\frac{1}{6}$ grain
Silver Oxide	0.06	Gm.	1 grain
Sodium Arsenate	0.005	Gm.	$\frac{1}{12}$ grain
Sodium Arsphenamine*	0.5	Gm.	8 grains
Sodium Bisulfite	0.5	Gm.	8 grains
Sodium Cyanide	0.008	Gm.	$\frac{1}{8}$ grain
Sodium Formate	0.04	Gm.	$\frac{2}{3}$ grain
Sodium Lactate	1	cc.	16 minims
Sodium Metavanadate	0.002	Gm.	$\frac{1}{30}$ grain
Sodium Nitrate	1	Gm.	15 grains
Sodium Phenolsulfonate	0.6	Gm.	10 grains
Sodium Pyrophosphate	1	Gm.	15 grains
Sodium Succinate	0.3	Gm.	5 grains
Sodium Sulfite	0.5	Gm.	8 grains
Sodium Valerate	0.2	Gm.	3 grains
Sodium Potassium Bismuthyl Tartrate**	0.1	Gm.	1$\frac{1}{2}$ grains
Solanum	4	Gm.	60 grains
Spigelia	4	Gm.	60 grains
Spleen, Dried	0.3	Gm.	5 grains
Stavesacre	0.06	Gm.	1 grain
Strontium Acetate	1	Gm.	15 grains
Strontium Arsenite	0.002	Gm.	$\frac{1}{30}$ grain
Strontium Carbonate	0.6	Gm.	10 grains
Strontium Iodide	0.3	Gm.	5 grains

	Metric		Apothecaries
Strontium Lactate	0.5	Gm.	8 grains
Strontium Phosphate	1	Gm.	15 grains
Strychnine Arsenate	0.001	Gm.	$\frac{1}{60}$ grain
Strychnine Valerate	0.0015	Gm.	$\frac{1}{40}$ grain
Sulfarsphenamine**	0.4	Gm.	6 grains
Suprarenals, Desiccated	0.2	Gm.	3 grains
Tamarind	15	Gm.	4 drachms
Tansy	2	Gm.	30 grains
Terebene	0.25	cc.	4 minims
Terpinol	0.2	cc.	3 minims
Testicular Substance, Dried	0.6	Gm.	10 grains
Teucrium	2	Gm.	30 grains
Theobromine	0.3	Gm.	5 grains
Theobromine Acetylsalicylate	0.5	Gm.	8 grains
Theobromine Salicylate	0.5	Gm.	8 grains
Theobromine Lithium Benzoate	0.5	Gm.	8 grains
Theobromine Sodium Acetate	0.5	Gm.	8 grains
Theobromine Sodium Benzoate	0.5	Gm.	8 grains
Theobromine Sodium Citrate	0.5	Gm.	8 grains
Theobromine Sodium Formate	0.5	Gm.	8 grains
Theobromine Sodium Iodide	0.5	Gm.	8 grains
Thuja	2	Gm.	30 grains
Thymus Gland, Dried	0.125	Gm.	2 grains
Thyresol (Methyl ether of santalol)	0.5	cc.	8 minims
Tilia Flowers	2	Gm.	30 grains
Tonga	2	Gm.	30 grains
Tribromophenol	0.2	Gm.	3 grains
Trypsin	0.5	Gm.	8 grains
Uranium Nitrate	0.01	Gm.	$\frac{1}{6}$ grain
Urea	1	Gm.	15 grains
Veronica	2	Gm.	30 grains
Xylene	0.5	cc.	8 minims
Yohimbine Hydrochloride	0.006	Gm.	$\frac{1}{10}$ grain
Zedoary	1	Gm.	15 grains
Zinc Bromide	0.125	Gm.	2 grains
Zinc Cyanide	0.015	Gm.	$\frac{1}{4}$ grain
Zinc Ferrocyanide	0.06	Gm.	1 grain
Zinc Lactate	0.03	Gm.	$\frac{1}{2}$ grain
Zinc Phosphide	0.003	Gm.	$\frac{1}{20}$ grain
Zinc Valerate	0.12	Gm.	2 grains

PART VII

SCHEDULE OF ANTIDOTES FOR POISONS*

In the following list, to avoid needless repetition, drugs which have a similar action are arranged in groups, the drug itself being named first, followed by its active constituents and preparations, e. g., Opium (Morphine, Codeine, Paregoric, Laudanum). In mentioning an alkaloid, etc., it is understood that its salts are included. No attempt has been made to give all the antidotes for each poison; only those deemed the most efficient and available are listed.

Poisons named are arranged in alphabetical order and are numbered; the antidote is placed opposite the poison. Where an antidote is recommended for several similar poisons a cross reference to the appropriate number has been inserted opposite each of the poisons named.

In the case of the caustic poisons due attention has been given to the Regulations of the U. S. Department of Agriculture. Those passages marked with an asterisk are quoted verbatim from the bulletin of the Department, issued April 9, 1928. In all cases, whether quoted or not, the recommended treatment is in harmony with the Federal regulations.

General Directions

Summon a Physician Immediately.—These suggestions are not intended to obviate the necessity of skilled medical attention, but merely to tell what to do while waiting for the physician to arrive. In most cases of poisoning the outcome will depend largely on how quickly the proper treatment is instituted. Begin your treatment at once but do not neglect to call the physician as soon as possible.

In the treatment of many poisonings the first step is to remove the poison from the stomach, before it can pass into the circulation, or to render it harmless by chemical neutralization. The poison can usually be removed from the stomach either by means of the stomach tube or by an emetic.

The stomach tube (stomach pump) requires considerable skill in its management —it is possible to kill a person through improper manipulation of this apparatus—and those unfamiliar with it should never attempt to use it.

Emetics.—(Substances which produce vomiting.) Perhaps the most generally useful emetic in toxicology is *Zinc Sulfate*, which may be given in doses of 20 grains dissolved in half a glassful of tepid water. If vomiting does not occur within 10 minutes the dose should be repeated. For the physician, *Apomorphine Hydrochloride*, $\frac{1}{10}$ grain, is the most certain and rapid emetic that we have but, as it must be administered hypodermically, it is not available for the laity. Since promptness of evacuation is of the utmost importance, no time should be wasted in seeking the ideal emetic; the one most readily to hand should be administered. *Powdered Mustard* is a

---

* Compiled by Horatio C. Wood, Jr., M.D., for the New Jersey Board of Pharmacy.

446

very prompt and efficient, although an unpleasant, emetic; 2 or 3 teaspoonfuls stirred in a glassful of warm (not hot) water may be given as a dose. If no other emetic is at hand, 1 tablespoonful of *Sodium Chloride* (common table salt) in a glassful of lukewarm water will usually cause vomiting, although not nearly so reliably. In some persons vomiting may be induced by touching the back of the throat with the fingers or a feather, but this frequently fails. Other drugs which may be used as emetics include *Cupric Sulfate* (5 grains), *Alum* (20 grains), *Ipecac* (Fluidextract 20 minims, or Syrup, 4 fluidrachms).

Emetics and stomach tube should be carefully avoided in cases of poisoning by strong mineral acids, caustic alkalies and strychnine.

Adsorbents.—(Certain fine powders have the property of adsorbing many toxic substances from their solutions and afford a sort of universal antidote.) The best of these is an activated *Charcoal* (such as Medicinal Charcoal, U.S.P. XII). The old-fashioned animal charcoal, although greatly inferior, is of some value. Powdered *Kaolin* has some value but is not so good as charcoal. Any of the above may be given in doses of several teaspoonfuls stirred in about half a glassful of water.

Demulcents.—(Substances to soothe mucous membranes, used after irritant and corrosive poisons have been taken.) There are three types of materials which may be used for this purpose: (1) Mucilaginous or gummy preparations, which include raw white of egg mixed with an equal quantity of water; mucilage of acacia; gelatin, 2 tablespoonfuls dissolved in a pint of lukewarm water. (2) Oils and fatty substances, including milk, butter, olive and salad oils. These must *not* be used in cases when they are likely to have solvent effects on the poison, or to promote its absorption. (3) Preparations of a starchy nature, which include gruels, made from cornstarch, wheat flour, potato flour, etc., by boiling 2 tablespoonfuls of the starchy substance with a pint of water; mashed potatoes; boiled rice; soft bread mixed to a thick paste with water. These must *never* be administered until they have been well cooled.

1. ACETANILID Antipyrine Aminopyrine (Pyramidon) Aspirin Phenacetin (Acetophenetidin) and most headache remedies	Empty the stomach by an emetic. Give *aromatic spirit of ammonia*, 1 teaspoonful, in half a glassful of water. Keep the patient warm. Inhalations of oxygen are useful if collapse symptoms develop. Alcohol is probably harmful, and coffee is of no use.
2. ACETOPHENETIDIN	See Acetanilid, No. 1.
3. ACID HYDROCYANIC	See Hydrocyanic Acid, No. 83.
4. ACID OXALIC	See Oxalic Acid, No. 119.
5. ACID PRUSSIC	See Hydrocyanic Acid, No. 83.

6. ACIDS, STRONG MINERAL Hydrochloric (Muriatic) Nitric Phosphoric Sulfuric (Oil of Vitriol)	Do NOT use emetics. The best antidote is *milk of magnesia*, of which 2 or 3 tablespoonfuls should be given. Useful also are *magnesium oxide* (calcined magnesia), 1 to 2 teaspoonfuls; *chalk*, 2 teaspoonfuls, although the evolution of carbonic acid gas is undesirable because of the possibility of rupture of the weakened walls of the stomach; in the absence of other antidotes, castile soap, about 2 teaspoonfuls, cut in small pieces and stirred up with warm water. If no alkali is at hand, give whites of 2 or 3 eggs, or 2 glassfuls of milk. *External Burns.* Wipe off the acid gently, immediately flood the surface with water, using soap freely, then cover with milk of magnesia or moist baking soda.
7. ACONITE Aconitine	These poisons act quickly. Treatment must be promptly given. Emetics, to be of any value, should be administered at once; if given too late they may fail and only exhaust the patient. Give *tannic acid*, about 20 grains, in a cupful of lukewarm water, followed by *medicinal charcoal* stirred in water. Keep patient in horizontal position, with head somewhat lower than the rest of the body. Sudden exertion may be fatal. The heart, circulation and respiration may be stimulated by teaspoonful doses of *aromatic spirit of ammonia*, well diluted, every 15 minutes as required. Also give *strychnine sulfate* hypodermically in $\frac{1}{20}$ grain doses every $\frac{1}{2}$ to 2 hours (this should be administered by the physician).
8. ALCOHOL Whisky Brandy Amyl Alcohol (Fusel Oil) and intoxicating beverages Paraldehyde	It is a great mistake to believe that acute alcohol poisoning is a trivial affair; many persons die of neglect. The stomach should be emptied by the use of an emetic or the stomach pump. Many believe that *ipecac* is the emetic of choice. Even if considerable time has elapsed since imbibing the alcohol, an emetic is still advisable as alcoholic beverages may remain in the stomach for 1 to 2 hours after their ingestion. After emptying the stomach, give *aromatic spirit of ammonia*, 1 teaspoonful in half a glassful of water, and a cup of hot black coffee. Keep the patient warm. The physician's efforts will be directed against the depressing influence of the alcohol by the use of such drugs as *strychnine, atropine*, etc.

9. ALKALIES	See Lye, No. 98.
10. ALLONAL	See Barbital, No. 24.
11. AMINOPYRINE	See Acetanilid, No. 1.
12. AMMONIA Ammonia Solution	The best antidote is *vinegar*, of which 1 tablespoonful may be given in a glassful of water. If vinegar is not at hand, give 2 oz. of *olive oil*. Other sources of organic acids, such as *orange juice* and *lemon juice*, if quickly available, are useful. *Diluted hydrochloric acid* may be employed in doses of 30 to 60 minims, well diluted, but is less desirable than those acids mentioned above. In ammonia poisoning there is likely to develop later swelling of the throat, leading to strangulation. As the only remedy for this is an immediate operation, the physician should remain at hand for at least 8 hours.
13. AMMONIATED MERCURY	See Mercury, No. 100.
14. AMYL ALCOHOL	See Alcohol, No. 8.
15. AMYTAL	See Barbital, No. 24.
16. ANTIMONY and its salts Tartar Emetic	These generally cause profuse vomiting, so that emetics are seldom needed. Give about 20 grains of *tannic acid* at once in a cupful of warm water. The tannic acid treatment should be repeated, in 5 grain doses, at intervals of about 30 minutes for 4 or 5 doses. Demulcents such as white of egg, milk, mucilage, oatmeal gruel, etc., may be of service to allay vomiting. If there is great depression use stimulants, such as *ammonia* or *strychnine sulfate*. In case of extreme irritation, *morphine sulfate* may be indicated (to be administered by physician only).
17. ANTIPYRINE	See Acetanilid, No. 1.
18. APOMORPHINE	Harmful effects usually due to exhaustion and collapse from excessive vomiting. Administer *aromatic spirit of ammonia* in water or give ammonia by inhalation. Keep patient recumbent and warmly covered.
19. ARNICA	The patient will usually have already vomited, but if not an emetic is indicated. There is no known chemical antidote, but *medicinal charcoal* may be given in tablespoonful doses, followed by demulcent drinks.

20. ARSENIC
    Fowler's Solution
    Paris Green
    "Rough on Rats"
    and other arsenic com-
      pounds and prepara-
      tions
	Give an emetic at once, *zinc sulfate*, 20 grains, or mustard water, or use a stomach pump. Follow with the *Arsenic Antidote* (*U.S.P. XI*), (Magma of Ferric Hydroxide). The druggist should keep the two component mixtures for making this antidote in separate containers in a box marked "Arsenic Antidote;" when needed they should be mixed according to the direction of the U.S.P. XI, preferably using milk of magnesia. If the official antidote is not at hand a useful substitute may be prepared rapidly by mixing 1 oz. diluted solution of ferric chloride with 5 oz. milk of magnesia (2 tablespoonfuls of sodium bicarbonate may be used if magnesia is not available). If iron solutions are not at hand, milk of magnesia alone has some antidotal effect. In arsenic poisoning the antidote should be followed by a saline cathartic, such as *Epsom Salt*. Later demulcent drinks and opiates may be required to check vomiting and diarrhea. After the patient has ceased vomiting he should be encouraged to drink water to replace the fluids lost from the alimentary canal.

21. ASPIRIN	See Acetanilid, No. 1.
22. ATROPINE	See Belladonna Group, No. 26.
23. AUTOMOBILE EXHAUST	See Gas, Illuminating, No. 75.

24. BARBITAL
    Amytal
    Allonal
    Veronal
    Luminal
    Peralga
    Phenobarbital
    and other barbituric
      acid derivatives
	There is no chemical antidote. Empty the stomach promptly, preferably by the stomach tube. If the patient is seen before becoming unconscious, emetics, such as *zinc sulfate*, 20 grains, or mustard, 2 drachms, should be administered. If the patient is already narcotized, the treatment can be conducted by a physician only. It should consist in the administration of strychnine, caffeine and other respiratory stimulants, the use of large amounts of water and diuretics to hasten elimination, and the meeting of such other symptoms as may arise.
	It should be noted that the continued use of these narcotics is likely to produce an addiction or chronic poisoning, which is very difficult to treat and which may end in permanent mental incapacity or in death.

25. BARIUM SALTS Barium Chloride Barium Sulfide Lead Salts Lead Acetate (Sugar of Lead)	Give at once *Epsom salt* (magnesium sulfate) or *Glauber's salt* (sodium sulfate), 2 tablespoonfuls in half a glassful of water. Follow by demulcents and stimulants as required.
26. BELLADONNA GROUP Belladonna Atropine Homatropine Hyoscyamus Hyoscyamine Hyoscine Stramonium Daturine Duboisine Scopola Scopolamine	The best chemical antidote is *aqueous solution of iodine* (Lugol's solution), 10 minims in half a glassful of water; *tannic acid*, 20 grains, is of less value. Medicinal charcoal, 2 teaspoonfuls, is useful. These may be followed by an emetic. Although the symptoms in these poisonings may be very alarming the mortality is low.
27. BENZIN	See Gasoline, No. 76.
28. BETAEUCAINE	See Cocaine, No. 45.
29. BLUE STONE Blue Vitriol	See Copper Salts, No. 51.
30. BRANDY	See Alcohol, No. 8.
31. CALABAR BEAN (Physostigma) Physostigmine (Eserine)	If the patient has not already vomited give an emetic, followed by *medicinal charcoal*, 1 tablespoonful, or *aqueous solution of iodine*, 10 minims in half a glassful of water. *Atropine* or *belladonna* is useful as a physiological antagonist. Respiratory stimulants, such as strychnine or caffeine, should be administered by the physician.
32. CAMPHOR Camphor and Soap Liniment	If the patient has not already vomited give an emetic, *zinc sulfate*, 20 grains, or *mustard water*. Follow by saline purge of *Epsom salt* about 1 oz. in water. Keep patient warm.
33. CANNABIS INDICA (Indian Hemp)	Give emetics, or wash out the stomach by a stomach tube, using plenty of lukewarm water. Stimulants, such as a cupful of strong black coffee, should be given every hour or two.

34. CANTHARIDES (Spanish Fly Chinese Blistering Beetle) Cantharidin	If the patient has not already vomited empty stomach by stomach tube or by use of emetics; afterwards give demulcent drinks, mucilage or gruel, with *opiates* (by physician) if necessary to quiet pain. There is no known chemical antidote. Patient should drink water freely. Pain in the kidneys may be mitigated by warm sitz baths, or by the application to the painful parts of cloths wrung out of hot water.
35. CARBOLIC ACID	See Phenol, No. 125.
36. CARBON MONOXIDE	See Gas, Illuminating, No. 75.
37. CARBON TETRA-CHLORIDE	See Ether, No. 66.
38. CAUSTIC POTASH Caustic Soda	See Lye, No. 98.
39. CHARCOAL FUMES	See Gas, Illuminating, No. 75.
40. CHINESE BLISTERING BEETLE	See Cantharides, No. 34.
41. CHLORAL HYDRATE	If the patient is not unconscious give an emetic or evacuate the stomach by means of a stomach tube. There is no known chemical antidote. Keep patient lying down; apply external heat to keep up the body temperature. Give stimulants such as coffee or *aromatic spirit of ammonia* (avoid alcohol); the physician will probably use *strychnine*. Artificial respiration may be needed.
42. CHLOROFORM	See Ether, No. 66.
43. CICUTA (Water Hemlock, Water Parsnip, Cowbane)	See Cocculus Indicus, No. 46.
44. CLEANING FLUIDS	Fluids used for cleaning clothes usually contain either benzin or carbon tetrachloride, or both. For treatment of benzin poisoning, see Gasoline, No. 76; the treatment of poisoning by carbon tetrachloride is the same as of that by Ether, No. 66.

45. COCAINE Eucaine (Betaeucaine)	If the cocaine has been taken by mouth (which is unusual) give as antidote *medicinal charcoal,* 2 teaspoonfuls or *Lugol's solution,* 10 minims, in water. Most emetics will fail to produce vomiting because of the action of the cocaine upon the nerve endings in the gastro-intestinal tract; the only efficient emetic is *apomorphine,* $\frac{1}{10}$ grain, hypodermically. When the poison has been injected there is, of course, no use for emetics. In the treatment of cocaine poisoning, especially after its hypodermic injection, the services of a skilled physician are absolutely essential. Treatment consists in the combating of convulsions by such drugs as *sodium amytal* or *chloroform,* and the use of stimulants, as *ammonia* and *epinephrine,* if circulatory collapse occurs.
46. COCCULUS INDICUS (Fish Berries) Picrotoxin Cicuta (Water Hemlock, Water Parsnip, Cowbane) Musquash Root	Empty the stomach with an emetic such as *zinc sulfate,* 20 grains, or *mustard;* follow by *medicinal charcoal,* 1 tablespoonful stirred in water. If convulsions occur, give inhalations of *chloroform.*
47. CODEINE	See Opium Group, No. 118.
48. COLCHICUM Colchicine	Should the patient not have vomited already, give a rapidly acting emetic, such as *zinc sulfate* or *mustard.* After the patient vomits give, as chemical antidote, *aqueous solution of iodine* (Lugol's solution), 10 minims in half a glassful of water, or *medicinal charcoal,* 1 teaspoonful. In the later management, *opium* is desirable to check the diarrhea and *strychnine* to combat collapse, but these should be used by a physician only.
49. CONIUM (Poison Hemlock) Coniine Gelsemium (Yellow Jasmin) Gelsemine	Conium is one of the most deadly plants growing in this country. Empty the stomach by the use of emetics, such as *zinc sulfate,* 20 grains, or *mustard.* Give *aqueous solution of iodine,* 10 minims, or *medicinal charcoal,* 2 teaspoonfuls, as antidotes. Subsequent treatment by a physician should consist in the use of stimulants, such as *ammonia* or *strychnine,* and artificial respiration if necessary.

THE PHARMACEUTICAL RECIPE BOOK

50. CONVALLARIA
    (Lily of the Valley)
    Convallamarin
	See Digitalis, No. 59.

51. COPPER SALTS
    Copper Sulfate
    (Blue Stone)
    Verdigris, etc.
	The best chemical antidote is *potassium ferro-cyanide*, 10 grain doses in warm water. If this is not available, give white of egg or milk freely, also plenty of water. CAUTION—*Avoid vinegar and oils.*

52. CORROSIVE SUBLIMATE	See Mercury, No. 100.
53. COWBANE	See Cocculus Indicus, No. 46.

54. CREOLIN
    Creosote
    Cresol
	See Phenol, No. 125.

55. CROTON OIL (Oleum Tiglii)	The patient will probably have vomited already, but if not emetics should be given. There is no known chemical antidote. Treatment should consist of administering milk freely, mucilaginous drinks to soothe the inflammation of the stomach and *opium* to control the diarrhea.
56. CYANIDES	See Hydrocyanic Acid, No. 83.
57. DATURINE	See Belladonna Group, No. 26.
58. DELPHINIUM	See Larkspur, No. 91.

59. DIGITALIS
    Digitalin
    Digitoxin
    Strophanthus
      Strophanthin
    Convallaria
    (Lily of the Valley)
      Convallamarin
    Scoparius
    Sparteine
	If the patient has not vomited thoroughly, empty the stomach by means of a stomach tube, using plenty of lukewarm water. There is no known chemical antidote. Keep patient in recumbent position and warm. Hot applications over the heart have been recommended.

60. DIONIN	See Opium Group, No. 118.
61. DOG BUTTONS	See Strychnine, No. 150.
62. DUBOISINE	See Belladonna Group, No. 26.
63. EMETINE	See Ipecac, No. 89.

64.	ERGOT	Evacuate the stomach with an emetic, such as *zinc sulfate*, 20 grains, or *mustard*, or with the stomach tube. Give 1 tablespoonful of *medicinal charcoal*. Keep the patient recumbent.
65.	ESERINE	See Calabar Bean, No. 31.
66.	ETHER (Ethyl Oxide) Chloroform Carbon Tetrachloride	If the ether has been taken by mouth and the patient is conscious enough to swallow, **give a** promptly acting emetic. When the ether is taken by inhalation emetics are, of course, of no value and may be harmful by exhausting the strength of the patient. Keep patient warm. Physician will give respiratory stimulants and artificial respiration.
67.	ETHYLMORPHINE HYDROCHLORIDE	See Opium Group, No. 118.
68.	EUCAINE	See Cocaine, No. 45.
69.	FISH BERRIES	See Cocculus Indicus, No. 46.
70.	FLUORIDES Sodium Fluoride Roach Poison	Sodium Fluoride is the basis of many insect poisons; it kills by depriving the system of calcium. Give at once *calcium chloride* or *calcium lactate*, 20 to 30 grains. If a soluble salt of calcium is not available, give chalk or lime water freely. Follow by giving an emetic or using the stomach pump. The calcium salts should be repeated at intervals until recovery is complete.
71.	FORMALDEHYDE Formalin	If the patient has not already vomited, give an emetic. Follow by a diluted solution of *ammonia*—such as *aromatic spirit of ammonia*, 1 teaspoonful, or *ammonia water*, ½ teaspoonful, in a glassful of water—as a chemical antidote. Then give demulcent drinks, mucilage or white of egg.
72.	FOWLER'S SOLUTION	See Arsenic, No. 20.
73.	FURNACE GAS	See Gas, Illuminating, No. 75.
74.	FUSEL OIL	See Alcohol, No. 8.
75.	GAS, ILLUMINATING Charcoal Fumes Automobile Exhaust Furnace Gas Carbon Monoxide	The gases of imperfect combustion owe their poisonous properties to the presence of carbon monoxide, which combines with the hemoglobin of the blood. The patient should be removed to fresh air at once, and if not breathing normally should receive artificial respiration. Summon a physician promptly; he will give oxygen inhalations and respiratory stimulants. Even if the patient survives, permanent disability may follow.

76. GASOLINE 　　Benzin 　　Kerosene	These are all narcotic poisons. The only treatment of any utility is prompt evacuation of the stomach before the poisons are absorbed. Use any of the customary emetics or the stomach tube.
77. GELSEMIUM 　　Gelsemine	See Conium, No. 49.
78. HAT BLEACH	See Oxalic Acid, No. 119.
79. HELLEBORE, WHITE	See Veratrum, No. 155.
80. HEROIN	See Opium Group, No. 118.
81. HOMATROPINE	See Belladonna Group, No. 26.
82. HYDROCHLORIC ACID	See Acids, Strong Mineral, No. 6.
83. HYDROCYANIC ACID 　　(Prussic Acid) 　　Cyanides 　　Potassium Cyanide 　　Sodium Cyanide 　　Oil of Bitter Almond, 　　　containing Hydrocyanic Acid	An extremely rapid poison, requiring quick action. The most useful chemical antidote is probably *Magma of Ferric Hydroxide*, U.S.P. XI (see under Arsenic, No. 20). If it is not at hand give a mixture of diluted solution of *ferric chloride*, 1 teaspoonful, with *milk of magnesia*, 2 tablespoonfuls. *Solution of hydrogen peroxide*, 2 teaspoonfuls in half a glassful of water, is also useful as an antidote. *Amyl nitrite* by inhalation may be useful. Emetics may fail to act. If a physician is available, he should empty the stomach by the use of a stomach tube. The subsequent treatment, which is carried out by the physician, will consist in the administration of circulatory and respiratory stimulants, as *strychnine* and *caffeine*, and the attempt to neutralize the poison in the blood by intravenous injection of *sodium nitrite, sodium thiosulfate*, or *methylthionine*.
84. HYOSCYAMUS 　　Hyoscyamine 　　Hyoscine	See Belladonna Group, No. 26.
85. IGNATIA	See Strychnine, No. 150.
86. INDIAN HEMP	See Cannabis Indica, No. 33.
87. INK ERADICATOR	See Oxalic Acid, No. 119.

88.	IODINE Tincture of Iodine Lugol's Solution	The best chemical antidote is *starch*. Stir rapidly 2 tablespoonfuls of flour with a tumblerful of water and give at once. Bread or other farinaceous food may be made up into a paste with water and taken freely. *Sodium thiosulfate*, 20 to 30 grains, is a very useful antidote, but is less likely to be available than starch. Unless patient has vomited follow the antidote with an emetic. The use of alkalies (sodium bicarbonate) has been recommended in the subsequent treatment (by the physician).
89.	IPECAC Emetine	As the patient has probably vomited already, emetics are unnecessary. Give large doses of *medicinal charcoal*, 1 tablespoonful, or *aqueous solution of iodine*, 10 minims. Keep the patient quiet and in a recumbent position. As soon as the vomiting has ceased, give *aromatic spirit of ammonia*, 1 teaspoonful in half a glassful of water. Other circulatory stimulants will be used by the physician. Opiates may be required to check excessive vomiting.
90.	KEROSENE	See Gasoline, No. 76.
91.	LARKSPUR (Delphinium, Staphisagria)	Accidental poisoning may occur from the use of one or the other species of delphinium as a hair wash. They are very active poisons, and treatment is not very satisfactory. Give *medicinal charcoal*, 1 tablespoonful, or *aqueous solution of iodine*, 10 minims, in water, followed by an emetic. Keep the patient quiet and in a horizontal position.
92.	LEAD SALTS	See Barium Salts, No. 25.
93.	LILY OF THE VALLEY	See Digitalis, No. 59.
94.	LOBELIA	See Nicotine, No. 107.
95.	LUGOL'S SOLUTION	See Iodine, No. 88.
96.	LUMINAL	See Barbital, No. 24.
97.	LUNAR CAUSTIC	See Silver Nitrate, No. 142.

98. LYE Caustic Potash Caustic Soda	Do NOT use emetics or the stomach pump. Give *vinegar*, 1 or 2 tablespoonfuls according to the amount of the poison imbibed, in a glassful of water. Other substances, as *lemon juice* or *orange juice*, are also useful but are not likely to be so quickly available. If no acid is immediately available, give 2 or 3 tablespoonfuls of *olive oil* or other salad oil. Follow the acid with 1 tablespoonful of olive oil or a tumblerful of cream. Keep patient warm and in recumbent posture. *External Burns.* Flood with water, then wash with vinegar.
99. LYSOL	See Phenol, No. 125.
100. MERCURY Mercury Bichloride (Corrosive Sublimate) Mercuric Oxide (Red Precipitate) Ammoniated Mercury (White Precipitate) and other irritant salts of Mercury	Corrosive sublimate is one of the most common and most deadly poisons. The efficient antidotes are rarely available in a hurry and promptness is of the utmost importance; the quickly available antidotes are of relatively little value. The most important thing is the immediate evacuation of the stomach by the use of any emetic measure at hand. *Zinc sulfate,* 30 grains in half a glassful of tepid water; *mustard,* 2 teaspoonfuls in a glassful of tepid water; or tickling the fauces with the fingers or a feather will usually cause vomiting. Between vomitings the patient must drink large amounts of luke warm water, containing a teaspoonful of salt to the tumblerful, to wash out the stomach. After the stomach is emptied, a chemical antidote may be administered. Of the useful chemical antidotes, the one most likely to be available is *medicinal charcoal,* 2 tablespoonfuls stirred in water. This is much superior to the commonly recommended white of egg. In the absence of other antidotes, *white of egg* is perhaps better than nothing. *Calcium sulfide,* 5 grains, is an efficient antidote, but is itself poisonous if given in a larger dose. Probably the most efficient chemical antidote for mercuric chloride is *sodium formaldehydesulfoxylate,* but this is rarely available. The answer to the question of whether to give the antidote or the emetic first will depend upon which is the more quickly available. If powdered charcoal is immediately at hand, give it first. The use of egg albumen is

100.	MERCURY (*Continued*)	likely to lessen the efficiency of the emetic. The subsequent treatment of mercury poisoning is directed towards the protection of the kidneys with large amounts of water and alkalizing drinks.
101.	METHYL ALCOHOL	See Wood Alcohol, No. 161.
102.	METHYL SALICYL-ATE	See Oil of Wintergreen, No. 117.
103.	MORPHINE	See Opium Group, No. 118.
104.	MURIATIC ACID	See Acids, Strong Mineral, No. 6.
105.	MUSHROOMS	If the patient has not vomited, give an emetic immediately—*zinc sulfate*, 20 grains, or *mustard water*—followed by *medicinal charcoal*, 1 tablespoonful. In poisoning by the fly agaric (Amanita muscaria), belladonna in full dose may be a life-saving measure, but it is not of great value in other types of mushroom poisoning.
106.	MUSQUASH ROOT	See Cocculus Indicus, No. 46.
107.	NICOTINE Lobelia	Severe cases of nicotine poisoning usually occur from its use as a horticultural insecticide. The treatment is unsatisfactory. If it has been swallowed, give a tablespoonful of *medicinal charcoal*, followed by an emetic, unless vomiting has already occurred. Keep the patient quiet and in a horizontal position. Give *aromatic spirit of ammonia* and other stimulants.
108.	NITRIC ACID	See Acids, Strong Mineral, No. 6.
109.	NITROGLYCERIN	This is a very rapidly acting poison; if taken in large dose the progress of symptoms is too rapid for any efficient treatment. Keep the patient recumbent and warm. The physician will probably use *epinephrine* by injection and other stimulants.
110.	NUX VOMICA	See Strychnine, No. 150.
111.	OIL OF BITTER AL-MOND, containing Hydrocyanic Acid	See Hydrocyanic Acid, No. 83.
112.	OIL OF PENNY-ROYAL	See Oil of Savin, No. 114.
113.	OIL OF RUE	See Oil of Savin, No. 114.

114. OIL OF SAVIN Oil of Pennyroyal Oil of Rue Oil of Tansy	If the patient has not vomited freely, wash out the stomach repeatedly, or give an emetic. A dose of *Epsom* salt should be given in case the bowels have not been moved freely. Then give demulcents—white of egg, oatmeal, gruel, arrowroot, etc. Stimulate heart and respiration, if needed, by strong black coffee. Morphine, $\frac{1}{4}$ grain doses, may be given for pain (by physician).
115. OIL OF TANSY	See Oil of Savin, No. 114.
116. OIL OF VITRIOL	See Acids, Strong Mineral, No. 6.
117. OIL OF WINTER- GREEN (Methyl Salicylate)	If the patient has not vomited give an emetic, or the physician will wash out the stomach with solution of *sodium bicarbonate.* Follow by *sodium bicarbonate*, 1 teaspoonful in water, or *milk of magnesia*, 1 tablespoonful, and demulcent drinks. Give water freely to encourage elimination. Keep patient recumbent.
118. OPIUM GROUP Opium Morphine Codeine Ethylmorphine Hydrochloride (Dionin) Heroin	Emetics usually fail to act if the patient has become narcotized but they may be used if he is seen before systemic symptoms are apparent. The best chemical antidote is *potassium permanganate*, about 10 grains in a pint of lukewarm water. Repeat the treatment in half an hour if necessary. Physiological antagonists: *caffeine*, in one or two cups of strong black coffee, *strychnine sulfate* and other respiratory stimulants should be given by physician. Patient should not be allowed to go to sleep; keep him awake by shouting, flipping with end of wet towel, or (best if available) by the use of the electric brush; avoid exercising him by walking. If he is not breathing properly, artificial respiration may be necessary.
119. OXALIC ACID Hat Bleach Ink Eradicator	Treatment must be prompt. Give at once 2 teaspoonfuls of *chalk* stirred up with water, or 2 fluidounces of *milk of magnesia*. (If neither is immediately at hand, remember most tooth powders and tooth pastes are made with a basis of chalk and may be used. Whiting, also, is a form of calcium carbonate.) The Federal regulations recommend following the antidote with an emetic.

120.	PARALDEHYDE	See Alcohol, No. 8.
121.	PARIS GREEN	See Arsenic, No. 20.
122.	PERALGA	See Barbital, No. 24.
123.	PHENACETIN	See Acetanilid, No. 1.
124.	PHENOBARBITAL	See Barbital, No. 24.
125.	PHENOL (Carbolic Acid) Creolin Creosote Cresol Lysol	There is no satisfactory chemical antidote. The only treatment of real value is the immediate evacuation of the stomach. Give *zinc sulfate*, 20 grains in half a glassful of tepid water, or *mustard*, 1 tablespoonful in a glassful of tepid water. After the patient has vomited, administer 2 tablespoonfuls of either *magnesium sulfate* (Epsom salt) or *sodium sulfate* (Glauber's salt), with a pint of water to clean out the intestines. The use of alcoholic liquids, such as brandy or whisky, while often advised, is injurious rather than beneficial. Follow the Epsom salt with demulcent drinks, such as white of egg or mucilage of acacia. AVOID THE USE OF OILS OR FATS. For external burns by phenol, wash the part with alcohol or whisky.
126.	PHOSPHORIC ACID	See Acids, Strong Mineral, No. 6.
127.	PHOSPHORUS Roach Poison	The best emetic is *cupric sulfate*, 5 grains, as it is a chemical antidote for phosphorus as well as an emetic. If it is not at hand, use other emetics followed by *potassium permanganate*, 10 grains in a glassful of water, or *solution of hydrogen peroxide*, 2 teaspoonfuls in water, as chemical antidotes. AVOID THE USE OF OILS OR FATS. Follow by saline cathartic, such as Epsom salt.
128.	PHYSOSTIGMA Physostigmine	See Calabar Bean, No. 31.
129.	PHYTOLACCA (Poke Root, Poke Berries)	Give emetic of *mustard* in warm water or use stomach tube if vomiting has not been produced by drug. Give *aromatic spirit of ammonia* diluted with water, or use *digitalis*. Give opium or morphine in small doses for pain (by physician only).
130.	PICROTOXIN	See Cocculus Indicus, No. 46.
131.	POISON HEMLOCK	See Conium, No. 49.

132.	POKE ROOT AND BERRIES	See Phytolacca, No. 129.
133.	POTASSIUM CYA-NIDE	See Hydrocyanic Acid, No. 83.
134.	POTASSIUM PER-MANGANATE	If the patient has not vomited give an emetic followed by white of egg and *medicinal charcoal*, 1 tablespoonful in water.
135.	PRUSSIC ACID	See Hydrocyanic Acid, No. 83.
136.	PYRAMIDON	See Acetanilid, No. 1.
137.	RED PRECIPITATE	See Mercury, No. 100.
138.	ROACH POISON	Most of the poison baits for roaches contain either Phosphorus or Sodium Fluoride; some contain both. See No. 127 and No. 70 for treatment.
139.	"ROUGH ON RATS"	See Arsenic, No. 20.
140.	SCOPARIUS	See Digitalis, No. 59.
141.	SCOPOLA Scopolamine	See Belladonna Group, No. 26.
142.	SILVER NITRATE (Lunar Caustic)	Give *sodium chloride* (common salt), 1 table-spoonful to a pint of water or milk (salt forms an insoluble and comparatively harmless com-pound). In the absence of salt, white of egg and large quantities of milk may be used. If there is pain and nervousness, morphine sulfate, $\frac{1}{4}$ grain, may be given hypodermically (by physi-cian). If there is great depressions, stimulants should be used.
143.	SODIUM CYANIDE	See Hydrocyanic Acid, No. 83.
144.	SODIUM FLUORIDE	See Fluorides, No. 70.
145.	SPANISH FLY	See Cantharides, No. 34.
146.	SPARTEINE	See Digitalis, No. 59.
147.	STAPHISAGRIA	See Larkspur, No. 91.
148.	STRAMONIUM	See Belladonna Group, No. 26.
149.	STROPHANTHUS Strophanthin	See Digitalis, No. 59.

150. **STRYCHNINE** Nux Vomica (Dog Buttons) Ignatia	Do NOT give emetics or use the stomach tube; any effort to empty the stomach is likely to cause a fatal convulsion. As a chemical antidote give *potassium permanganate*, 10 grains in a tumblerful of water, or *medicinal charcoal*, 1 tablespoonful. If the convulsions become violent, attempts to control them may be made by inhalations of *chloroform*, in the same manner as for anesthesia. Other drugs useful for the convulsions are *sodium amytal*, 5 grains, *sodium pentobarbital*, 5 grains, or *chloral hydrate* 20 grains, but these should be used by a physician only as they are best given by injection.
151. **SUGAR OF LEAD**	See Barium Salts, No. 25.
152. **SULFURIC ACID**	See Acids, Strong Mineral, No. 6.
153. **TARTAR EMETIC**	See Antimony, No. 16.
154. **TINCTURE OF IODINE**	See Iodine, No. 88.
155. **VERATRUM** (Veratrum Viride) White Hellebore	This drug, while it is a powerful poison acting like aconite, is seldom fatal because it is an active emetic. If there has not been free vomiting, siphon out the stomach or use an emetic, *mustard*, 4 tablespoonfuls to a tumblerful of lukewarm water, or *zinc sulfate*, 20 grains. Follow by *medicinal charcoal*, 1 tablespoonful in water, or *aqueous solution of iodine*, 10 minims in a half glass of water, as the best available antidotes. Keep patient in a horizontal position, head somewhat lower than the rest of the body. Atropine is the best physiological antagonist (to be given by the physician). Other stimulants, as *aromatic spirit of ammonia* or *strychnine sulfate*, may also be of service.
156. **VERDIGRIS**	See Copper Salts, No. 51.
157. **VERONAL**	See Barbital, No. 24.
158. **WATER HEMLOCK** (Water Parsnip)	See Cocculus Indicus, No. 46.
159. **WHISKY**	See Alcohol, No. 8.
160. **WHITE PRECIPITATE**	See Mercury, No. 100.

161. **WOOD ALCOHOL** (Methyl Alcohol)	This is a dangerous poison; even if not fatal, it may cause permanent blindness. Poisoning may occur either from inhaling the fumes or from swallowing the alcohol. In the latter case give an emetic, as *zinc sulfate* or *mustard*, at once or wash out the stomach by means of a stomach tube. After the stomach is thoroughly cleansed give *sodium bicarbonate*, 60 grains, and make the patient drink water freely. Keep the patient warm. *Aromatic spirit of ammonia* may be used, if stimulation seems necessary.
162. **YELLOW JASMIN**	See Conium, No. 49.
163. **ZINC SALTS** Zinc Acetate Zinc Chloride Zinc Sulfate	Patient has probably vomited. Give *medicinal charcoal*, 1 tablespoonful in water, or *white of egg*. Follow with *sodium bicarbonate*, 1 teaspoonful in water. Give water freely. Physician will use stimulants and opiates as necessary.

PART VIII

TABLE OF SOLUBILITIES

The figures given represent the *number of cc. of solvent* in which *1 Gm.* of the substance dissolves at *25° C.* or the temperature otherwise stated.

ABBREVIATIONS

abs.	absolute
dec.	decomposed
dehyd.	dehydrated
fr. sol.	freely soluble (from 1 to 10 cc.)
insol.	insoluble
misc.	miscible
mod. sol.	moderately soluble
m. r. sol.	more readily soluble
part. sol.	partially soluble
pr. insol.	practically insoluble (in more than 10,000 cc.)
read. sol.	readily soluble
sl. sol.	slightly soluble (from 100 to 1000 cc.)
slow. sol.	slowly soluble
sol.	soluble (from 10 to 30 cc.)
sp. sol.	sparingly soluble (from 30 to 100 cc.)
v. sl. sol.	very slightly soluble (from 1000 to 10,000 cc.)
v. slow. sol.	very slowly soluble
v. sol.	very soluble (less than 1 cc.)

TABLE OF SOLUBILITIES

	25° C.	Water 100° C. or Stated Temp:	Alcohol	Chloroform	Ether	Glycerin
Acetanilidum	190	20	3.5	4	17	5
Acetophenetidinum	1300	85	15	15	130	..
Acidum acetyl-salicylicum	300	..	5	17	10–15	..
Acidum amino-aceticum	2	..	v. sl. sol.	..	..	..
Acidum ascorbicum	3	..	30	insol.	insol.	..
Acidum benzoicum	275	20	3	5	3	..
Acidum boricum	18	4	18	..	..	4
Acidum citricum	0.5	0.5	2	..	30	..
Acidum lacticum	misc.	misc.	misc.	insol.	misc.	..

465

	25° C.	Water 100° C. or Stated Temp.	Alcohol	Chloroform	Ether	Glycerin
Acidum mandelicum	6.5	..	fr. sol.	..	fr. sol.	..
Acidum nicotinicum	60	fr. sol.	sol.	..	insol.	..
Acidum salicylicum	460	15	3	45	3	..
Acidum stearicum	insol.	..	20	2	3	..
Acidum tannicum	v. sol.	v. sol.	v. sol.	pr. insol.	pr insol.	1
Acidum tartaricum	0.8	0.5	3	pr. insol.	sl. sol.	..
Acidum trichlor- aceticum	0.1	..	sol.	..	sol.	..
Acriflavina	3	..	pr. insol.	insol.	insol.	
Acriflavinæ hydro- chloridum	3	..	sol.	insol.	insol.	
Æther	12	..	misc.	misc.	..	
Æthylhydrocupreinæ hydrochloridum	2	..	5	2.5	pr. insol.	..
Æthylis acetas	10	..	misc.	..	misc.	..
Æthylis amino- benzoas	2500	..	5	2	4	..
Æthylis carbamas	0.5	..	1	1	2	3
Æthylmorphinæ hydrochloridum	10	..	25	sl. sol.	sl. sol.	..
Alcohol	misc.	misc.	..	misc.	misc.	..
Alumen:						
(ammonium)	7	0.3	insol.	..	..	fr. sol.
(potassium)	7.5	0.3	insol.	..	..	fr. sol.
exsiccatum	20 v. slow	2	insol.	..	..	..
Alumini:						
chloridum	0.5	..	4	..	..	sol.
sulfas	1	11.3	insol.	..	..	..
Aminopyrina	18	..	1.5	1	13	..
Ammonii:						
benzoas	10	..	35.5	..	..	8
bromidum	1.3	0.9	12	..	..	..
carbonas	4 v. slow	dec.	part. sol.	..	..	..
chloridum	2.6	1.4	100	..	..	8
hypophosphis	1	v. sol.	20	..	..	..
iodidum	0.6	0.5	3.7	..	..	1.5
salicylas	1	..	3	..	..	..
valeras acidus	0.3	..	0.6	..	sol.	..
Anethol	pr. insol.	pr. insol.	2	read. sol.	read. sol.	..
Antimonii et po- tassii tartras	12	3	insol.	..	..	15
Antipyrina	1	..	1.3	1	43	..
Apomorphinæ hy- drochloridum	50	20 (80)	50	v. sl. sol.	v. sl. sol.	..

	25° C.	Water 100° C. or Stated Temp.	Alcohol	Chloroform	Ether	Glycerin
Arecolinæ hydro-bromidum	1	..	10	sl. sol.	sl. sol.	..
Argenti nitras	0.4	0.1	30	..	sl. sol.	..
Argentum-proteini-cum forte	fr. sol.	fr. sol.	pr. insol.	pr. insol.	pr. insol.	..
Argentum-proteini-cum mite	fr. sol.	fr. sol.	pr. insol.	pr. insol.	pr. insol.	..
Arseni triiodidum	12	..	sol.	sol.	sol.	..
Arseni trioxidum	slow. sol.	..	sl. sol.	...	sl. sol.	fr. sol.
Arsphenamina	sol.	..	sol.	v. sl. sol.	v. sl. sol.	sol.
Atropina	460	90 (80)	2	1	25	27
Atropinæ sulfas	0.5	..	5	420	3000	2.5
Barbitalum	130	13	15	75	35	..
Barbitalum sodium	5	2.5	sl. sol.	..	insol.	..
Barii sulfas	insol.	..	insol.	..	..	..
Bentonitum	insol.	..	..	..	..	..
Benzaldehydum	350	..	misc.	..	misc.	..
Betanaphthol	1000	80	1	17	1.5	sol.
Bismuthi:						
subcarbonas	insol.	insol.	insol.	..	..	..
subgallas	pr. insol.	..	pr. insol.	..	pr. insol.	..
subnitras	pr. insol.	pr. insol.	insol.	..	..	..
subsalicylas	pr. insol.	pr. insol.	..	..	..	..
et potassii tartras	2	..	insol.	insol.	insol.	..
Bromum	90	..	fr. sol.	fr. sol.	fr. sol.	..
Brucinæ sulfas	70	v. sol.	sp. sol.	..	..	..
Butacaina	v. sol.	..	v. sol. (warm)	sl. sol.	insol.	..
Butylis amino-benzoas	7000	..	sol.	sol.	sol.	..
Caffeina	50	6 (80)	70	6	550	..
Caffeina citrata	..	4 (warm)	..	..	..	..
Caffeinæ cum sodium benzoate	1.2	..	30	part. sol.	..	..
Calcii:						
bromidum	0.7	0.4	1.3	insol.	insol.	..
chloridum	1.2	0.7	10	..	..	..
creosotas	part. sol.	..	..	..	..	..
gluconas	30	5	insol.	..	..	..
glycerophosphas	50	..	insol.	..	..	..
hypophosphis	6.5	..	insol.	..	..	..
iodobehenas	insol.	..	v. sl. sol.	fr. sol. (warm)	v. sl. sol.	..

	25° C.	Water 100° C. or Stated Temp.	Alcohol	Chloroform	Ether	Glycerin
Calcii:						
lactas	20	..	pr. insol.	..	..	..
mandelas	sl. sol.	80	insol.	..	..	..
Calx	840	1740	insol.	..	..	sol.
Camphora	800	..	1	0.5	1	..
Camphora mono-						
bromata	pr. insol.	..	6.5	0.5	1.6	..
Carbarsonum	sl. sol.	..	sl. sol.	pr. insol.	pr. insol.	..
Carbonei tetra-						
chloridum	2000	..	misc.	misc.	misc.	
Carbromalum	3000	..	18	3	14	..
Cerii oxalas	insol.	..	insol.	..	insol.	
Chloralis hydras	0.25	..	1.3	2	1.5	
Chloramina-T	7	2	dec.	insol.	insol.	..
Chlorobutanol	125	..	1	read. sol.	read. sol.	10
Chloroformum	210	..	misc.	..	misc.	..
Chlorothymol	pr. insol.	..	0.5	2	1.5	..
Chrysarobinum	v. sl. sol.	v. sl. sol.	400	15	160	..
Cinchonidinæ sulfas	65	22 (80)	90	620	pr. insol.	..
Cinchoninæ sulfas	60	33 (80)	12.5	47	3230	..
Cinchophenum	pr. insol.	pr. insol.	120	400	100	..
Cocaina	600	270 (80)	7	1	3.5	..
Cocainæ hydro-						
chloridum	0.5	..	3.5	15	insol.	sol.
Codeina	120	..	2	0.5	50	..
Codeinæ phosphas	2.5	0.5 (80)	325	4500	1875	..
Codeinæ sulfas	30	6.5 (80)	1280	insol.	insol.	..
Colchicina	25	..	fr. sol.	fr. sol.	220	..
Cotarninæ chloridum	1	v. sol.	v. sol.	..	..	..
Coumarinum	400	50	fr. sol.	fr. sol.	fr. sol.	..
Creosoti carbonas	insol.	..	fr. sol.	misc.	..	..
Creosotum	sl. sol.	sl. sol.	misc.	..	misc.	..
Cresol	50	..	misc.	..	misc.	misc.
Cupri sulfas	3	0.5	500	..	..	2.8
Dextrinum album	part. sol.	3	..	..	..	..
Dextrosum	1	..	60	..	..	..
Dichloramina-T	pr. insol.	pr. insol.	dec.	1	..	..
Dihydromorphinonæ						
hydrochloridum	3	..	sp. sol.	..	insol.	..
Diphenylhydanto-						
inum sodicum	fr. sol.	..	sol.	pr. insol.	pr. insol.	..
Emetinæ hydro-						
chloridum	fr. sol.	fr. sol.	fr. sol.	..	..	..
Ephedrinæ hydro-						
chloridum	3	..	14	..	insol.	..

	25° C.	Water 100° C. or Stated Temp.	Alcohol	Chloroform	Ether	Glycerin
Ephedrinæ sulfas	fr. sol.	..	fr. sol. (hot)	..	..	..
Epinephrina	v. sl. sol.	v. sl. sol.	v. sl. sol.	insol.	insol.	..
Ergonovinæ maleas	36	..	120	insol.	insol.	..
Ergotaminæ tartras	500	..	500	..	..	..
Estradiolis benzoas	pr. insol.	..	sol.	..	sl. sol.	..
Estronum	sl. sol.	..	sol.	..	..	..
Eucainæ hydro- chloridum	30	m. r. sol.	35	6	..	..
Eucalyptol	v. sl. sol.	v. sl. sol.	misc.	misc.	misc.	..
Eucatropinæ hy- drochloridum	v. sol.	..	fr. sol.	fr. sol.	insol.	..
Eugenol	sl. sol.	sl. sol.	misc.	misc.	misc.	..
Ferri:						
chloridum	0.2	..	fr. sol.	..	sol.	sol.
et ammonii cit.	read. sol.	read. sol.	insol.	..	..	..
glycerophosphas	2	..	insol.	..	..	..
hypophosphis	2300	1200	..	..	..	..
phosphas solub.	fr. sol.	fr. sol.	insol.	..	..	..
pyrophosphas solubilis	10	fr. sol.	insol.	..	..	..
sulfas	1.5	0.5	insol.	..	..	..
Ferrum:						
peptonatum	fr. sol.	fr. sol.	pr. insol.	..	..	..
Fluoresceinum so- dicum	fr. sol.	..	sp. sol.	..	..	..
Glucosum	v. sol.	v. sol.	sp. sol.	..	..	..
Glycerinum	misc.	misc.	misc.	insol.	insol.	..
Guaiacol	60–70	..	misc.	misc.	misc.	1
Guaiacolis car- bonas	insol.	insol.	60	1	18	sl. sol.
Hexylresorcinol	2000	..	fr sol.	fr. sol.	fr. sol.	fr. sol.
Histaminæ phosphas	4	..	..	..	..	..
Homatropinæ hy- drobromidum	6	..	40	420	insol.	..
Hydrargyri:						
bichloridum	13.5	2.1	3.8	..	25	12
chloridum mite	insol.	insol.	insol.	insol.	insol.	..
iodidum flavum	pr. insol.	pr. insol.	insol.	..	insol.	..
iodidum rubrum	pr. insol.	pr. insol.	115	910	120	..
oxidum flavum	pr. insol.	pr. insol.	insol.	..	..	..
oxidum rubrum	pr. insol.	pr. insol.	insol.	..	..	..
salicylas	pr. insol.	pr. insol.	pr. insol.	..	..	..

	25° C.	Water 100° C. or Stated Temp.	Alcohol	Chloroform	Ether	Glycerin
Hydrargyri:						
succinimidum	20	5	sl. sol.	..	insol.	..
Hydrarg. ammon.	insol.	insol.	insol.	..	..	..
Hydrastinæ hydro-						
chloridum	v. sol.	v. sol.	v. sol.	sl. sol.	v. sl. sol.	..
Iodoformum	pr. insol.	pr. insol.	60	10	7.5	80
Iodophthaleinum						
sodicum	7	..	sl. sol.	..	..	..
Iodum	2950	..	13	fr. sol.	fr. sol.	80
Lactosum	5	2.6	v. sl. sol.	insol.	insol.	..
Lithii:						
benzoas	3	..	16	..	..	..
bromidum	0.6	0.4	fr. sol.	..	sol.	..
carbonas	78	140	pr. insol.	..	..	..
citras	1.4	..	v. sl. sol.	..	..	..
salicylas	v. sol.	v. sol.	v. sol.	..	..	..
Magnesii:						
carbonas	pr. insol.	pr. insol.	insol.	..	..	..
oxidum	pr. insol.	pr. insol.	insol.	..	..	..
sulfas	1	0.2	sp. sol.	..	..	1
Mangani citras						
solubilis	4	..	pr. insol.	..	..	..
Mangani glycero-						
phosphas sol.	sl. sol.	..	insol.	..	..	..
Mangani hypoph.	6.5	6	insol.	..	..	..
Menadionum	pr. insol.	..	60	mod. sol.	..	..
Menthol	sl. sol.	sl. sol.	v. sol.	v. sol.	v. sol.	..
Merbrominum	fr. sol.	..	pr. insol.	insol.	insol.	..
Mersalyl	1	..	2	insol.	insol.	..
Methenamina	1.5	..	12.5	10	..	..
Methylis parahy-						
droxy benzoas	400	..	2.4	..	8	..
Methylis salicylas	sl. sol.	sl. sol.	misc.	misc.	misc.	..
Methylrosanilæ						
chloridum	30–40	..	10	sol.	insol.	15
Methylthioninæ						
chloridum	25	fr. sol.	65	sol.	..	..
Morphinæ hydro-						
chloridum	17.5	0.5	52	insol.	insol.	sol.
Morphinæ sulfas	16	0.7 (80)	565	insol.	insol.	..
Neoarsphenamina	v. sol.	v. sol.	sl. sol.	pr. insol.	pr. insol.	sol.
Neocinchophenum	pr. insol.	..	sol. (hot)	v. sol.	v. sol.	..

	25° C.	Water 100° C. or Stated Temp.	Alcohol	Chloroform	Ether	Glycerin
Neostigminæ						
bromidum	1	..	sol.	..	..	..
methylsulfas	10	..	less sol.	..	..	..
Nicotinamidum	1	..	1.5	..	..	10
Ouabainum	75	..	100	..	..	..
Pamaquinæ						
naphthoas	insol.	..	sol.	..	..	..
Pancreatinum	slow. sol.	..	insol.	..	..	..
Papaverinæ hydro-						
chloridum	40	..	sol.	sol.	pr. insol.	..
Paraldehydum	8	17	misc.	misc.	misc.	..
Pectinum	sol.	..	insol.	insol.	insol.	..
Pelletierinæ tannas	250	..	sol.	insol.	sl. sol.	..
Pentobarbitalum						
sodicum	v. sol.	..	fr. sol.	..	pr. insol.	..
Pepsinum	fr. sol.	fr. sol.	pr. insol.	pr. insol.	pr. insol.	..
Phenacainæ hydro-						
chloridum	50	..	fr. sol.	fr. sol.	insol.	..
Phenobarbitalum	1000	..	10	40	15	..
sodicum	v. sol.	..	sol.	pr. insol.	pr. insol.	..
Phenol	15	..	v. sol.	v. sol.	v. sol.	v. sol.
Phenolphthal-						
einum	pr. insol.	pr. insol.	15	..	75	..
Phenolsulfon-						
phthaleinum	1300	..	350	pr. insol.	pr. insol.	..
Phenothiazina	insol.	..	75	..	..	..
Phenylis salicylas	6770	..	6	v. sol.	v. sol.	..
Phosphorus	pr. insol.	pr. insol.	400 (dehyd.)	40	102 (abs.)	..
Physostigminæ						
salicylas	75	16 (80)	16	6	250	..
Pilocarpinæ hydro-						
chloridum	0.3	..	3	366	insol.	..
Pilocarpinæ nitras	4	..	75	insol.	insol.	..
Plumbi acetas	1.6	0.5	30	..	..	fr. sol.
Potassa sulfurata	2	v. sol.	part. sol.	..	..	..
Potassii:						
acetas	0.5	0.2	3	..	..	..
bicarbonas	2.8	2 (50)	pr. insol.	..	..	..
bitartras	165	16	8820	..	..	..
bromidum	1.5	1	250	..	..	4.6
carbonas	1	0.7	insol.	..	..	..
chloras	16.5	1.8	pr. insol.	..	..	sol.
chloridum	2.8	2	insol.	..	..	..

	25° C.	Water 100° C. or Stated Temp.	Alcohol	Chloroform	Ether	Glycerin
Potassii:						
citras	1	..	pr. insol.	..	..	fr. sol.
et sodii tartras	1	..	pr. insol.	..	..	..
guaiacolsulfonas	7.5	..	insol.	..	insol.	..
hydroxidum	1	0.6	3	..	..	2.5
hypophosphis	0.6	0.4	9	..	..	..
iodidum	0.7	0.5	22	..	..	2
nitras	3	0.5	620	..	..	sol.
permanganas	15	3.5	dec.	..	..	..
sulfas	10	4	insol.	..	..	..
thiocyanas	0.5	0.2	12	..	..	..
Procainæ hydro-chloridum	1	..	30	sl. sol.	pr. insol.	..
Pyrogallol	2	v. sol.	1.5	..	2	..
Quinacrinæ hydro-chloridum	30	..	sol.	..	..	..
Quinidinæ sulfas	100	15	10	sol.	pr. insol.	..
Quinina	1560	800	1	1	sol.	..
Quininæ æthyl-carbonas	sl. sol.	sl. sol.	3	1	10	..
bisulfas	10	0.7	25	625	2500	15
dihydro-chloridum	0.6	..	12	sl. sol.	v. sl. sol.	..
et ureæ hydrochloridum	1	..	3	..	..	..
hydrobromidum	40	3.2 (80)	1	1	25	7
hydrochloridum	16	0.5 (80)	1	1	350	7
phosphas	600	60	..	..	..	..
salicylas	sl. sol.	..	15	25	160	13
sulfas	810	47 (80)	120	sl. sol.	sl. sol.	30
Resorcinol	1	0.2 (80)	1	sl. sol.	fr. sol.	fr. sol.
Resorcinol fuscum	15	..	sol.	..	sp. sol.	sol.
Riboflavinum	v. sl. sol.	..	pr. insol.	insol.	insol.	..
Rubrum scarlatinum	insol.	..	sl. sol.	15	..	..
Saccharinum	290	25	31	v. sl. sol.	v. sl. sol.	..
Saccharinum sodicum	1.5	..	50	..	..	..
Salicinum	25	3.3 (80)	90	insol.	insol.	..
Santoninum	pr. insol.	sl. sol.	45	2	110	..
Scopolaminæ hydro-bromidum	1.5	..	20	sl. sol.	insol.	..

	25° C.	Water 100° C. or Stated Temp.	Alcohol	Chloroform	Ether	Glycerin
Sodii:						
acetas	0.8	..	19	..	..	..
arsenas	1.5	1	sl. sol.	..	..	..
arsenas exsiccatus	3.5	1.5	sl. sol.	..	..	..
benzoas	2	1.4	61	..	..	..
bicarbonas	10	..	insol.	..	..	
biphosphas	fr. sol.	fr. sol.	pr. insol.	pr. insol.	pr. insol.	.
boras	16	1	insol.	..	..	1
bromidum	1.2	..	16	..	..	..
cacodylas	0.5	..	2.5	..	..	..
carbonas mono- hydratus	3	1.8	insol.	..	..	7
chloridum	2.8	2.7	sl. sol.	..	..	10
citras	1.5	0.6	insol.	..	..	..
glycerophosphas	1.5	v. sol.	pr. insol.	..	..	..
hydroxidum	1	0.3	v. sol.	..	..	..
hypophosphis	1	0.2	sol.	..	..	fr. sol.
indigotindisul- fonas	sp. sol.	sp. sol.	pr. insol.	..	..	..
iodidum	0.6	0.4	2	..	..	1
nitris	1.5	v. sol.	sp. sol.	..	..	..
perboras	40	sol.	..	..	..	sol.
phophas	4	..	v. sl. sol.	.,	..	..
phosphas exsiccatus	8	1.1	insol.	..	..	..
salicylas	1	v. sol.	10	..	..	4
sulfas	1.5	..	insol.	..	..	sol.
sulfas exsiccatus	3.6	2.6	insol.	..	..	..
sulfis exsiccatus	4	..	sp. sol.	..	..	..
thiocyanas	0.7	v. sol.	4	..	..	..
thiosulfas	0.5	..	insol.	..	..	sol.
Sparteinæ sulfas	1.1	..	3	insol.	insol.	..
Strontii bromidum	0.35	..	sol.	..	insol.	..
salicylas	19	3.7	61	..	..	..
Strophanthinum	sol.	sol.	sol.	pr. insol.	pr. insol.	..
Strychnina	6420	3100	136	5	v. sl. sol.	..
Strychninæ nitras	45	10	150	105	insol.	50
phosphas	30	..	sl. sol.	..	..	..
sulfas	35	7	85	220	insol.	fr. sol.
Sucrosum	0.5	0.2	170	insol.	insol.	..
Sulfanilamidum	125	..	37	insol.	insol.	sol.
Sulfapyridinum	3500	..	440	..	..	..
Sulfapyridinum sodicum	1.5	..	10	..	..	..
Sulfarsphenamina	v. sol.	..	sl. sol.	..	insol.	..
Sulfathiazolum	1700	..	200	..	..	..

	25° C.	Water 100° C. or Stated Temp.	Alcohol	Chloroform	Ether	Glycerin
Sulfobromophthal- einum sodicum	sol.	..	insol.	..	..	..
Sulfonmethyl- methanum	200	m. r. sol.	12	..	sol.	..
Sulfonmethanum	365	16	60	11	64	..
Terebenum	pr. insol.	pr. insol.	3	misc.	misc.	..
Terpini hydras	200	35	13	135	140	..
Tetracainæ hydro- chloridum	v. sol.	..	sol.	..	insol.	..
Tetrachlor- æthylenum	pr. insol.	..	misc.	misc.	misc.	..
Theobromina sodio- acetas	1.5	..	sl. sol.	..	..	..
cum sodii salicylate	1	..	sl. sol.	insol.	insol.	..
Theophyllina	120	m. r. sol.	80	..	sp. sol.	..
æthylenedi- aminica	5	..	insol.	..	insol.	..
sodioacetas	25	..	insol.	insol.	insol.	..
Thiaminæ hydro- chloridum	1	..	100	..	insol.	insol.
Thymol	1000	..	1	1	1.5	..
Thymolis iodidum	insol.	insol.	sl. sol.	read. sol.	read. sol.	insol.
Thyroxinum	insol.	insol.	pr. insol.	pr. insol.	pr. insol.	..
Totaquina	insol.	..	sol. (warm)	sol.	part. sol.	..
Tribromoæthanol	35	..	..	..	..	..
Trichloro- æthylenum	pr. insol.	..	misc.	misc.	misc.	..
Trinitrophenol	80	15	12	35	65	..
Tryparsamidum	2	..	sl. sol.	insol.	insol.	..
Urea	1.5	..	10	insol.	insol.	..
Vanillinum	100	20 (80)	fr. sol.	fr. sol.	fr. sol.	20
Zinci:						
acetas	2.5	1.6	30	..	..	..
chloridum	0.5	..	1.5	..	..	2
iodidum	v. sol.	..	fr. sol.	..	sol.	..
phenolsulfonas	1.6	0.4	1.8	..	..	..
sulfas	0.6	..	insol.	..	..	2.5

TABLES FOR MAKING PERCENTAGE SOLUTIONS FOR PRESCRIPTIONS

The U.S.P. XII specifies, "When the expression 'per cent' is used in prescriptions without further qualification, it is to be interpreted to mean that:

for solutions of solids in liquids, per cent weight in volume;
for solutions of liquids in liquids, per cent volume in volume;
for solutions of gases in liquids, per cent weight in volume."

Tables for Weight in Volume (Solids)—Volume in Volume (Liquids) Percentage Solutions

The following table gives the amount of material to be used with enough of the solvent to make the volume at the top of the column. Multiples or fractions of these volumes may be calculated from these figures.

Percentage Strength of Solution Desired	For Solids, Weight in Volume		For Liquids, Volume in Volume	
	Dissolve the grains specified below in solvent q. s. to make 1 fl. oz.	Dissolve the grams specified below in solvent q. s. to make 100 cc.	Add minims specified below to solvent q. s. to make 1 fl. oz.	Add cc. specified below to solvent q. s. to make 100 cc.
0.1% (1:1000)	0.45 (½) gr.	0.1 Gm.	0.48 ♏	0.1 cc.
0.25% (1:400)	1.14 gr.	0.25 Gm.	1.2 ♏	0.25 cc.
0.5% (1:200)	2.28 gr.	0.5 Gm.	2.4 ♏	0.5 cc.
1%	4.56 gr.	1 Gm.	4.8 ♏	1 cc.
2%	9.12 gr.	2 Gm.	9.6 ♏	2 cc.
3%	13.68 gr.	3 Gm.	14.4 ♏	3 cc.
4%	18.24 gr.	4 Gm.	19.2 ♏	4 cc.
5%	22.8 gr.	5 Gm.	24 ♏	5 cc.
10%	45.6 gr.	10 Gm.	48 ♏	10 cc.
15%	68.4 gr.	15 Gm.	72 ♏	15 cc.
20%	91.2 gr.	20 Gm.	96 ♏	20 cc.
25%	114 gr.	25 Gm.	120 ♏	25 cc.
40%	182.4 gr.	40 Gm.	192 ♏	40 cc.
50%	228 gr.	50 Gm.	240 ♏	50 cc.

The following formulas may be used to calculate the amounts of material, solid or liquid, to be used to make percentage solutions for prescriptions.

For solids—weight in volume:

$4.5 \times$ % desired $\times$ no. of fl. oz. desired = grains of material to be dissolved in the solvent q. s.

For liquids—volume in volume:

$4.8 \times$ % desired $\times$ no. of fl. oz. desired = minims of material to be dissolved in the solvent q. s.

METRIC EQUIVALENTS

Many of the equivalents below are approximate only, but are perfectly safe and are chosen with the view of facilitating calculations as needed.

Metric Weights, Gm.	Apothecaries' Weight and Measure, Grains or Minims	Metric Measures, cc.
0.00054	$\frac{1}{120}$	0.00051
0.001	$\frac{1}{64}$	0.00096
0.0011	$\frac{1}{60}$	0.001
0.0016	$\frac{1}{40}$	0.0015
0.0022	$\frac{1}{30}$	0.002
0.004	$\frac{1}{16}$	0.0038
0.0065	$\frac{1}{10}$	0.006
0.008	$\frac{1}{8}$	0.0077
0.011	$\frac{1}{6}$	0.01
0.016	$\frac{1}{4}$	0.015
0.0325	$\frac{1}{2}$	0.03
0.065	1	0.06
0.13	2	0.12
0.2	3	0.18
0.26	4	0.25
0.325	5	0.3
0.65	10	0.62
1.3	20	1.25
1.95	30	1.85
3.25	50	3.10
6.5	100	6.0
	Drams or Fluid Drams	
3.9	1	3.7
7.8	2	7.4
15.5	4	14.8
23.3	6	22.2
31.1	8	29.6
	Apothecaries' Ounce or Fluid Ounce	
31.1	1	29.6
62.2	2	59.0
124.4	4	118.3
248.8	8	236.6
373	12	354.8
497.6	16	473

1 Gm.   = 15.432 Grains or approximately 15.5 Grains.
1 cc.   = 16.23   Minims or approximately 16 Minims.
1 Kgm. = 2.2   Avoirdupois lbs. = 2.6 Apothecary lbs.
1 L.   = 2.11   Pints or 1.057 Quarts.

PART IX
TABLE OF SYNONYMS

Aabam	Lead
Abies Bark	Hemlock Spruce Bark
Abric	Sulfur
Aceite de Beleno	Oil of Hyoscyamus
Acid of Sugar	Oxalic Acid
Acor Meconicus	Morphine
Acorn Sugar	d-Quercitol
Adermin	Vitamin B₆
Adipsos	Licorice
Agave	American Aloe
Agotan	Cinchophen
Ague Salt	Quinine Sulfate
Alan-Gilan	Cananga Oil, Ylang Ylang Oil
Alcohol of Vinegar	Glacial Acetic Acid
Alkalized Mercury	Mercury with Chalk, Gray Powder, Hive Powder
Alkargen	Cacodylic Acid
Alphozone	Succinyl Peroxide
Anise Camphor	Anethol
Antifungin	Magnesium Borate
Apple Oil	Iso-amyl-iso-valerate
Aqua Dulcis	Chloroform Water
Aqua Fortis	Nitric Acid
Aqua Sicca	Mercury
Argillaceous Earth	Kaolin
Argillicum	Aluminum
Asa Dulcis	Benzoin, Benjamin
Asthma Weed	Lobelia, Bladder Pod, Vomit Wort
Bahia Powder	Goa Powder, Araroba
Baker's Salt	Ammonium Carbonate
Balsam of Life	Compound Decoction of Aloes
Balsam of Sulfur	Sulfurated Linseed Oil
Banewort	Belladonna Leaves, Death's Herb, Dwale
Banks Oil	Cod Liver Oil
Bassora Gum	False Tragacanth
Benne Oil	Sesame Oil
Benzinoform	Carbon Tetrachloride
Bertoni's Ether	Tertiary Amyl Nitrite
Betel Nuts	Areca Nuts
Bismuth White	Bismuth Subnitrate, Spanish White, Flake White

Bitter Bark — Alstonia, Dita Bark

Bitter Salt — Magnesium Sulfate, Epsom Salt, Hair Salt, Salts of England

Black Balsam — Peru Balsam, China Oil, Balsam St. Salvadore

Black Drops — Acetum Opii, Vinegar of Opium

Black Jam — Confection of Senna

Blanc de Troyes — Prepared Chalk

Blessed Thistle — Centaurea

Bogbean — Menyanthes, Water-Shamrock

Brandy Bitters — Compound Tincture of Gentian

Bran Oil — Furfural, Artificial Oil of Ants

Brazilian Cocoa — Guarana

Broadbent's Mixture — Compound Quinine Mixture

Brompton Blacks — Compound Glycyrrhiza Troches

Brown Acid — Brown Oil of Vitriol

Bur Oil — Oil of Burdock

Butter of Arsenic — Arsenic Trichloride, Caustic Oil of Arsenic

Butter Oil — Cotton Seed Oil, Sweet Nut Oil

Butterfly Weed — Asclepias

Button Bush — Cephalanthus

Cadie Gum — Cambogia

Camelina Oil — German Sesame Oil

Camphor Julep — Camphor Water

Canelle — Bismarck Brown

Caoutchouc — Rubber

Caustic Alcohol — Solution Sodium Ethylate

Caustic Barley — Sabadilla

Ceratum Epuloticum — Calamine Ointment

Chameleon Mineral — Potassium Permanganate

Chelsea Pensioner — Compound Confection of Guaiac

Chilli Pasta — Capsicum Ointment

China Bark — Quillaja, Soap Bark, Panama Bark, Murilla Bark

Chinese Isinglass — Agar-Agar

Chittem Bark — Cascara Bark

Chloramide of Mercury — Ammoniated Mercury, Lemery's White Precipitate

Chloric Ether — Spirit of Chloroform

Chloroazotic Acid — Nitrohydrochloric Acid, Aqua Regia

Chloroform — Formyl Trichloride

Chop or Split Nut — Physostigma

Christopher Root — Actæa spicata

Cibozol — European word for Sulfathiazole

Cibus Deorum — Asafœtida, Food of the Gods, Lachryma Syriaca

Climbing Staff Tree	Celastrus, False Bittersweet
Cochia Pills	Compound Pills of Colocynth
Colza Oil	Rapeseed Oil
Concentrated Opium	Pantopon
Condy's Fluid	Solution Potassium Permanganate
Confectio Cardiaca	Aromatic Chalk Powder
Confection of Hips	Confection of Rose Fruit
Coryfin	Menthyl Ethylglycollate
Cosmetic Bismuth	Bismuth Oxychloride
Count Palmer's Powder	Magnesium Carbonate
Crespigny's Pill	Pills of Aloe and Mastic, Thomson's Antibilious Pills
Crocus Saturnis	Red Lead
Crow-Fig	Nux Vomica
Daffy's Elixir	Compound Tincture of Senna, Elixir Salutis
Dagenan	Sulfapyridine
Dakin's Oil	Chlorcosane
Deer's Tongue	Liatus, Vanilla Plant
Denver Mud	Kaolin Cataplasm
Derosne's Salt	Narcotine
Deseptyl	Sulfanilamide, Stramid, Streptocid
Dice Ore	Lead Sulfide, Tesselated Ore, Galena
Dippel's Oil	Rectified Animal Oil
Dippel's Acid Elixir	Aromatic Sulfuric Acid
Diuretic Salt	Potassium Acetate
Draco Venenatus	Mercuric Chloride
Drago Mitigatus	Calomel, Manna Metallorum, Aquila Alba
Dragon Gum	Gum Tragacanth, Fiddle Gum, Gum Hog
Duck's Foot	Mandrake
Dulcified Spirit of Salt	Spirit of Hydrochloric Ether
Dutch Liquid	Ethylene Dichloride
Eau de Broccherai	Solution of Creosote
Eau de Luce	Aromatic Spirit of Ammonia
Eau de Naphe	Orange Flower Water
Emulsio Communis	Mistura Amygdalae
English Salt	Smelling Salt
Essence of Bigarade	Oil of Bitter Orange Peel
Essoral	Menthyl Borate
Ethal	Cetylic Acid
Ethiops Mineral	Black Mercuric Sulfide
Eunatrol	Sodium Oleate
European Tea	Veronica
Everlasting Pills	Pills of Metallic Antimony

Extract of Quinquinami — Extract of Cinchona
Extract of Thebiaci — Extract of Opium

Febrifuge Salt — Potassium Chloride
Fever Drops — Compound Tincture of Cinchona
Fever Tree — Eucalyptus Leaves
Field Balm — Catnip, Oatmint
Flowers of Antimony — Antimony Oxide
Flowers of Arsenic — Arsenic Trioxide, Arsenious Acid
Flowers of Benjamin — Benzoic Acid
Flowers of Zinc — Zinc Oxide
Fluidextract Tang-kui — Eumenol
Fool's Gold — Iron Pyrites
Formosa Camphor — Camphor from China
Friar's Cowl — Aconite, Mousebane
Fringe Tree — Chionanthus
Frost Balsam — Lin, Iodo-Camphoratum
Fuller's Herb — Saponaria, Bouncing Bet
Fuming Spirit of Libavius — Stannic Chloride
Fusible Salt of Urine — Sodium Ammonium Hydrogen Phosphate, Microcosmic Salt

G. D. D. Liniment — Compound Liniment of Aconite and Chloroform
Galen's Cerate — Cold Cream
Garden Balm — Melissa, Lemon Balm
Gardenal — Phenobarbital
Gilbert's Syrup — Syrup Mercuric Iodide
Gingelly Oil — Sesame Oil, Teel Oil (also see Benne Oil)
Gipsy Wort — Lycopys Virginicus, Water Bugle
Glymol — Liquid Petrolatum
Goa Powder — Chrysarobin
Godfrey's Cordial — Mixture Sassafras and Opium
God's Grace — Haarlem Oil
Golden Ointment — Yellow Mercurial Ointment
Gooroo Nuts — Kola Seeds, Bissy Nuts, Gurn Nuts
Goulard's Extract — Strong Solution Lead Subacetate
Ground Apple — Roman Chamomile
Gumbo — Bentonite, Soap Clay

Haarlem Oil — Sulfurated Spirit Turpentine
Harle's Solution — Solution Sodium Arsenite
Hawthorn — Crataegus
Heberden's Ink — Mistura Ferri Aromatica
Hebra's Ointment — Ointment Lead Oleate, Diachylon Ointment

Hemisine — Epinephrine
Herapath's Salt — Quinine-iodo-sulfate
Hexal — Methenamine Sulfosalicylate

Hiera Picra	Powder of Aloe and Canella
Hippo Wine	Ipecacuanha Wine
Hjerne's Testament Drops	Elixir Long Life, Swedish Bitters
Homberg's Sedative Salt	Boric Acid, Sedative Salt
Hot Drops	Tincture of Capsicum and Myrrh
Hungary Water	Compound Spirit Rosemary
Hunn's Drops	Compound Mixture Cajeput
Hydralit	Sodium Formaldehyde Sulfoxylate
Hydrocarbon Oil	Liquid Paraffin, Terraline, Mineral Glycerin, Usoline
Jaggary	Crude Sugar
Jamaica Wood	Logwood, Steam Black, Campeachy Wood
Java Pepper	Tailed Pepper Cubeb
Jeffersonia Diphylla	Twin Leaf, Rheumatic Root
Jequirty	Seeds of Abrus Pecatorius, Prayer Beads, Jumble Beads
Julin's Carbon Chloride	Hexachlorobenzene
Juniper Gum	Sandarac
Kautschin	Limonene
Kermes Mineral	Sulfurated Antimony
Khordofan Gum	Gum Arabic, Turkey Gum
Kinder Pulver	Compound Powder Rhubarb
Kineurine	Quinine Glycerophosphate
Klee's Salt	Acid Potassium Oxalate, Salt of Lemons, Salt of Sorrel
Koji	Takadiastase
Kyapootic Oil	Oil of Cajeput
Lactucarium	Lettuce Opium
Lambkin's Cream	Inj. Hydrargyri, Oleum Cinereum
Laughing Gas	Nitrous Oxide
Laurel Nut Oil	Calophyllum Oil, Domba Oil, Poonseed Oil, Calaba Oil
Layor Carang	Agar
Lengibel	Ginger
Lenicet	Powdered Aluminum Acetate
Levant Wormseed	Santonica
Liquor Aquilegius	Spirit of Wine
Lister's Antiseptic	Mercuric Zinc Cyanide
Lixivium Sapona Rium	Liquor Potassæ
Looch Blanc	Emulsion of Sweet Almond
Loxa Bark	Pale Cinchona Bark
Luedecks's Mixture	Antacid Mixture
Luna Cornea	Silver Chloride
Lund's Oil	Lubricant Oil, Catheter Oil
Lung Tonic	Elixir Pectorale

Lutz's Ointment — Ointment Mercuric and Potassium Iodides

Lysoform — Liquor Formaldehydi Saponati
Lytta — Cantharides

Macquer's Salt — Potassium Arsenite
Mad Weed — Scutellaria, Plue Pimpernel, Scullcap Herb

Magistery of Bismuth — Basic Bismuth Nitrate, Blanc de Fard
Malarine — Acetophenone-Phenetidine
Mallebrein — Aluminum Chlorate
Marc Brandy Oil — Fusel Oil, Potato Oil
Marignac's Salt — Potassium Stannosulfate
Marine Acid — Hydrochloric Acid
Maté — Paraguay Tea, Jesuits' Tea, St. Bartholomew's Tea

Maw Seeds — Black Poppy Seeds
Meadow Saffron — Colchicum Corm
Meconium — Opium
Mephitic Air — Nitrogen
Mescal Buttons — Seeds of Anhalonium Lewinii
Mexican Tea — Chenopodium
Mexico Seeds — Castor Oil Seeds
Milk Ipecac — Apocynum Androsæmifolium
Mineral Solution — Solution Potassium Arsenite
Mirabilite — Sodium Sulfate, Glauber's Salt
Mohr's Salt — Ferrous Ammonium Sulfate
Moss Starch — Lichenin
Mother's Friend — Carminative Mixture, Infants' Preservative

Mountain Flour — Infusorial Earth, Tripolite

Nageli's Solution — Solution Zinc Chloride and Iodide
Nanny Berry — Viburnum Prunifolium
Neapolitan Ointment — Mercury Ointment
Noah's Ark — Cypripedium

Oesipos — Anhydrous Lanolin, Agnin
Oil of Chinese Cinnamon — Oil of Cassia
Oil of Curled Mint — Oil of Spearmint
Oil of Duty — Oil of Rhodium
Oil of Earthnut — Oil of Arachis, Peanut Oil
Oil of Infernal Regions — Very impure Olive Oil
Oil of Man — Oil of Cornu Cervi, Oil of Hartshorn, Dippel's Oil

Oil of Mirbane — Nitrobenzene
Oil of Niobé — Methyl Benzoate
Oil of Origanum — Oil of Thyme
Oil of Palma Christi — Castor Oil

Oil of Partridge Berry	Oil of Wintergreen, Methyl Salicylate, Oil of Teaberry
Oil of Poley	Oil of Pennyroyal, Oil of Pulegium
Oil of Portugal	Oil of Sweet Orange Peel
Oil of Tar	Deliquescent Potassium Carbonate
Oil of Vitriol	Concentrated Sulfuric Acid
Olefiant Gas	Ethylene
Oleum	Fuming Sulfuric Acid, Nordhausen Sulfuric Acid
Oleum Badianae	Oil of Star Anise
Oleum Rusci	Swedish Birch Tar
Ortiga Blanca	Spanish name for White Nettle
Oryzanin	Vitamin B$_1$ hydrochloride, Torulin
Paramorphine	Thebaine—alkaloid of Opium
Paranephrine	Epinephrine
Parsley Camphor	Apiol
Pelosine	Berberine
Pepperidge Bush	Barberry Bark, Sour-spine
Peppermint Camphor	Menthol
Petrosulfal	Artificial substitutes for Ammonium-ichtho-sulfonates, Tumenol, Thiol
Phenazone	Antipyrine, Pyracine
Philosopher's Wool	Zinc Oxide
Phocenic Acid	Isovaleric Acid
Phospho-lutein	Lecithin
Phosphoric Ether	Ethyl Oxide, Sulfuric Ether
Piedra Infernal	Spanish name for Silver Nitrate
Pigeon Berry	Phytolacca
Piral	Pyrogallol
Plummer's Pills	Compound Pills of Mercurous Chloride
Pod Pepper	Capsicum
Poho Oil	Oil of Peppermint
Pompholix	Zinc Oxide, Philosopher's Wool, Flowers of Zinc
Potato Spirit Oil	Amylic Alcohol, Grain Oil
Poudre de Reglisse	Powdered Licorice
Poudre de Savory	Seidlitz Powder
Prince's Pine	Chimaphila
Propanone	Acetone
Pudding Pipe	Cassia Fistula
Puff Ball	Dandelion Root, Lion's Tooth
Putty Powder	Gray Tin Oxide, Tin Stone, Tin Ash
Pyraloxin	Pyrogallol oxidized
Quebrachine	Yohimbine
Quevenne's Iron	Iron by Hydrogen
Quinine Elixir	Aromatic Elixir of Licorice

Rattlesnake Root	Senega
Red Lavender	Compound Tincture of Lavender
Redoxon	Ascorbic Acid
Rest Harrow Root	Ononis Root
Royal Powder	Compound Scammony Powder
Rufus Pills	Pills of Aloe and Myrrh
Sailor's Pepper	Cubeb
Salaigugl	Olibanum
Sal Chalybdis	Iron Sulfate
Sal de Duobus	Potassium Sulfate, Sal Polychrest
Sal Enixum	Bisulfate of Potassium
Salmester	Mesotan, Ericin
Salmiak	Ammonium Chloride
Salt of Alembroth	Compound of Mercury and Ammonium Chloride
of Amber	Succinic Acid
of Saturn	Lead Acetate, Sugar of Saturn
of Steel	Ferrous Sulfate
of Wisdom	Compound of Mercuric and Ammonium Chloride, Salt of Alembroth, White Precipitate
Salt of Wormwood	Potassium Carbonate
Salzburg Vitriol	Cupric sulfate
Sand-Brier	Solanum
Sanluol	Arsphenamine
Sapocarbol	Lysol
Saponis Aromaticus	Linimentum Saponatus Camphoratum
Scabwort	Inula, Horse-heal, Elfwort
Scotch Paregoric	Ammoniated Tincture of Opium
Scott's Dressing	Compound Ointment of Mercury
Scott's Liniment	Liniment of Mercury
Sea Onion	Squill
Seignette's Salt	Sodium Potassium Tartrate, Tartrated Soda
Seven Barks	Hydrangea
Sipiri Bark	Bebeeru Bark, Greenheart
Sodaic Powders	Effervescing Powders
Soldier's Herb	Matico Leaves
Soldier's Ointment	Ung. Hydrarg. Mite
Solomon's Seal	Polygonatum
Soothing Ointment	Compound Resorcin Ointment
Spirit of Alum	Sulfuric Acid
of Sweet Wine	Ethyl Chloride
of Verdigris	Acetic Acid
Spurge Flax	Mezereum, Paradise Plant
Starch Sugar	Dextrose

Stone Wax	Carnauba Wax
Steel Drops	Tr. Iron Perchloride, Tr. Steel
Sugar of Gelatin	Amino Acetic Acid, Glycocoll
Sundew	Drosera
Sweet Oriental Gum	Storax
Sweet Spirit of Vitriol	Spirit of Ether
Sycose	Saccharin
Talbor's Powder	Cinchona Powder, Lugo's Powder, Countess Powder
Tallow Seed Oil	Stillingia Oil
Tasteless Salts	Sodium Phosphate
Teamster's Tea	Ephedra
Teli	Sassy Bark, Bondou, Doom Bark, Red Water Tree Bark
Tennant's Salt	Chlorinated Lime
Theinum	Caffeine
Thiersch's Solution	Boro-salicylated solution
Thiery's Solution	Solution Picric Acid
Thomas Balsam	Tolu Balsam, Opobalsam
Thomsonian No. 6	Tr. Capsicum and Myrrh
Thridace	French Lactucarium
Tilleul	French name for Tilia or Linden Flowers
Tincture Cato	Tincture Catechu
Tobacco Wood	Hamamelis, Winter Bloom
Toothache Seed	Henbane Seed
Tournesol	Litmus
Town's Specific	Mixture Belladonna, Xanthoxylum and Hyoscyamus
Trebizond Opium	Persian Opium
Tree of Heaven	Ailanthus glandulosa, Chinese Sumac
Tree of Life	Thuja, False White Cedar
Trumpet-Weed	Eupatorium purpureum, Queen of the Meadow
Trypaflavine	Acriflavine
Tully's Powder	Compound Morphine Powder
Tung Oil	Chinese Wood Oil
Turkey Corn	Corydalis, Squirrel Corn
Turlington's Drops	Compound Tincture Benzoin, Wade's Drops, Traumatic Balsam, Horse Tincture, Friar's Balsam, Balm Drops, Commander's Balsam
Turpentine Camphor	Bornyl Chloride
Turps	Oil of Turpentine, Turpentine Spirit
Tyratol	Thymol Carbonate
Urari	Curare, Woorari
Urisol	Methenamine

Van Swieten's Solution — Solution Mercuric and Ammonium Chloride

Vegetable Calomel — Podophyllum
Vegetable Mercury — Manaca, Mururé
Vegetable Pepsin — Papain
Vegetable Sulfur — Lycopodium
Vesipyrin — Phenyl Acetylsalicylate
Vinegar Naphtha — Ethyl Acetate
Vomiting Salt — Zinc Sulfate

Waken-beggar — Pulv. Hellebore Alba
Ward's Essence — Ammoniated Camphor Liniment
Water Pepper — Polygonum, Smartweed
Westrosal — Trichloroethylene
Whitewood Bark — Canella
Wilson's Ointment — Zinc Ointment
Wind Water — Carminative Water, Gripe Drops
Winter's Bark — Drimyswinteri, Pepper Bark
Wood Sugar — Xylose

Xaxa — Aspirin, Helicon
Xaxaquin — Quinine Acetylsalicylate
Xyloidin — Pyroxylin

Yajeine — Harmine, Banisterine, Telepathine
Yatren — Chinofon Powder
Yaw Root — Stillingia, Silver Leaf
Yellow Parilla — Menispermum, Canadian Moonseed
Yellow Puccoon — Hydrastis, Indian Turmeric
Yerba Santa — Eriodictyon, Consumptive's Weed, Gum Plant
Ypadre — Coca Leaves
Yperite — Dichloro-diethyl-sulfide, Mustard Gas

Zaccatila — Black Cochineal
Zeller's Ointment — Ammoniated Mercury Ointment
Zinkspath — Calamine
Zootic Acid — Hydrocyanic Acid
Zylonite — Celluloid

PART X

LATIN ABBREVIATIONS

This section on Latin terms and abbreviations represents a small part of the Latin vocabulary used in the practice of pharmacy. For a more complete coverage of all Latin terms and abbreviations used, consult any one of the standard Latin textbooks available in libraries or in the Colleges of Pharmacy.

A. c.	ante cibos,	before eating.
Aa.	ana,	of each.
Abs. febr.	abstente febre,	in the absence of fever.
Add.	adde,	add (thou).
Ad aur. dext.	ad auris dextra,	to the right ear.
Ad aur. laev.	ad auris laeva,	to the left ear.
Ad lib.	ad libitum,	as much as you please, at pleasure
Ad sat.	ad saturandum,	to saturation.
Admov.	admoveatur,	let it be applied.
Ads. febr.	adstante febre,	while fever is on.
Aggr. febr.	aggrediente febre,	while the fever is coming on.
Agit.	agitatur,	let it be shaken.
Altern. dieb.	alternus diebus,	every other day.
Altern. hor.	alternis horis,	every other hour.
Altern. noc.	alternis noctibus,	every other night.
Ant. jentac.	ante jentaculum,	before breakfast.
Ant. prand.	ante prandium,	before dinner.
Applic.	applicetur,	let it be applied.
Aq. bull.	aqua bulliens,	boiling water.
Aq. calid.	aqua calida,	hot water.
Aq. dest.	aqua destillata,	distilled water.
Aq. ferv.	aqua fervens,	warm water.
Aq. font.	aqua fontana,	spring or tap water.
Aq. pur.	aqua pura,	pure water.
Aurib.	auribus,	to or for the ears.
Auristill.	auristillæ,	ear drops.
B.	bis,	twice, two.
B. i. d.	bis in die,	twice a day.
Bol.	bolus,	a large pill.
B.P.		British Pharmacopœia.
B.P.C.		British Pharmaceutical Codex.
Bib.	bibe,	drink.
Butyr.	butyrum,	butter.

C.*	centum,	a hundred.
	congius,	a gallon.
	cum,	with.
C. m. s.	cras mane sumendus,	to be taken tomorrow morning.
Cap.	cape, capiat,	take (thou), let him take.
Cap. amylac.	capsula amylacea,	a cachet, Konseal.
Cap. gelat.	capsula gelatina,	a gelatin capsule.
Catapl.	cataplasma,	a poultice.
Cereol.	cereolus,	a urethral suppository or bougie.
Chart. cerat.	charta cerata,	a waxed paper.
Chartul.	chartula,	a small paper.
Cito disp.	cito dispensetur,	let it be dispensed quickly.
Clar.	clarus, a, um,	clear, bright.
Coch. { amp. mag. max.	cochleare amplum, cochleare magnum, cochleare maximum,	a tablespoon or tablespoonful.
Coch. { med. mod.	cochleare medium, cochleare modicum,	a dessertspoon or dessertspoonful.
Coch. { min. parv.	cochleare minimum, cochleare parvum,	a teaspoon or teaspoonful.
Coch. cum.	cochleare cumulatum,	a heaped spoonful.
Col.	cola, colatura,	strain, the strained portion.
Collun.	collunarium,	a nosewash, nasal wash.
Collut.	collutorium,	a mouthwash, oral wash.
Collyr.	collyrium,	an eye wash, eye lotion.
Conf.	confectio,	a confection.
Cong.	congius,	a gallon.
Cont., contus.	contusus,	bruised.
Cyath.	cyathus,	a glass.
D. in dup.	detur in duplo,	let twice as much be given.
D. in p. æq.	divide in partes æquales,	divide into equal parts.
D. t. d.	dentur tales doses,	let such doses be given.
Dec., decant.	decanta,	pour off, decant.
Decub. hor.	decubitus hora,	at bedtime.
Deglut.	deglutiatur,	let it be swallowed.
Dext. lat.	dextro lateri,	to the right side.
Dieb. alt.	diebus alternis,	every other day.
Dim.	dimidius, a, um,	the half, one-half.
Dolent. part.	dolente parte,	to the painful part.
Dulc.	dulcis,	sweet.
Dur. dol.	durante dolore,	while the pain lasts.
E. m. p.	ex modo praescripto,	in the manner prescribed.
Ejusd.	ejusdem,	of the same.

* C. has several meanings determined from its context.

Elect.	electuarium,	an electuary.
Extend.	extende,	spread.

F., ft.	fac, fiat, fiant,	make (thou). let it be made. let them be made.
F. l. a.	fiat lege artis,	let it be made according to art (rule).
Frust.	frustillatim,	little by little, small pieces.
Ft. pulv. subtil.	fiat pulvis subtilis,	let a fine powder be made.
Fusc.	fuscus, a, um,	brown.

Garg.	gargarisma,	a gargle.
G., Gm., Grm.	gramme, grammata,	a gramme, grammes (a gram, grams).
gr.	granum, grana,	a grain, grains.
Gtt.	gutta, guttae,	a drop, drops.
Guttat.	guttatim,	drop by drop.
Gutt. applic.	gutturi applicandus,	to be applied to the throat.

H.	hora,	hour, at the hour of.
H. d.	hora decubitus,	at bedtime, at hour of sleep.
H. s.	hora somni,	at bedtime, before retiring.
H. s. s.	hora somni sumendus,	to be taken at bedtime.
H. noc.	hac nocte,	tonight.
Hirud.	hirudo, hirudines,	a leech, leeches.
Hor. un. spat.	horæ unius spatio,	at the end of an hour.

I. c.	inter cibos,	between meals.
Id.	idem,	the same.
In p. æq.	in partes æquales,	in equal parts.
In phial. obtur.	in phiala obturata,	in a stoppered bottle.
In scat.	in scatula,	in a box.
Inj.	injectio,	injection.
Insip.	insipidus,	tasteless.
Insp.	inspissus,	thickened.
Int. noc.	inter noctem,	during the night.

Jent.	jentaculum,	breakfast.
Jusc.	jusculum,	broth.

L.	lac,	milk.
Lb. ov., L. vac.	lac bovinum, lac vaccæ,	cow's milk.
Lat. dol.	lateri dolente,	to the affected side.
Luc. p.	luce prima,	early in the morning.

	mane,	in the morning.
	massa,	a pill mass.
	mille,	one thousand.
M.*	minimum,	a minum.
	misce,	mix (thou).
	mistura,	a mixture.
	mitte,	send (thou).
M. d.	more dicto,	as directed.
M. et v.	mane et vespere,	morning and evening.
M. s., mor. sol.	more solito,	in the usual manner.
Mit.	mitis,	mild.
Man.	manus,	the hand.
Mens.	mensura,	by measure.
N., noc.	nocte,	at night.
N. et m.	nocte et mane,	night and morning.
Nas.	nasus,	nose.
Neb.	nebula,	a spray.
Nov.	novus, a, um,	new.
Nux, nuc.	nux, nucis,	nut.
O.	octarius,	a pint.
O. m.	omne mane,	every morning.
O. n.	omne nocte,	every night.
Obduc.	obduc, obducatur,	coat, cover, let it be coated.
Oblat.	oblatum,	a cachet, Konseal.
Ocul.	oculus,	the eye.
Om. bid.	omne biduo,	every two days.
Om. quadr. hor.	omne quadrante horæ,	every quarter of an hour.
Op.	ope,	by means of.
Op. pen.	ope pencilli,	with a camel-hair brush.
Opt.	optimus,	the best.
P.	pondere,	by weight.
P. aur.	pone aurem,	behind the ear.
P. p. a.	phiala prius agitata,	the bottle being previously shaken.
P. r. n.	pro re nata,	as occasion arises, occasionally.
Panis	panis,	bread.
Parv.	parvus, a, um,	small.
Pediluv.	pediluvium,	a foot bath.
Per. fist. vitr.	per fistulam vitreum,	through a glass tube.
Phial.	phiala,	a vial, a bottle.
Post cib.	post cibos,	after meals.
Pulv. consper.	pulvis conspersus,	a dusting powder.
Pulv. tenu.	pulvis tenuissimus,	a very fine powder.

* M. has several meanings, determined from its context.

Q. h.	quartis horis,	every four hours.
Q. l.	quantum libet,	as much as you please.
Q. p.	quantum placet,	as much as is desired.
Qq.	quaque,	every.
Quart. qq. hor.	quarta quaque hora,	every fourth hour.
Q. s.	quantum sufficiat, quantum sufficiens, quantum satis est,	a sufficient quantity, as much as is sufficient.
Quart.	quartus,	the fourth.
Quat.	quater,	four times.
Quotid.	quotidie,	daily.
Q. O. S.	quoties opus sit,	as often as necessary.

R, Rx.	recipe,	take (thou).
Rad.	radix,	a root.
Rec.	recens,	recent, fresh.
Rect.	rectificatus,	rectified.
Red. in pulv.	redactus in pulverem,	reduce to a powder.

S.*	signa, signetur, sine, solve, sumat,	label (thou). let it be labeled. without. dissolve. let him (the patient) take.
S. a.	secundem artem,	with pharmaceutical skill, according to art or custom.
S. G., Sp. Gr., s/g.		specific gravity.
S. O. S.	si opus sit,	if occasion requires, if needed.
Scat.	scatula,	a box.
Sec. hor.	secundis horis,	every two hours.
Semih.	semihora,	half an hour.
Sem., s., ss.	semis, semissis,	one-half.
Sesq.	sesqui,	one and a half.
Sesquih.	sesquihora,	an hour and a half.
S. s. n.	signetur suo nomine,	let it be labeled with its own name.
Som.	somnus,	sleep.
St.	stet,	let it stand.
Subtil.	subtilis,	a fine powder.
Syr. fusc.	syrupus fuscus,	brown syrup, molasses.

T.	ter,	three times, thrice.
T. i. d.	ter in die,	three times a day.
T. q. d.	ter quaterve die,	three or four times a day.
Tal.	talis,	of such, like this.

* S. has several meanings, determined from its context.

Tars. ocul.	tarsis oculorum,	to the eyelids.
Temp. dext.	tempore dextro,	to the right temple.
Temp. læv.	tempore lævo,	to the left temple.
Teren.	terendus, a, um,	to be rubbed.
Tunic.	tunicentur,	let them be varnished.
Tunic. c. gelat.	tunicentur cum gelatino,	let them be coated with gelatin.
Tuss.	tussis,	a cough.
Ult.	ultime,	at last, finally.
Ung. cærul.	unguentum cæruleum,	blue ointment.
Ust.	ustus, a, um,	burnt.
Ut dict.	ut dictum,	as directed.
Ut supr.	ut supra,	as above.
Utend. mor. sol.	utendus more solito,	to be used in the usual manner.
V., vesp.	vespere,	in the evening.
Vase claus.	vase clauso,	in a closed container or vessel.
Virid.	viridis,	green.
Vitell. ovi	vitellus ovi,	yolk of egg.
Vit.	vitrum,	glass.
Vom. urg.	vomitione urgente,	when vomiting is troublesome.

NUMERALS

Arabic No.	Roman Symbol	Cardinals	Ordinals
1	I	unus	primus, a, um.
2	II	duo	secundus
3	III	tres	tertius
4	IV	quattuor	quartus
5	V	quinque	quintus
6	VI	sex	sextus
7	VII	septem	septimus
8	VIII	octo	octavus
9	IX	novem	nonus
10	X	decem	decimus
11	XI	undecim	undecimus
12	XII	duodecim	duodecimus
13	XIII	tredecim	tresdecimus
14	XIV	quattuordecim	
15	XV	quindecim	
16	XVI	sedecim	
17	XVII	septemdecim	
18	XVIII	duodeviginti	
19	XIX	undeviginti	
20	XX	viginti	
21	XXI	unus et viginti or viginti unus	
22	XXII	duo et viginti or viginti duo	
23	XXIII	tres et viginti or viginti tres	
28	XXVIII	duodetriginta	
29	XXIX	undetriginta	
30	XXX	triginta	
40	XL	quadraginta	
50	L	quinquaginta	
60	LX	sexaginta	
70	LXX	septuaginta	
80	LXXX	octoginta	
90	XC	nonaginta	
100	C	centum	
200	CC	ducenti	

PART XI

VITAMIN REVIEW

NAME	SYNONYMS	DESCRIPTION and PROPERTIES
Vitamin A	Fat-soluble A. Anti-xerophthalmic Vitamin. Anti-keratinizing Vitamin.	A pale viscous liquid; soluble in fat solvents; loses its activity on oxidation and exposure to high temperature especially in presence of rancid fat.
Vitamin B_1	Thiamine Hydrochloride. Thiamin Chloride. Vitamin B_1 hydrochloride. Water-soluble Vitamin. Anti-neuritic Vitamin. Anti-beriberi Vitamin. Thiamin. Torulin.	White crystals or powder with a characteristic odor; very soluble in water and fairly soluble in alcohol; stable in air and in dilute acids or acid solutions; decomposed by alkalies, sulfites, excessive heat and ultra-violet radiation.
Vitamn B_2 (G)	Riboflavin. Vitamin G. Water-soluble B_2.	Orange-yellow crystalline powder slightly soluble in water and alcohol; stable in air but slowly deteriorates in light; practically odorless; gradually destroyed in alkaline solutions.
Nicotinic Acid and Amide	Pellagra - Preventive Factor. P-P. Factor. Niacin.	Acid—white, odorless crystalline powder having a slightly tart taste; 1 Gm. is soluble in 60 cc. of water and in 80 cc. of alcohol. Stable when dry and in solution. Amide—white crystaline powder, slightly bitter taste; 1 Gm. is soluble in 1 cc. of water and very soluble in alcohol; stable when dry and in aqueous solution.

SOURCE	DEFICIENCY EFFECTS	AVERAGE DAILY REQUIREMENTS
Fish liver oil, liver, eggs, butter and cream, yellow plants, carrots, sweet potatoes, etc.	Night blindness. Xerophthalmia. Hyperkeratosis of the skin and mucous membranes.	Infants (under 1 yr.) 1500 I.U. Children 2000–4500 I.U. Adolescents 5000 I.U. Adults 5000 I.U. Nursing mothers 8000 I.U.
Seeds, grains, bran, nuts, legumes, meat, yeast, milk, eggs, fruits and vegetables.	Beriberi, polyneuritis of alcoholism, pregnancy, and pellagra. Certain cardio-vascular disturbances. Anorexia, suboptimal growth in infants and children.	Infants (under 1 yr.) 0.4 mg. Children 0.6–1.2 mg. Adolescents 1.2–2.0 mg. Adults 1.2–2.0 mg. Nursing mothers 2.3 mg.
Milk, cheese, liver, eggs, yeast, wheat germ, meat and leafy vegetables.	Cheilosis (lesions at the corners of the lips). Glossitis. Seborrheic lesions about the eyes and nose. Vascularizing keratitis. Photophobia. Loss of hair, lack of vigor.	Infants (under 1 yr.) 0.6 mg. Children 0.9–1.8 mg. Adolescents 1.8–3.0 mg. Adults 1.8–3.0 mg. Nursing mothers 3.0 mg.
Liver, bran, eggs, fish, yeast, wheat germ, several leafy green vegetables, organs and muscles of many animals.	Factor in development of pellagra in man. Skin eruptions; thickening, inflammation, and lesions of the back of the hand, feet, forearms, and neck. Derangement of the central nervous system.	Infants (under 1 yr.) 4 mg. Children 6–12 mg. Adolescents 12–20 mg. Adults 12–23 mg. Nursing mothers 23 mg.

NAME	SYNONYMS	DESCRIPTION and PROPERTIES
Vitamin B_6	Pyridoxine. Adermin. "anti-acrodynia factor."	White crystalline powder, salty in taste and odorless. One Gm. is soluble in 5 cc. of water and in about 100 cc. of alcohol; aqueous solution is acid; fairly stable to light and air, the stability decreasing with increase in pH.
Pantothenic Acid	Referred to as "Filtrate Factor" or as Factor II. "Chick Antidermatitis Factor." Pantothen.	Available as the calcium salt; white crystalline powder; dissolves freely in water; sweet taste and odorless; relatively stable in aqueous solution; decomposed with excessive heat, incompatible with strong acids, alkalies, ferric salts, sulfates, carbonates, phosphates and tartrates.
Vitamin C	Ascorbic Acid. Anti-scorbutic Vitamin. Cevitamic Acid. Water-soluble C.	White crystalline powder; odorless. One Gm. is soluble in 3 cc. of water and about 25 cc. of alcohol and 100 cc. of glycerin; insoluble in oils. Stable in dry state, but rapidly deteriorates in aqueous solution in presence of air. More stable in acid than in alkalies. Incompatible with oxidizing agents and copper salts.
Vitamin D	Anti-rachitic Vitamin. Fat-soluble D. Sunshine Vitamin. Calciferol or D_2.	D_2 is formed by irradiation of ergosterol. D_3 is formed by irradiation of 7-dehydrocholesterol. White odorless crystals, soluble in oils and fat solvents; stable to heat and oxidation although prolonged exposure to light may cause some destruction.

SOURCE	DEFICIENCY EFFECTS	AVERAGE DAILY REQUIREMENTS
Whole grain cereals, liver, yeast, egg yolk, crude cane molasses.	Significance in human nutrition not established as yet; thought to be necessary for the prevention of dermatitis in humans.	Not determined.
Yeast, liver, eggs, crude cane molasses and wheat germ are among the better sources of pantothenic acid.	Significance in human nutrition not definitely established. Dermatitis in chicks. Hemorrhagic adrenals and achromotrichia in rats.	Not determined.
Citrus fruits, tomatoes, green peppers and various other fresh vegetables.	Scurvy, prescorbutic conditions. Defective dentition anorexia, anemia, slow wound healing, weakened capillaries and susceptibility to infection may be concomitant of ascorbic acid deficiency.	Infants (under 1 yr.) 30 mg. Children 35– 75 mg. Adolescents 80–100 mg. Adults 75 mg. Nursing mothers 150 mg.
Fish liver oils, eggs, liver, butter and cream.	Rickets, spasmophilia, osteomalacia.	Infants (under 1 yr.) 500 I.U. Children 700 I.U. Adolescents 700 I.U. Adults 700 I.U. Nursing mothers 1000 I.U.

NAME	SYNONYMS	DESCRIPTION and PROPERTIES
Vitamin E	Alpha-tocopherol. Anti-sterility Vitamin. Fertility Vitamin. Reproductive Factor. Muscular Dystrophy Factor. Fat-soluble E.	Light yellow, viscous, oily liquid odorless but oily taste, soluble in fats and fat solvents but insoluble in water. Not affected by acids, alkalies or hydrogenation; slowly oxidized by air. Rapidly oxidized by ferric salts, silver nitrate and other oxidizing agents.
Vitamin K	Anti-hemorrhagic Vitamin. Coagulation Vitamin. 2-methyl-3-phytyl-1,4-naphthoquinone.	Viscous liquid, soluble in oils, insoluble in water and moderately soluble in alcohol. Pure vitamin and its solutions are fairly stable in the dark but are rapidly decomposed on exposure to light and alkalies and reducing agents.
2-Methyl-1,4-naphtho-quinone (Vitamin K active)	Menadione.	Yellow, crystalline powder, practically odorless; slightly soluble in water and sparingly soluble in alcohol; freely soluble in oils. Stable in air and moisture when protected from light. Decomposed by alkalies and incompatible with reducing agents, halogens and alkalies.

Miscellaneous Postulated Vitamins

Vitamin B_3	Now believed to be pantothenic acid. Concerned with growth and nutrition of pigeons.
Vitamin B_4	Necessary for a specific paralysis in rats and chicks.
Vitamin B_5	Now believed to be vitamin B_6. Required for the maintenance of weight in pigeons.
Choline	Considered to have a function similar to that of vitamins. Essential in fat metabolism.
Vitamin H or Biotin	A growth factor essential for yeast and certain microorganisms. Prevents so-called "egg white injury" in rats.

SOURCE	DEFICIENCY EFFECTS	AVERAGE DAILY REQUIREMENTS
Wheat germ oil, cottonseed oil, green leafy vegetables, milk, eggs and grain.	Significance in human nutrition not established as yet. Suggest limited value in certain cases of muscular dystrophy and amyotrophic lateral sclerosis. Some clinical value in overcoming certain cases of sterility in both sexes.	Not determined.
Alfalfa, spinach, cabbage and other green vegetables.	Prothrombin deficiency, prolonged clotting time, hemorrhagic diathesis in newborn and in certain types of hepatic and biliary disease.	Not determined.
No evidence that this compound occurs in natural foods.	See Vitamin K.	Not determined. U.S.P. dose 1.0 mg.

MISCELLANEOUS POSTULATED VITAMINS (*Continued*)

Inositol — Essential in fat metabolism. Prevents loss of hair in mice.

Para-Amino-benzoic Acid — Reported to be a chromotrichia factor for the rat, and a growth factor for the chick and certain bacteria.

Vitamin P or Citrin — A substance found in citrus fruits. Reported to be associated with vitamin C, and to be of value in maintaining normal capillary resistance and permeability.

Factor W — A water-soluble, heat-labile factor, necessary for the growth of rats and dogs.

Factors L_1 and L_2 — These factors are reported as being necessary for lactation in rats.

INDEX

501